Transesophageal echocardiography in congenital heart disease

Transesophageal echocardiography in congenital heart disease

Edited by

Oliver Stümper MD
Senior Registrar in Paediatric Cardiology, Heart Unit, The Children's Hospital, Birmingham.

and

George R. Sutherland MRCP
British Heart Foundation Senior Research Fellow and Honorary Consultant Cardiologist at the Western General Hospital, Edinburgh.

Co-editors
J. R. T. C. Roelandt and J. Hess

Edward Arnold
A member of the Hodder Headline Group
LONDON   MELBOURNE   AUCKLAND

© 1994 Edward Arnold

First published in Great Britain 1994

Distributed in the Americas by Little, Brown and Company,
134 Beacon Street, Boston, MA 02108

British Library Cataloguing in Publication Data
Stümper, O.
    Transesophageal Echocariography in
    Congenital Heart Disease
    I. Title
    616.1

    ISBN 0-340-55653-6

Whilst the advice and information in this book is believed to be true
and accurate at the date of going to press, neither the author nor the
publisher can accept any legal responsibility or liability for any errors
or omissions that may be made. In particular (but without limiting
the generality of the preceding disclaimer) every effort has been
made to check drug dosages; however, it is still possible that errors
have been missed. Furthermore, dosage schedules are constantly
being revised and new side effects recognised. For these reasons the
reader is strongly urged to consult the drug companies' printed
instructions before administering any of the drugs recommended in
this book.

Photoset in Linotron 202 Bembo by
Rowland Phototypesetting Limited, Bury St Edmunds, Suffolk.
Printed and bound in Hong Kong for Edward Arnold, a division
of Hodder Headline PLC, 338 Euston Road, London N1 3BH by
Butler and Tanner Ltd, Frome, Somerset.

Preface

Over the past five years, transesophageal echocardiography (TEE) has become firmly established as a routine diagnostic technique within the practice of cardiology. In the adult patient with acquired cardiac disease, the technique allows for both a superior image quality when compared with transthoracic ultrasound examination, and the visualisation of posterior cardiac structures not normally well visualised from the precordium. This has led to the general acceptance of transesophageal studies as the diagnostic technique of choice in the evaluation of potential cardiac sources of embolism, native and prosthetic valve disease, endocarditis and thoracic aortic disease. In comparison, the use of the technique in the evaluation of patients with congenital heart disease has been limited.

It was only with the introduction of dedicated paediatric transesophageal ultrasound transducers that such studies became feasible and safe in children. Currently the technique is becoming increasingly used as a complementary diagnostic and monitoring technique to precordial imaging in paediatric cardiology. However, more and more children with cardiac defects are growing up and presenting as adolescents and adults with a complex range of problems to the adult cardiologist. The complexity of lesions and the sequelae of prior surgical repairs performed in these patients mean that newer imaging techniques are required for their evaluation. Transesophageal echocardiography, in our experience, represents a most valuable new investigative tool in this patient population.

The aim of this book is to present a concise overview of the current practice of transesophageal echocardiography in the assessment of congenital heart disease. The text provides guidance both to the paediatric cardiologist who is aware of the complexities of congenital cardiac lesions (but unfamiliar with transesophageal imaging) and to the adult cardiologist who is familiar with the technique, but to a lesser extent with the specific questions and problems surrounding the ultrasound evaluation of congenital heart disease.

Oliver Stümper
George R. Sutherland
1993

Contributors

Professor JRTC Roelandt
Head, Division of Cardiology, Thoraxcenter, Erasmus Universiteit, Rotterdam, Postbus 1738, 3000 DR Rotterdam, THE NETHERLANDS

Dr George R Sutherland
Consultant Cardiologist, Western General Hospital, Crewe Road, EDINBURGH EH4 2XU

Dr Oliver Stumper
Department of Cardiology, The Children's Hospital, Ladywood Middleway, BIRMINGHAM B16 8ET

Dr Naryswamy Sreeram
Heart Clinic, Royal Liverpool Children's Hospital, Alder Hey, Eaton Road, LIVERPOOL L12 2AP

Dr Piotr Hoffman
National Institute of Cardiology, Warszawa 04-628, Alpejska 42, POLAND

Dr J Hess
Division of Paediatric Cardiology, Sophia Childrens Hospital, Gordelweg 160, NL-3038 GE Rotterdam, THE NETHERLANDS

Dr Achi Ludomirsky
Division of Pediatric Cardiology, CS Mott Children's Hospital, F1310 MCHC, Box 0204, Ann Arbor, Michigan 48109-0204, USA

Dr Alan G Fraser
Department of Cardiology, University Hospital of Wales, College of Medicine, Heath Park, CARDIFF CF4 4XN

Contents

ABBREVIATIONS

Ao   aorta
AoV   aortic valve
DAo   descending aorta
IVC   inferior caval vein
LA   left atrium
LLPV   left lower pulmonary vein
LPA   left pulmonary artery
LV   left ventricle
LUPV   left upper pulmonary vein
MV   mitral valve
PA   pulmonary artery
PV   pulmonary valve
RA   right atrium
RLPV   right lower pulmonary vein
RPA   right pulmonary artery
RV   right ventricle
RUPV   right upper pulmonary vein
SVC   superior caval vein
TV   tricuspid valve

CHAPTER 1

The development of TEE: A historical review

J. Roelandt and J. Souquet

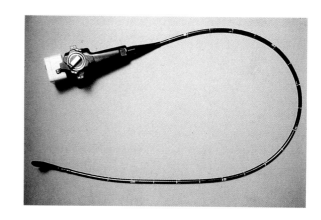

INTRODUCTION

The difficulties encountered in obtaining good quality cardiac ultrasound signals through the chest wall when using the early insensitive precordial transducers stimulated many investigators to search for alternative ultrasound windows. Interestingly, at that time, most investigators directed their thoughts towards developing intravascular and intracardiac imaging as the logical alternative approach to defining cardiac structure and function. As early as 1960, Cieszynski mounted a single element on a catheter which could be introduced into the jugular vein. Using this catheter, echoes in the amplitude mode were obtained from cardiac structures in dogs (1). Three years later, Omoto et al.(2) obtained static cross-sectional images in patients, with a slowly rotating single element transducer mounted at the tip of a sonde which was introduced into the right atrium via either the femoral or jugular vein. A device used to monitor the dynamic behaviour of intracardiac dimensions using a single element mounted at the tip of a catheter capable of scanning in all directions, was reported in 1968 by Carleton and Clark (3). In 1970, Eggleton constructed a catheter with four elements at its tip (4) and produced the first cross-sectional images of intracardiac structures. The images were reconstructed by computer using slow rotation and electrocardiographic triggering. Two years later, Bom et al.(5) from the Thoraxcentre of the Erasmus University in Rotterdam described a real-time intracardiac scanner using an electronically phased circular array of 32 elements at the tip of a 9F catheter.

However, the intrinsic problems encountered in manufacturing catheter systems which allowed a rapid real-time acquisition of cross-sectional images of good resolution, led to a fading of interest in these innovative alternative approaches. In addition, the original impetus for their development also became less important as developments in transducer technology resulted in a marked improvement in the quality of the images that could be obtained by transthoracic echocardiography.

In 1968, a new generation of gastroscopes became available with a steerable tip, which allowed direct contact between the esophageal wall and an ultrasonic transducer mounted at the tip. The first cardiac investigations with ultrasound via the oesophagus using such a gastroscope were reported by Side and Gosling in 1971 (6). They used a dual element construction mounted on a standard gastroscope to obtain continuous wave Doppler information about the velocity of cardiac blood flow.

Subsequently, Olson and Shelton in 1972 (7,8) measured displacement of the walls of the thoracic aorta and pulmonary artery. Pulsed wave Doppler interrogation from within the oesophagus was described by Duck et al.(9) and Daigle et al.(10) in 1975.

Transesophageal echocardiography in an embryonic form was initially introduced by Frazin et al. in 1976 (11). They, and others (12), recorded M-mode echocardiograms of the left ventricle, and used the changes in its dimensions thus measured to monitor its function (Fig. 1.1). However, their work did not attract the attention of clinicians. One factor responsible for this was the problems associated

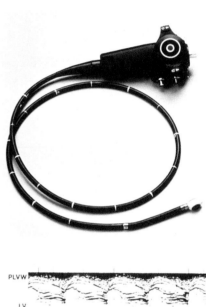

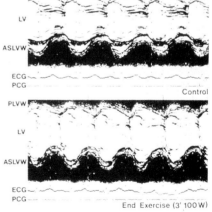

Figure 1.1 *A transesophageal M-mode echo transducer system and an M-mode echocardiogram of the left ventricle. The upper tracing shows the control M-mode tracing recorded at rest and the lower panel the ventricular dimensions and contraction pattern at the end of a three-minute period of exercise at 100 watts workload. PLVW = posterior and ALVW = anterior left ventricular wall. ECG = electrocardiogram and PCG = phonocardiogram. Reproduced by permission of Matsumoto et al.(32).*

with conscious patients swallowing the probe. Since this was less of a problem for anaesthetists, further research was then directed towards the intraoperative monitoring of left ventricular performance. This work was undertaken mainly by Japanese investigators and especially by Matsumoto and colleagues (13).

Cross-sectional real-time imaging was first reported in 1977 by Hisanaga *et al.*(14). They constructed a scanning device which consisted of a rotating single element in an oil-filled balloon mounted at the tip of a gastroscope. Much later, in 1984, a similar system was described by Bertini *et al.*(15). One year after their first report, Hisanaga *et al.*(16) also described a linear mechanical scanner suitable for transesophageal echocardiographic studies. A single element was moved parallel to the long axis of the gastroscope and 8–20 images were obtained.

The development of single transverse plane transesophageal imaging

The introduction of electronic scanners marked the next, and most important, step in the development of transesophageal echocardiography. DiMagno *et al.*(1980) constructed a high-frequency (10 MHz) linear array, which was originally designed for scanning the gastrointestinal tract (17). However, it was the electronic phased-array transducer introduced by Souquet *et al.*(18) in Hamburg in 1982 which marked the definitive breakthrough for the transesophageal approach. The frequency of this phased-array transducer was 3.5 MHz, the same as that of the standard precordial transducers of that era (Fig. 1.2).

The initial applications of the new transesophageal probes differed between Europe and America. In the United States of America, the main applications were in the intraoperative monitoring of regional myocardial function in high risk non-cardiac surgical patients, and in the recognition of intracardiac air during neurosurgical procedures (19). In Europe, investigators adopted a different approach and used the system for the diagnosis of cardiac disease in the outpatient clinic (20). This resulted in the technique rapidly becoming integrated into diagnostic practice, because of its unique

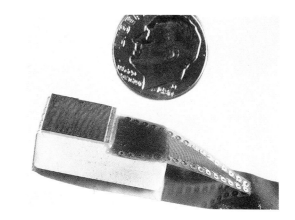

Figure 1.2 *First 32-element 3.5 MHz phased-array transducer developed by J. Souquet which was fitted on an Olympus gastroscope by J. Souquet.*

Table 1.1 *Advantages of transesophageal over transthoracic echocardiography*

No obstruction to ultrasound by chest wall structures, or lung tissue
Different imaging approach allows the visualisation of structures not seen from the precordium
Improved signal-to-noise ratio allows better detection of poor echo-reflective structures (intracardiac tumour, thrombi)
Higher ultrasound frequencies can be used, providing higher image resolution
Reduced target range for pulsed Doppler, and higher sensitivity of colour flow imaging, when studying posterior cardiac structures

advantages over conventional precordial echocardiography (Table 1.1).

Subsequently, specific clinical applications evolved which stimulated the production of newer higher resolution transducers. In our institution, the first phased-array transducer for use via the esophagus was constructed in 1982. Improvements in micro-miniature cutting and bonding technology subsequently resulted in the production of a series of transducers in which image quality was progressively improved. The final design was a transverse array of 64 elements with a frequency of 5.6 MHz, which exhibited an extremely low level of artefacts (grating lobes) combined with superior lateral and axial resolution (21) (Figs 1.3 and 1.4). Of the wide range of single plane transducers commercially available, this is now the most widely used.

Another important breakthrough for transesophageal imaging occurred in 1987, when colour flow mapping was combined with high-resolution

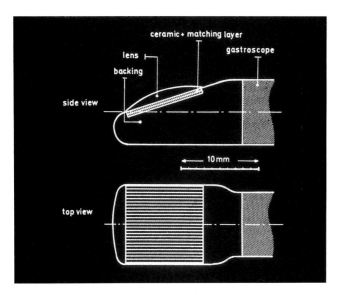

Figure 1.3 *A schematic diagram of a transesophageal assembly. The lateral view shows the different parts. For focusing the transverse beam a silicon rubber lens is positioned in front of the ceramic transducer elements.*

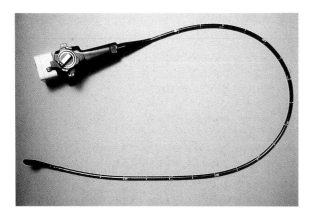

Figure 1.4 *First transesophageal 5 MHz transducer system for adult use developed at the Thoraxcentre. The external controls for flexion-extension and sideways movement can be seen.*

imaging. This combination led to an almost immediate worldwide increase in the application of transesophageal echocardiography. Subsequent developments have included the development of mechanically driven high-frequency transducers with an annular array, providing both high-resolution imaging and the capability for continuous wave Doppler interrogation (22,23). Continuous wave Doppler facilities have also been incorporated into the majority of current generation transverse plane phased-array probes.

BIPLANE TRANSESOPHAGEAL IMAGING

A biplane transesophageal probe had been proposed as early as 1982 by Souquet *et al.* in order to overcome the lack of versatility associated with imaging structures only in the transverse plane (24) (Table 1.2).

Table 1.2 *Advantages of (biplane) transesophageal echocardiography*

Longitudinally aligned structures are better visualised than in the transverse planes (venae cavae, right ventricular outflow tract, aortic valve, left ventricular apex, thoracic aorta)
Facilitates three-dimensional conceptualisation of the heart and complex structures (e.g. mitral valve apparatus)
Reduces probe manipulation

In such a transducer, two phased-array transducers were to be mounted at the tip of the gastroscope at right angles to each other, thus providing the capability for imaging both transverse and longitudinal planes. The first assembly of this type was composed of two transducers each having 32 elements and operating at 3.5 MHz (Fig. 1.5). The next generation biplane transesophageal systems utilised transducers operating at higher frequencies (typically 5.0 MHz) thus providing improved image resolution. In addition, a concomitant significant reduction in the size of the rigid section located at

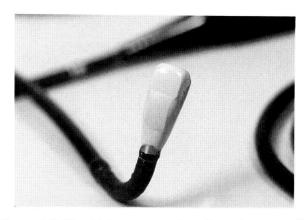

Figure 1.5 *First biplane transesophageal transducer assembly made in 1982 by J. Souquet. Two phased-array transducers are mounted on an Olympus gastroscope – the more apical one for imaging in the transverse plane and the proximal one for imaging in the longitudinal plane.*

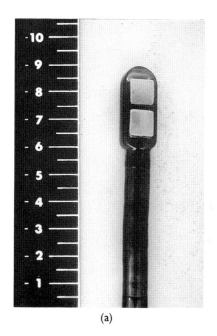

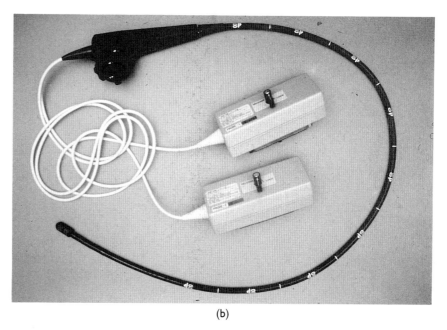

(a)　　　　　　　　　　　　　　　　　　　(b)

Figure 1.6 *The tip of a current biplane imaging system (a) and the biplane probe itself (b). Note the two sets of connectors to the ultrasound machine. Biplane real-time imaging is not possible, but this may be simulated by recording one plane into the cine-loop and subsequently displaying this in a side by side manner with the second plane using a split screen format.*

the tip of the gastroscope meant that the patient had less difficulty in swallowing the probe (Fig. 1.6). Clinical experience with the first biplane probe was published by Hanrath *et al.*(20) in 1982. However, an extensive clinical evaluation of the biplane approach was only reported many years later by Omoto *et al.*(25). One problem encountered with the standard biplane probe is that the distance between the centres of the two transducers is about 1 cm. As a result, minimal repositioning of the shaft of the probe is required in order to visualise exactly the same cardiac segment. The need for repositioning has been overcome by the recently developed biplane phased-array matrix which allows orthogonal biplane scanning from the one transducer array kept at a constant position (26).

MULTIPLANE TRANSESOPHAGEAL IMAGING

Multiplane imaging is another important development in TEE and was proposed by Harui and Souquet in 1985 (27). This system provides an infinite number of planes over a full 180° rotation of a single phased-array transducer. Advantages of this new approach are indicated in Table 1.3.

Table 1.3 *Advantages of multiplane transesophageal echocardiography*

Best for three-dimensional reconstruction
Transitional (oblique) planes reduce interpretation problems of both single and biplane TEE
Minimal repositioning facilitates and shortens examinations
Optimisation of imaging and Doppler flow mapping

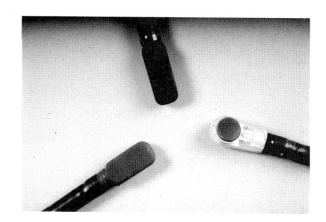

Figure 1.7 *Three transesophageal probes developed at the Thoraxcentre by Brommersma et al. The multiplane (Varioplane) transducer is shown at right. From a transverse imaging position, the transducer can be rotated 90 degrees leftwards and rightwards allowing full 180 degree rotation. At left the single plane and above the biplane probes are shown.*

A prototype multiplane transducer (Varioplane) developed at the Thoraxcentre by Brommersma *et al.* is shown in Fig. 1.7 and initial experience has been reported (28). Recently, a 'variomatrix' probe was introduced combining the rotating capabilities of the multiplane probe and the simultaneous, side-by-side matrix probe (26,29).

PAEDIATRIC TRANSESOPHAGEAL IMAGING

The size of standard adult transesophageal transducers and gastroscopes is a major limitation to the application of transesophageal echocardiography in paediatric cardiology. This is especially the case for infants. Size also limits the use of the technique for prolonged monitoring of patients in the intensive care unit. Thus, efforts have been directed towards both the further miniaturisation of phased-array transducers and the provision of higher frequencies for improved resolution, so that probes can be used in small children and infants (Fig. 1.8). Such systems clearly extend the range of clinical applications of transesophageal echocardiography (28). It is possible to use standard adult transesophageal probes in children larger than 20 kilograms in weight, if they are anaesthetised, but below this size, only small probes should be used. The development of paediatric transesophageal probes has also influenced probe design in other areas of echocardiography, such as the development of miniature finger-tip transducers for intraoperative imaging from the epicardial surface (31).

Recently, standard adult transesophageal probes

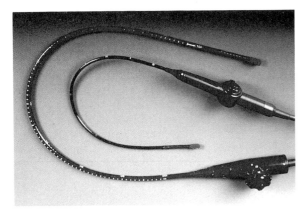

Figure 1.8 *The paediatric transesophageal 5 MHz transducer system developed at the Thoraxcentre is shown together with a standard monoplane transducer system.*

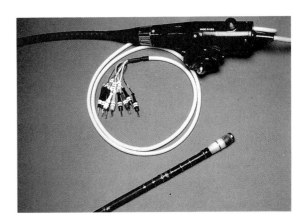

Figure 1.9 *Standard transesophageal probe with a series of electrodes for atrial pacing.*

have been modified to incorporate a series of electrodes which can be used for atrial pacing (Fig. 1.9). Left ventricular wall motion can be monitored during the onset of ischaemia induced by increasing heart rate by transesophageal atrial pacing.

THE CHARACTERISTICS OF TRANSESOPHAGEAL SYSTEMS

The basic construction of all transesophageal transducers is similar. A commercially available gastroscope or bronchoscope is adapted, by fitting a phased-array transducer at its tip for imaging in the transverse axis. The fibreoptics together with the channels used for suction and biopsy are removed, to provide space for the electronic connections for the transducer, but the normal guidance controls are retained, giving the tip at least 90 degrees of antero-posterior mobility and more than 70 degrees of lateral mobility in each direction. In one early probe (Toshiba/Mashida), the fibreoptics and a channel for insufflating air were retained, so that the transducer could be positioned under direct endoscopic control. The probe could not be used for a simultaneous upper gastrointestinal endoscopy, since it had no channels for suction or for taking biopsies. Most investigators agree, however, that fibreoptics are unnecessary when performing transesophageal echocardiography.

Most modern transducers provide images with a sector of 90 degrees. The number of elements varies, but the operating frequency is typically centred around 5 MHz. In one system (Vingmed), an annular phased-array transducer and a miniature motor for its mechanical rotation, are both incorporated in the tip of the gastroscope. Mechanical annular phased-array transducers are capable of providing frequencies up to 7.5 MHz, and continuous wave Doppler (22,23).

The length of adult gastroscopes varies between 70 and 110 centimetres. The shaft is marked at intervals of ten centimetres. A longer cable is often desirable when the probe is being used for intraoperative monitoring or in the intensive care unit, so that access to the patient for other purposes is not impeded by the echocardiographic machine.

TRANSESOPHAGEAL COLOUR FLOW MAPPING

The basic advantages of the use of the transesophageal approach include a reduced target range for many structures when compared with the transthoracic approach. This results in an improvement in the sensitivity of colour flow mapping when compared with the precordial approach and an ability to encode a wider range of velocities, without causing aliasing. Within this range, however, the same limitations apply as are present during colour flow mapping from the praecordium. Since there are constraints on the time available for processing the signals from the transducer, a compromise has to be made between the frame rate, the density of the scan lines, the frequency of resolution, and the depth of scanning. Thus, to obtain the optimal colour flow maps of a particular area of interest, the depth of scanning should be reduced to the minimum required to include that area, and the sector of the colour encoding should be kept as narrow as possible.

More detailed information about the optimisation of colour flow maps is available in other published texts (32–34). Some other specific technical points are discussed throughout the text of this book when appropriate.

SAFETY CONSIDERATIONS

Considerations for safety include the control of electrical hazards and probe temperature. Between studies, the probe should be washed and cleaned, and then 'sterilised' or disinfected according to the manufacturer's guidelines and similar to the practice with standard endoscopes. Alternatively, the probe can be inserted into a long rubber sheath containing some ultrasound gel at its tip. If this is done, full sterilisation of the probe between successive examinations is not required, but should still be performed as a precaution at the end of each day. The maximum allowable electrical leakage current of the ultrasound system, including machine and probe, is set down in international standards (IEC601). Next to this system test, which is too complex to perform daily, it is useful to do a routine inspection of the TEE-probes for bitemarks and other damage. In addition, a DC-leakage-current measurement should be carried out each day prior to probe use. This test is far more sensitive than just a visual inspection.

The generation of acoustic energy is attended with some thermal energy. This will cause a small increase of temperature of the tip, especially when the probe is used in Doppler-mode or with maximum driving voltage. A thermocouple has been added in the tip of some transducers to monitor temperature. When the limit of 41°C is reached, transmitting power will be switched off or a warning appears on the screen. The probe will then only be re-activated when the probe temperature has fallen to a clinically acceptable level.

A multicenter study including 10,419 TEE examinations in adults has been published indicating that the risk of a transesophageal study for this age range in experienced hands and under proper safety conditions is low (35).

REFERENCES

1. CIESZYNSKI T. Intracardiac method for the investigation of structure of the heart with the aid of ultrasonics. *Arch Immum Ter Dosw* 1960; **8:** 551–7.
2. OMOTO R, ATSUMI K, SUMA K, TOYODA T, SAKURAI Y, MUROI T, FUJIMORI Y, IDEZUKI Y, TSUNEMOTO M, SUGIWURA M, SAUGUSA M. Ultrasonic intravenous sonde – 2nd report. *Med Ultrason (Jpn)* 1963; **1:** 11.
3. CARLETON RA, CLARK JG. Measurements of left ventricular diameter in the dog by cardiac catheterisation. Validation and physiologic meaningfulness of an ultrasonic technique. *Circ Res* 1968; **22:** 545–8.
4. EGGLETON RC, TOWNSEND C, HERRICK J, TEMPLETON G, MITCHELL JH. Ultrasonic visualisation of left ventricular dynamics. *Ultrasonics* 1970; **17:** 143–53.

5. BOM N, LANCÉE CT, VAN EGMOND FC. An ultrasonic intracardiac scanner. *Ultrasonics* 1972; **10:** 72–6.

6. SIDE CG, GOSLING RG. Non-surgical assessment of cardiac function. *Nature* 1971; **232:** 335.

7. OLSON RM, SHELTON DK. A nondestructive technique to measure wall displacement in the thoracic aorta. *J Appl Physiol* 1972; **32:** 147–51.

8. SHELTON DK, OLSON RM. A nondestructive technique to measure pulmonary artery diameter and its pulsatile variations. *J Appl Physiol* 1972; **33:** 542–4.

9. DUCK FA, HODSON CJ, POMLIN PJ. Esophageal Doppler probe for aortic flow velocity monitoring. *Ultrasound Med & Biol* 1975; **1:** 233–41.

10. DAIGLE RE, MILLER CW, HISTAND MB, MCLEOD FD, HOKANSON DE. Nontraumatic aortic blood flow sensing using an ultrasonic esophageal probe. *J Appl Physiol* 1975; **38:** 6.

11. FRAZIN L, TALANO JV, STEPHANIDES L, LOEB HS, KOPEL L, GUNNAR RM. Esophageal echocardiography. *Circulation* 1976; **54:** 102.

12. HANRATH P, KREMER P, LANGESTEIN BA, MATSUMOTO M, BLEIFELD W. Transösophageale Eckokardiographie: Ein neues Verfahren zur dynamischen Ventrikel-funktionanalyse. *Dtsch Med Wochenschr* 1981; **106:** 523–5.

13. MATSUMOTO M, OKA Y, STROM J, et al. Application of transoesophageal echocardiography to continuous intraoperative monitoring of left ventricular performance. *Am J Cardiol* 1980; **46:** 95–105.

14. HISANAGA K, HISANAGA A, NAGATA K, YOSHIDA S. A new transoesophageal real-time two-dimensional echocardiographic system using a flexible tube and its clinical application. *Proc Jpn Soc of Ultrasonics in Med* 1977; **32:** 43–4.

15. BERTINI A, MASOTTI L, ZUPPIROLI A, CECCHI F. Rotating probe for transoesophageal cross-sectional echocardiography. *J Nucl Med Allied Sci* 1984; **28:** 115–21.

16. HISANAGA K, HISANAGA A, ICHIE Y. A new transoesophageal real-time linear scanner and initial clinical results. *Proc Jpn Soc of Ultrasonics in Med* 1978; **35:** 115–16.

17. DIMAGNO EP, BUXTON JL, REGAN PT, HATTERY RR, WILSON DA, SUAREZ JR, GREEN PS. Ultrasonic endoscope. *Lancet* 1980; **1:** 629.

18. SOUQUET J, HANRATH P, ZITELLI L, et al. Transoesophageal phased array for imaging the heart. *IEEE Trans Biomed Engineer* 1982; **29:** 707.

19. KREMER P, SCHWARTZ L, CAHALAN MK, GUTMAN J, SCHILLER NB. Intraoperative monitoring of left ventricular performance by transoesophageal M-mode and 2-D echocardiography (abstract). *Am J Cardiol* 1982; **49:** 956.

20. HANRATH P, SCHLÜTER M, LANGESTEIN BA, POLSTER J, ENGELS S. Transoesophageal horizontal and sagittal imaging of the heart with a phase array system: initial clinical results. In Hanrath P, Bleifeld W (eds), *Cardiovascular Diagnosis by Ultrasound.* The Hague: Martinus Nijhoff Publishers, 1982: 251–9.

21. LANCÉE CT, DE JONG N, BOM N. Design and construction of an esophageal phased array probe. *Med Prog Technol* 1988; **13:** 139–48.

22. ANGELSEN BAJ, HOEM J, DORUM S, CHAPMAN J, GRUBE E, GERCKENS U, VISSER VA, VANDENBOGAERDE J. High-frequency annular array transoesophageal probe for high-resolution imaging and continuous wave Doppler measurements. In: Erbel R, et al. (eds), *Transoesophageal Echocardiography.* Berlin: Springer-Verlag, 1989.

23. CHAPMAN JV, VANDENBOGAERDE J, EVERAERT JA, ANGELSEN BAJ. The initial clinical evaluation of a transoesophageal system with pulsed Doppler, continuous wave Doppler, and colour flow imaging based on an annular array technology. *Int J Card Im* 1989; **5:** 9–16.

24. SOUQUET J. Phased array transducer technology for transoesophageal imaging of the heart: current status and future aspects. In: Hanrath, et al. (eds), *Cardiovascular diagnosis by ultrasound.* London: Martinus Nijhoff, 1982: 251–9.

25. OMOTO R, KYO S, MATSUMURA M, SHAH P, ADACHI H, MATSUNAKA T, TACHIKAWA K. Recent technological progress in transoesophageal colour Doppler flow imaging with special reference to newly developed biplane and paediatric probes. In: Erbel R, et al. (eds), *Transoesophageal Echocardiography.* Berlin: Springer-Verlag, 1989.

26. OMOTO R, KYOS S, MATSUMURA M, ADACHI H, MARUYAMA M, MATSUNAKA T. New direction of biplane transoesophageal echocardiography with special emphasis on real-time biplane imaging and matrix phased-array biplane transducer. *Echocardiography* 1980; **7:** 691–8.

27. HARUI N, SOUQUET J. Transoesophageal echocardiography scanhead. United States Patent No. 4.543.960, October 1, 1985.

28. ROELANDT JRTC, THOMSON IR, VLETTER WB, BROMMERSMA P, BOM N, LINKER DT. Multiplane transesophageal echocardiography: latest evolution in an imaging revolution. *J Am Soc Echocardiogr* 1992; **5:** 361–7.

29. OMOTO R, KYO S, MATSUMURA M, YAMADA E, MATSUNAKA T. Variomatrix – A newly developed transesophageal echocardiography probe with a rotating matrix biplane transducer: technological aspects and initial clinical experience. *Echocardiology* 1993; **10:** 79–90.

30. STÜMPER O, KANITZ R, ELZENGA NJ, BOM N, ROELANDT J, HESS J, SUTHERLAND GR. The value of transoesophageal echocardiography in children with congenital heart disease. *J Am Soc Echo* 1991; **4:** 164–76.

31. SMYLLIE J, VAN HERWERDEN L, BROMMERSMA P, DE JONG J, BOM N, BOS E, GUSSENHOVEN E, ROELANDT J, SUTHERLAND GR. Intraoperative epicardial echocardiography: early experience with a newly developed small surgical transducer. *J Am Soc Echo* 1991; **4:** 147–54.

32. KISSLO J, ADAMS DB, BELKIN RN. *Doppler colour flow imaging.* New York: Churchill Livingstone, 1988.

33. OMOTO R (ed.). *Colour atlas of real-time two-dimensional Doppler echocardiography.* 2nd ed. Tokyo: Shinan-To Chiryo Co., 1987.

34. MATSUMOTO M, HANRATH P, KREMER P, BLEIFELT W,

Moeda T, Yasui K, Abe H. The evaluation of left ventricular function by transoesophageal M-mode exercise echocardiography. In: Hanrath P, Bleifelt W, Souquet J (eds), *Cardiovascular diagnosis by ultrasound.* London: Martinuus Nijhoff, 1982: 227–36.

35. Daniel WG, Erbel R, Kasper W, Visser CA, Engberding R, Sutherland GR. Safety of transesophageal echocardiography. A multicenter survey of 10,419 examinations. *Circulation* 1991; **83:** 817–21.

CHAPTER 2

Technology and techniques

O. Stümper and G. R. Sutherland

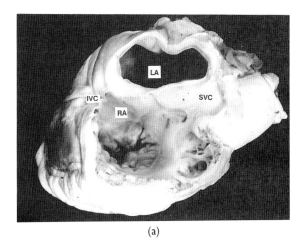

(a)

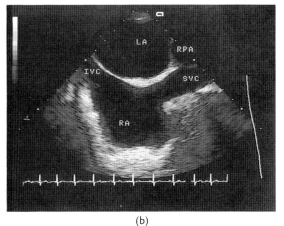

(b)

INTRODUCTION

The first clinical transesophageal echocardiographic studies, performed by Frazin and associates (1), provided only M-mode recordings of the heart and were obtained from either the oesophagus or the stomach. Clearly such studies were very limited in their applications. In 1981/2, Souquet, Hanrath and colleagues developed and clinically evaluated transesophageal two-dimensional phased-array imaging systems (2,3), which used a 2.5 MHz phased-array ultrasound transducer mounted at the tip of an endoscope. Over the next four years, a number of publications demonstrated the feasibility and potential advantages of the technique in a series of adult patients (3,4). However, clinical interest in the technique remained limited as image quality was poor and only morphologic information could be obtained. It was not until the introduction in 1986/7 of the second generation of single (transverse) plane transesophageal probes which provided the combination of high-resolution imaging (centred around 5.0 MHz) and colour flow mapping that this technique became accepted as a major new diagnostic technique in a number of European institutions. Since then, transesophageal echocardiography has become widely acknowledged to be an essential addition to cardiac investigation in the adult patient over a wide spectrum of acquired heart disease. The most common current indications for a transesophageal study in adult acquired heart disease are listed in Table 2.1.

Table 2.1 *Main clinical indications for a transesophageal study in adult acquired heart disease*

Aortic dissection
Mitral prosthesis function
Endocarditis
Cardiac source of emboli
Native mitral valve disease
Failed precordial study

Probe development continues to proceed at a rapid pace and at present is focused on (1) providing higher resolution imaging, (2) the development of smaller probes for studies in children, (3) the incorporation of additional imaging planes and Doppler facilities and (4) the development of ultrasound generated three-dimensional reconstruction of cardiac structure. The following section will attempt to provide an overview of the scanning equipment currently available, both for adult and for paediatric use, and will outline some of the recent developments currently under clinical evaluation.

THE CHANGING TECHNOLOGY OF TRANSESOPHAGEAL PROBES

Transesophageal probes consist essentially of an ultrasound transducer (or transducers) mounted at the tip of a flexible endoscope. Major differences between the various available probe designs include (1) the maximal dimensions of the shaft and the transducer tip and (2) the number of imaging elements and the design of the ultrasound transducer. The sub-division of the range of transesophageal probes currently available into adult and paediatric probes is to some extent arbitrary and is based essentially on the maximal overall dimensions of the various probes.

Adult transesophageal scanning equipment

The most widely used transesophageal probes in adult cardiology are systems built on an endoscope that has a maximal shaft diameter of some 10–11 mm, and a total shaft length of some 110 cm. The steering facilities of these probes normally provide both anterior/posterior and right/left lateral tip angulation. The length of the flexible portion of these probes measures some 10 cm. The distance from the maximal point of angulation to the very tip of the endoscope is normally some 7 cm. The ultrasound transducer itself is embedded in the most distal rectangular segment of the probe. The length of the tip normally measures some 23 mm, the maximal height most often 12–13 mm and the maximal width some 14–15 mm. Thus, the maximal tip circumference [2 × (height + width)] often exceeds 52 mm. Modifications in transducer tip design include a rounding of the rectangular shape. This appears to facilitate the swallowing of the probe by the awake patient.

The majority of current generation single-plane probes use an imaging frequency centred around 5 or 5.6 MHz and have a phased-array transducer containing 64 elements. The ultrasound elements are mounted at the flexible tip so as to provide transverse plane images of the heart; that is their scan plane is at right angles to the shaft of the endoscope. Cross-sectional imaging, in combination with colour flow mapping and pulsed wave Doppler interrogation, is provided on all currently available probes. More recently continuous wave Doppler facilities have become available on selected phased-array transesophageal probes. In addition, one annular array mechanical system is available, that allows a dynamic shift in imaging frequency from 5 to 7.5 MHz in combination with both high pulse repetition frequency Doppler and continuous wave Doppler.

In 1989, Omoto and colleagues (5) introduced the first biplane transesophageal probe for use in adult patients. Current generation biplane probes have two separate ultrasound transducer element arrays mounted at the tip of the scope so as to provide both transverse axis and longitudinal axis images of the heart and the great vessels. Conventionally, the more distal transducer provides the standard transverse axis images. By switching a button on the ultrasound system the more proximal transducer is activated and generates longitudinal plane images. Subsequent attempts to use the same set of ultrasound crystals to generate both imaging planes (using a matrix array format) have met with limited success so far. Since the advantages of biplane transesophageal imaging have become increasingly apparent over the last two years (6,7), more manufacturers have turned to this technology. In fact, with miniaturisation in transducer design it is now possible to construct biplane transesophageal probes with two sets of 64-element channels, which have similar dimensions to the current standard 64-element single-plane probes.

The ultimate goal in transesophageal probe design, however, remains the construction of high-resolution multiplane imaging probes. Such probes are currently under development (8). In these probes, a 48 or 64-element phased-array transducer is mounted on a circular footprint, which can be rotated from 0 degrees (transverse plane) through 90 degrees (longitudinal plane) to almost 180 degrees (reversed transverse plane). Such systems have many theoretical and practical advantages. Since in clinical practice lateral angulation of an endoscope within the oesophagus beyond 30 degrees is rarely possible without causing considerable discomfort to the patient, this multiplane approach can provide a number of additional imaging planes not normally available using standard biplane probes. A further advantage of this system is that all the required im-

aging planes can normally be obtained from the one transducer position within the oesophagus. Initial clinical studies have documented that, firstly, such a transducer design is feasible and, secondly, that several advantages are provided over biplane imaging alone (8). These include (1) the potential three-dimensional reconstruction of cardiac anatomy, (2) a better insight into certain aspects of mitral valve morphology and function, (3) a better evaluation of left ventricular morphology and function and (4) a more detailed assessment of the atrial septum and the great arteries. To a large extent, this probe design liberates transesophageal imaging from the constraints of a tomographic imaging technique. Structures can be followed and connected by unlimited rotation of the probe, in a manner comparable to precordial imaging.

Paediatric transesophageal scanning equipment

The term 'paediatric scanning equipment' in the context of transesophageal imaging, is chosen to imply that the maximal dimensions of these probes will allow the safe investigation of small children. The first such paediatric probe was developed in late 1988, and an initial clinical experience with its use was reported by Omoto and colleagues (9). The original design featured a 5 MHz 24-element phased-array transducer mounted at the tip of a paediatric gastroscope. The maximal shaft diameter measured just under 7 mm. This miniaturisation could only be accomplished by a reduction in the number of ultrasound crystals (and hence connecting wires), as well as by sacrificing the lateral steering mechanism. Adapted to paediatric use, the total shaft length measured some 70 cm. The tip of the transducer measured roughly 7 mm in maximal width and 8 mm in maximal height. Thus transducer tip circumference was just under 30 mm.

Until recently, this particular probe was the only dedicated paediatric transesophageal probe which was commercially available. However, with the rapid evolution of paediatric transesophageal imaging as an adjunct to the diagnostic armamentarium in paediatric cardiology, several further probe designs have become available. These include a 48-element 5 MHz phased-array single-plane probe, which evolved from the prototype probe engineered at the Thoraxcentre in Rotterdam (10). Although this probe has slightly larger dimensions than the probe developed by Omoto et al, it allows safe studies in children down to 3.5 kilograms bodyweight. In this new probe, cross-sectional imaging resolution was considerably improved, the near field artefact reduced, and the depth at which both colour and pulsed wave Doppler studies could be carried out was improved. At least one further similar probe design, which also incorporates continuous wave Doppler facilities, is now under evaluation.

Mechanical probes have also been developed for paediatric imaging and annular array systems have become available in two sizes with an 11.5 and 9 mm transducer tip diameter. Both probes provide a dynamic shift in imaging frequency from 5 to 7.5 MHz and continuous wave Doppler facilities.

Finally, a dedicated neonatal transesophageal probe has been developed which allows studies in premature infants. The maximal shaft diameter of this probe measures just 4 mm and the tip a mere 4 × 5 mm. However, because of the considerable reduction of the total number of ultrasound elements to 17, this probe does not provide high-resolution cross-sectional imaging. Nonetheless, the probe allows for the acquisition of high-quality Doppler and colour flow mapping information in either the critically ill neonate or after neonatal cardiac surgery.

In order to overcome the shortcomings of single-plane transverse axis imaging in the assessment of lesions involving the right ventricular outflow tract and the ventriculo-arterial junction, a single-plane longitudinal axis transducer had been developed for use in children. Although this approach offers several advantages in the evaluation of outflow tract lesions, the longitudinal imaging plane proved to be only an adjunct to transverse axis imaging rather than a viable alternative. At the time of writing, a number of biplane paediatric transesophageal probes are being introduced into clinical paediatric practice. However, as with many current generation adult imaging probes, biplane technology can currently only be achieved at the expense of image quality in each plane. Our current requirements for the ideal configuration of a paediatric transesophageal probe are listed in Table 2.2. The compromises which must be considered in the design of such a probe are listed in Table 2.3.

Table 2.2 *The ideal paediatric transesophageal transducer*

Tip circumference less than 30mm
Bi- or multi-plane with 48 channels in each imaging plane
Multi-hertz capability with imaging at either 5.0 or 7.0 mHz
Integrated continuous wave and high PRF Doppler
The incorporation of both antero-posterior and lateral
   steering capabilities

Table 2.3 *Compromises in transducer design for paediatric transesophageal echocardiography*

Transducer size versus element number
Patient weight range (3–70 kg)
Imaging frequency versus Doppler information
Transverse versus longitudinal plane
Single plane versus biplane versus multiplane
Steering mechanism

ANATOMY OF TRANSESOPHAGEAL IMAGING

A detailed understanding of the normal anatomy of the cardiac chambers and great vessels, as seen from within the oesophagus, is essential to the assessment of congenital cardiac lesions by transesophageal ultrasound studies. In this section, the correlations between standard transesophageal cross-sectional images and the corresponding anatomic sections will be described.

To date, in routine clinical practice, only standard 90 degree ultrasound images can be obtained. However, the relationships of one structure to another within a much wider arc of interrogation can be simply understood by appropriate rotation of the probe.

Transverse axis imaging planes

The scan plane of conventional single-array transesophageal transducers is mounted at right angles to the shaft of the scope, thus producing transverse axis images. With the transducer positioned in the oesophagus, transverse (i.e. short) axis images of the heart are obtained from an intraesophageal position posterior to the left atrium. The anatomic relationship between the thoracic aorta and the oesophagus is complex and is such that the ascending aorta and proximal aortic arch are anterior and to the right of the upper oesophagus, and the descending thoracic aorta spirals downwards almost posterior to the oesophagus. Thus, a gradual leftward rotation has to be carried out to visualise the entire thoracic aorta from the arch down to below the diaphragm.

When transesophageal imaging was first introduced there was disagreement on how best to display the images. Some groups favoured displaying the left aspects of the heart to the left of the operator and with the image inverted. However, over the past few years almost universal agreement has settled on the following image orientation (11,12). The posterior aspects of the heart are displayed at the top of the screen and the anterior aspects on the bottom. The left sided aspects of the heart are displayed to the right of the operator, and the right sided to the left. This image orientation of transverse axis images will be used throughout this book.

We now focus on a more detailed description of seven standard transverse imaging sections through the heart. The corresponding transesophageal cross-sectional images were obtained by rotation of the probe so as to visualise the lateral aspects of the heart; no lateral probe angulation was used, as this would alter the sectioning plane.

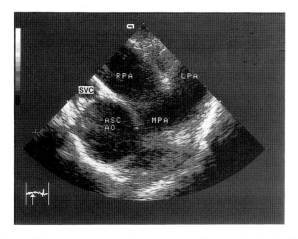

Figure 2.1 *A transverse plane image taken at the level of the pulmonary arteries. The main pulmonary artery is seen to the left of the proximal ascending aorta. In this plane, the bifurcation of the main pulmonary artery into left and right pulmonary arteries is well visualised. The superior vena cava is seen sectioned in short axis lying between the mid right pulmonary artery and ascending aorta.*

1. THE PLANE OF THE PULMONARY ARTERIES

With the probe positioned in the mid oesophagus, at a level just below the bifurcation of the trachea, the central pulmonary artery system is visualised. The pulmonary trunk is seen to the left of the proximal ascending aorta (Fig. 2.1). The bifurcation of the pulmonary trunk is seen on top of the screen and slight rotation of the probe from this position will demonstrate the origin of both the right and the left pulmonary arteries. Lying anterior to the right pulmonary artery, the distal segment of the superior caval vein will be visualised in short axis. Posterior to the left pulmonary artery a cross-section of the descending aorta is obtained. Owing to interposition of the bronchial tree between the oesophagus and the left pulmonary artery, visualisation of the entire central pulmonary arterial system is frequently difficult to achieve. In particular, only the proximal portion of the left pulmonary artery will be visualised near the pulmonary artery bifurcation, and a short, more distal segment may be visualised immediately anterior to the descending aorta. Slight advancement of the probe from plane 1 to an intermediate scan position will visualise the relationships of the superior vena cava, proximal ascending aorta, left atrial cavity and appendage to each other (Fig. 2.2).

2. THE PLANE OF THE AORTIC VALVE

Further advancement of the probe in the oesophagus from sectioning plane 1 will allow visualisation of the aortic valve in its characteristic wedged position between the two fibrous atrioventricular valve rings (Fig. 2.3). Posteriorly a superior portion of the left atrial cavity is seen, and anteriorly the distal portion of the right ventricular outflow tract and the pulmonary valve are visualised. To the left of the aortic valve the left atrial appendage is demonstrated. The appendage is separated posteriorly by a rim of muscular atrial tissue from the left upper pulmonary vein. Further rotation of the probe to the left will bring a cross-section of the descending aorta into view. To the right of the aortic valve and the proximal ascending aorta the superior caval vein and its junction with the right atrial cavity is seen. Anteriorly the upper portion of the right atrial appendage can be visualised. Posterior to the junction of the superior vena cava with the right atrium, the distal segment of the right upper pulmonary vein and its connection with the left atrium is visualised. The transesophageal approach to the visualisation of all four pulmonary veins is described fully in Chapter 3.3

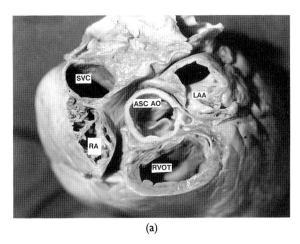

(a)

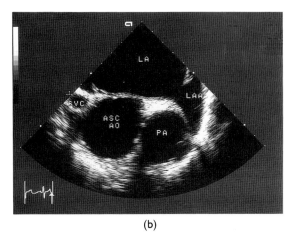

(b)

Figure 2.2 (a) *A morphologic specimen of a heart cut in the transverse plane at the level of the superior vena cava–right atrial junction. This plane is slightly inferior to that of the plane of the pulmonary arteries which is shown in Fig. 2.1.* **(b)** *The corresponding transverse plane transesophageal image. In this section, the relationship of the inferior portion of the superior vena cava, ascending aorta, pulmonary artery, left atrium and left atrial appendage are well documented.*

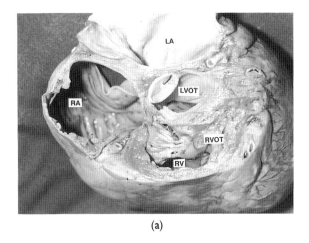

(a)

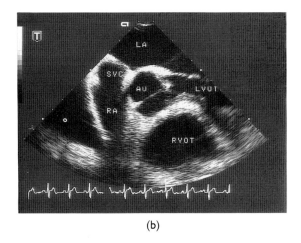

(b)

Figure 2.3 (a) *A morphologic specimen sectioned at the level of the aortic valve to simulate the corresponding transverse transesophageal plane.* **(b)** *The corresponding transverse plane transesophageal image. This transesophageal image has been taken precisely at the superior vena cava right atrial junction and demonstrates well the relationship of the two atria, the aortic valve, the left ventricular outflow tract and the right ventricular outflow tract. Further rotation of the probe to the left from this cross-section would bring the descending aorta into view.*

3. THE PLANE OF THE LEFT VENTRICULAR OUTFLOW TRACT

The next imaging plane, obtained by further insertion of the probe, is a transverse cut through the left ventricular outflow tract (Fig. 2.4). The non-coronary cusp of the aortic valve is frequently visualised in this cut moving in and out of the scan plane. Anteriorly the muscular outlet septum is demonstrated and the septomarginal trabecula can be seen within the right ventricular outflow tract. The cavity of the left atrium is seen posteriorly. To the left the superior portion of the atrial septum is demonstrated as is a superior section of the right atrium. At this level, there is frequently an apparent thickening of the atrial septum due to fibrous fatty tissue within Waterston's groove.

4. THE PLANE OF THE CENTRAL ATRIAL SEPTUM

Minimal further advancement of the probe from plane 3 allows the visualisation of the central aspect of the atrial septum, i.e. the oval fossa. This fibrous structure is in continuity with both the anterior and the posterior muscular portion of the atrial septum. Anteriorly the aortic (anterior) leaflet of the mitral valve is demonstrated, and to the right of the left ventricular outflow tract the membranous portion of the atrioventricular septum is demonstrated. The attachment of the septal leaflet of the tricuspid valve and a portion of the right ventricular cavity can usually be demonstrated in the same scan plane.

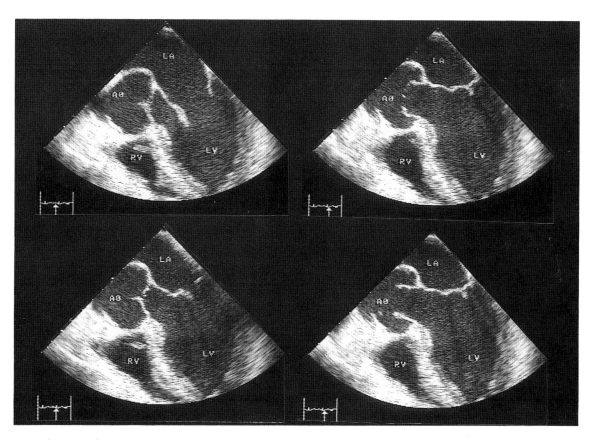

Figure 2.4 *The normal systolic and diastolic opening and closing patterns of the mitral and aortic valve leaflets is well demonstrated.*

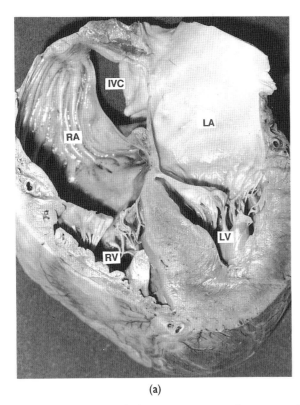

(a)

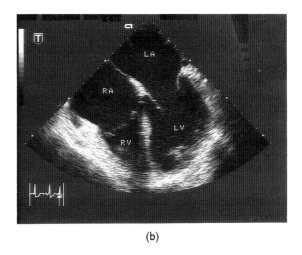

(b)

Figure 2.5 (a) *A morphologic section cut in the transesophageal transverse plane at the level of the atrioventricular junction. In this section, the normal arrangement of offsetting of the atrioventricular valves as they insert into the central fibrous body is well visualised.* **(b)** *The corresponding transverse plane transesophageal image of the atrioventricular junction. The morphologic features shown in (a) are well seen in this transesophageal image (see text).*

5. THE PLANE OF THE ATRIOVENTRICULAR JUNCTION

This imaging plane is often referred to as being the standard transesophageal four chamber view. However, unlike the apical four chamber view obtained by precordial imaging, this transverse axis view does not demonstrate the entire left ventricular cavity. In fact, the sections of the left ventricle obtained are always foreshortened and the true left ventricular apex rarely is visualised (Fig. 2.5). Posteriorly the inferior portion of the atrial septum is visualised. The fibrous tissue of the oval fossa may extend down to this level. Anterior to this, the muscular 'primum' septum is seen. The extension and the attachment of the Eustachian valve to this structure can be demonstrated. Further apically the membranous portion of the inlet ventricular septum is clearly visualised, as are the differing levels of attachment of the septal leaflet of the tricuspid valve and the anterior leaflet of the mitral valve to the crux cordis. Depending on the degree of probe tip angulation and the dimensions of the cardiac chambers variable amounts of the ventricular cavities and

the muscular ventricular septum are visualised. Posteriorly and to the left, the site of connection of the left lower pulmonary vein to the left atrial cavity can be visualised in the majority of cases. To the right the site of connection of the right lower pulmonary vein to the left atrium can be demonstrated.

6. THE FLOOR OF THE ATRIAL CHAMBERS

From a scan position near to the esophageal hiatus, the floor of both atrial cavities and the site of connection of the inferior caval vein with the right atrium can be visualised. In addition, the proximal portion of the coronary sinus can consistently be seen as it runs in the floor of the left atrium to drain into the right atrium. The Thebesian valve, which guards its orifice in the right atrium, is not well appreciated on cross-sectional imaging. Anteriorly the postero-medial commissure of the mitral valve is sectioned in parallel (see Fig. 2.6).

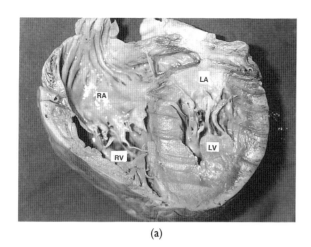

(a)

Figure 2.6 *A transverse plane transesophageal image of the left ventricular outflow tract. In this section, the atrial septum is not visualised. Slight probe withdrawal and rotation of the probe to the right would bring this structure into view.*

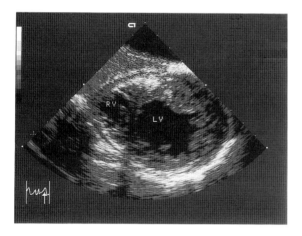

Figure 2.7 *A transverse plane transgastric image demonstrating a short axis cut of the left ventricle taken just below papillary muscle level (for other transgastric images, see Chapter 3.8).*

7. TRANSGASTRIC IMAGING PLANES

With the transducer positioned in the stomach, short axis images of the ventricular chambers are obtained (Fig. 2.7). It is noteworthy that using this transducer position, the inferior aspects of the ventricles are displayed at the top of the screen. Thus, the postero-medial papillary muscle of the mitral valve is displayed above the antero-lateral papillary muscle. The mitral valve apparatus can normally be examined in close detail, whereas this is difficult for the tricuspid valve.

Recently we have expanded the use of transgastric imaging in the assessment of congenital heart disease. With further introduction of the probe, a true four or five chamber view of the heart can be obtained when maximal anteflexion of the probe is employed. Rotation of the probe together with gradual withdrawal provides images which are similar to subxiphoid precordial imaging. Such views are of particular value in the assessment of lesions involving either the ventricular outflow tract (see Chapter 3.8) or in patients with complete transposition.

Longitudinal axis imaging planes

The additional longitudinal imaging planes that are available on biplane transesophageal transducers have proved to be a definite advantage in the evaluation of certain aspects of acquired heart disease. This is especially true for the assessment of complex congenital cardiac lesions. New insights have been gained into lesions of the atrial septum, the atrioventricular valves, the right and left ventricular outflow tracts, the aortic valve, the ventriculo-arterial junction and the thoracic aorta.

Because of the short period during which the technique has been available, confusion on how to display these images persists. It is our opinion that as in the standard display of precordial long axis images of the heart, the superior aspects of the heart should be displayed to the right of the operator and the inferior aspects to the left (13). In contrast, Seward and colleagues (14) have favoured an inversion of the images on the screen, i.e. to display the posterior aspects at the bottom of the screen. The rationale behind this was that the images thus obtained appear to be similar to precordial images. However, the majority of sections obtained are, in fact, quite different. In addition, the constant inversion of the images during a full biplane study is both time consuming and frequently confusing. Finally, biplane imaging is likely to be a transitional step to multiplane imaging, which will display the posterior aspects of the heart at the top of the screen. Thus we proposed the following image orientation for longitudinal plane transesophageal imaging: the posterior aspects are displayed on top of the screen, the anterior aspects on the bottom. The superior aspects are displayed to the left, the inferior aspects to the right of the operator. This orientation is in agreement with other recently published papers from other groups (15–17). However, controversy still surrounds this matter (18,19).

In the following the anatomic basis of the standard longitudinal imaging planes will be described in detail together with the corresponding cross-sectional images. The anatomic sections are displayed in the same orientation as the cross-sectional images which are displayed as described above. The standard transducer position is within the oesophagus posterior to the left atrium. The different sections are obtained by gradual rotation of the probe around its long axis.

1. THE PLANE OF THE CAVAL VEINS

With the probe positioned at mid esophageal level and the scanning plane orientated towards the right aspects of the heart, the right sided pulmonary veins will be visualised entering the left atrium. Slight

further rotation will then show the supra cardiac portion of the superior vena cava and its connection to the right atrium Fig. 2.8. Posterior to the superior vena cava the right pulmonary artery is sectioned in short axis. Anteriorly the right atrial appendage and right atrial cavity are visualised. Posteriorly the left atrial cavity is sectioned. This plane cuts through the atrial septum at the level of the oval fossa, which is seen as a thin membrane-like structure. The muscular portion of the atrial septum (which extends all the way around the oval fossa) and the fibrous fatty tissue within Waterston's groove result in apparent thickening of the remaining atrial septum. The inferior caval vein can be visualised entering the right atrium when the probe is advanced slightly. The Eustachian valve, guarding the inferior caval orifice, is normally well seen in this imaging plane.

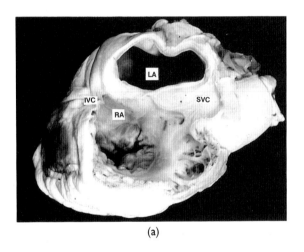

(a)

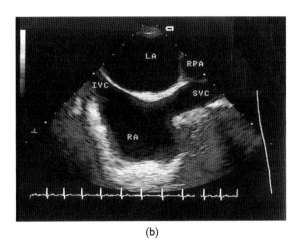

(b)

Figure 2.8 (a) *A morphologic specimen sectioned to represent the transesophageal longitudinal plane which images the caval veins, atrial septum and right atrial appendage.* **(b)** *The corresponding transesophageal longitudinal image of the plane of the caval veins.*

2. THE PLANE OF THE ASCENDING AORTA

Slight counter-clockwise rotation of the probe from plane 1 will bring the ascending aorta into view anteriorly. The cavity of the left atrium is seen posteriorly (Fig. 2.9). Both the fibrous and the muscular portions of the anterior aspect of the atrial septum are sectioned. The scan plane cuts through the lateral portion of the tricuspid valve, demonstrating the antero-superior and the inferior leaflet.

Frequently a lateral segment of the right ventricle is demonstrated in the same plane. In a subset of patients using minimal rotation from this scan position, it is possible to demonstrate the origin of the right coronary artery as it arises from the aorta. Using full lateral angulation of the transducer tip, it is possible to image the aortic valve in a true cross-section. All three leaflets will be well imaged as will the valve orifice. This longitudinal view (using full lateral tip angulation) is increasingly being used to define aortic valve orifice area.

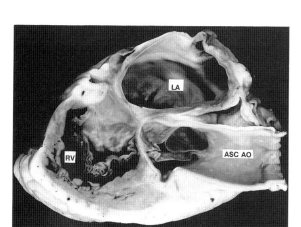

(a)

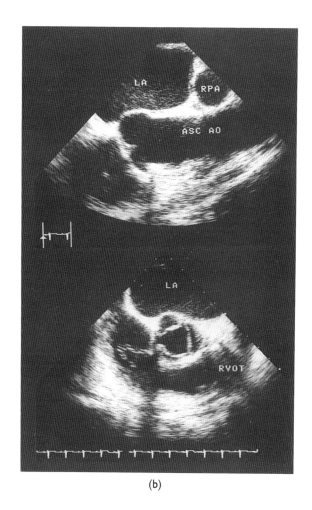

(b)

Figure 2.9 (a) *A morphologic specimen sectioned to simulate the transesophageal longitudinal plane which visualises the ascending aorta.* **(b)** *(Upper panel) The transesophageal longitudinal image taken in the plane of the ascending aorta. In this view, the aortic valve, aortic sinuses and first 4–5 cm of the ascending aorta are well imaged in the long axis. By counter-clockwise rotation of the lateral steering mechanism, a short axis view of the aortic valve in the longitudinal plane will be imaged. It is our experience that this is the best view for imaging the true aortic valve orifice and aortic valve leaflet morphology. (Lower panel) The image thus obtained. Note the tricuspid nature of the aortic valve is clearly imaged.*

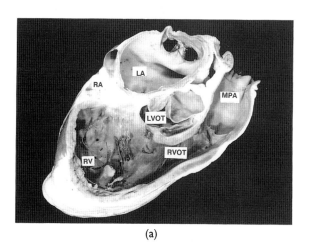

(a)

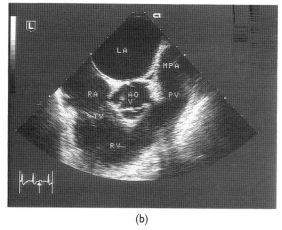

(b)

Figure 2.10 (a) *A morphologic specimen sectioned in the plane of the right ventricular outflow tract. This image is obtained by rotating the transducer to the patient's left from Fig. 2.9(b) upper panel.* **(b)** *The corresponding longitudinal plane image of the right ventricular outflow tract.*

3. THE PLANE OF THE RIGHT VENTRICULAR OUTFLOW TRACT

Further rotation and rightward angulation of the probe from plane 2 will open up the right ventricular cavity and the right ventricular outflow tract (Fig. 2.10). These structures lie in the far field of imaging. To the right of the operator the pulmonary valve and the pulmonary trunk are visualised. Centrally the aortic root is sectioned obliquely. The right coronary cusp of the aortic valve is displayed to the operator's left. The septal leaflet of the tricuspid valve and the superior portion of the atrial septum are also often demonstrated in this scan plane.

4. THE PLANE OF THE VENTRICULAR SEPTUM

With the probe back in a neutral position (i.e. with no lateral angulation) and using further counterclockwise rotation the ventricular septum can be scanned (Fig. 2.11). These longitudinal planes cut through the septum obliquely, and thus result in apparent thickening of the muscular septum. Anteriorly the apical portion of the right ventricular cavity is demonstrated. Inferiorly the coronary sinus and the postero-medial commissure of the mitral valve are sectioned in short axis.

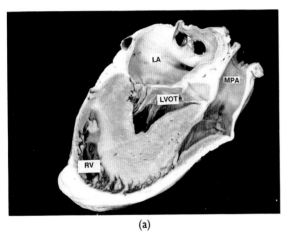
(a)

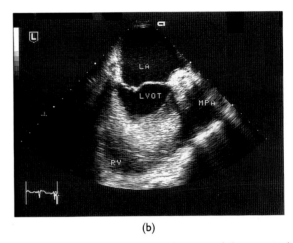
(b)

Figure 2.11 (a) *A morphologic specimen sectioned to simulate the longitudinal plane transesophageal image of the ventricular septum. Note that the oblique cut of the septum in this plane produces the false impression of increased septal thickening.*
(b) *The corresponding transesophageal longitudinal plane image of the ventricular septum.*

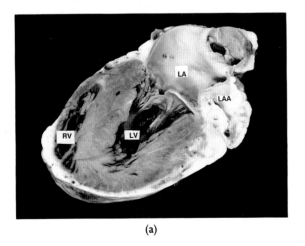
(a)

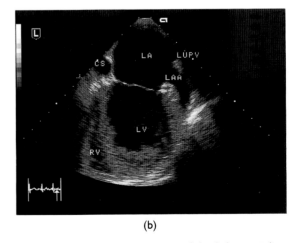
(b)

Figure 2.12 (a) *A morphologic specimen sectioned to simulate the longitudinal plane of the long axis of the left ventricle. This is the only transesophageal plane (either esophageal or transgastric) which images the apex of the left ventricle. The ventricular apex can also be imaged from a transgastric position (see Fig. 2.15).* **(b)** *The corresponding longitudinal plane transesophageal image of the left ventricle.*

5. THE PLANE OF THE LEFT VENTRICLE

Further rotation of the probe will section the left ventricle in its long axis (Fig. 2.12). The true left ventricular apex is visualised for the first time from the oesophagus. The lateral aspects of the mitral valve and the papillary muscles are demonstrated in detail. Superiorly the left atrial appendage can be seen together with a cross-section through the left pulmonary artery. Posteriorly the left sided pulmonary veins are demonstrated. When the probe is rotated even further postero-laterally and is gradually withdrawn, the whole descending thoracic aorta can be examined in its long axis.

6. TRANSGASTRIC LONGITUDINAL PLANE IMAGING

The transgastric longitudinal plane may provide valuable new information on the inferior vena cava (Fig. 2.13), the right ventricular outflow tract (Fig. 2.14), the left ventricular apex (Fig. 2.15) and the mitral valve (Fig. 2.16).

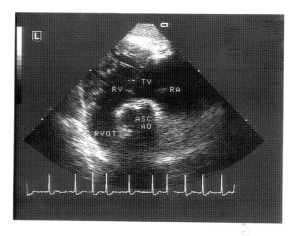

Figure 2.14 *A transgastric long axis view of the right ventricular inflow and outflow tracts. This image is obtained by rotating the probe to the left of the patient from the imaging plane demonstrated in Fig. 2.13.*

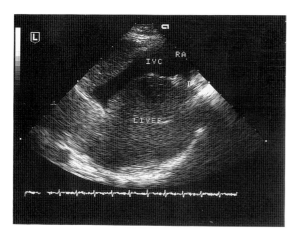

Figure 2.13 *A longitudinal plane transgastric image demonstrating the intrahepatic portion of the inferior vena cava and its junction with the right atrium.*

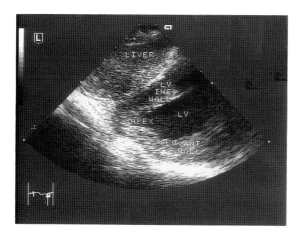

Figure 2.15 *A transgastric longitudinal plane image demonstrating the apex of the left ventricle.*

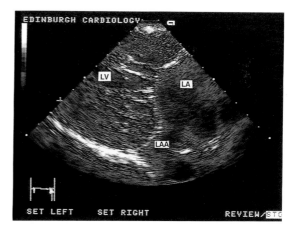

Figure 2.16 *A transgastric longitudinal plane image demonstrating the mitral valve. It is the transgastric longitudinal plane which best separates out the two papillary muscles and the primary and secondary chordae. This view may be difficult to obtain. It does however contain some of the most useful information on the dynamic function of the mitral valve which may be obtained using the esophageal approach.*

STANDARD EXAMINATION TECHNIQUE

The physician who undertakes transesophageal studies should either have a sound experience in gastroenterology or be trained specifically to perform esophageal intubation. It is our opinion that sufficient experience can be acquired by observing some 20 gastroscopies and thereafter by performing another 20 to 40 esophageal intubations under supervision.

All adult patients who are scheduled for a transesophageal echocardiographic study should have a history taken concerning current or previous upper gastrointestinal disease, spinal disease and bleeding disorders. The procedure should be explained in detail to the patient, as should be the reasons why such a study is undertaken. Appropriate modifications in this pro forma should be made for paediatric patients. Written consent from the patients or their parents should be obtained. Patients should be fasted at least four hours prior to the procedure and any dental prosthesis should be removed.

Probe preparation

Prior to all studies the investigator should check on the proper function of the probe, both in terms of probe mechanics and transducer performance. The probe may then be inserted into a long plastic sheath, if that is the policy of the operator. The sheath should contain a sufficient amount of ultrasound gel at its tip. Care must be taken that there are no air bubbles left at the level of the transducer. As the sheath can cause discomfort to the patient, we and others prefer to perform studies without the use of a sheath. In such cases, the shaft of the probe should be well lubricated. The probe must be carefully disinfected between studies.

Sterilisation is carried out by thorough washing of the probe and by subsequent emersion in a Cidex solution for 20 minutes. Alcohol should not be used for disinfection since it may degrade the silicon material used to cover the ultrasound transducer. All transesophageal probes should be routinely checked for electrical safety, as this may be compromised by even microscopic cracks in the coating material.

Adolescents and adult studies in the outpatient clinic

The procedure should be explained to the patient in detail and reassurance given. Local anaesthesia (lignocaine spray) is applied to the hypopharynx and tongue, and the patient is then asked to swallow. Venous access should be established in all patients, and electrocardiographic leads connected to allow continuous ECG monitoring. Sedation should be used more liberally in adolescents and young adults with congenital heart disease, than in the older patient with acquired cardiac disease. This is, firstly, because transesophageal studies in complex congenital heart disease tend to be more time consuming, and, secondly, patient tolerance towards esophageal intubation is relatively poorer in the younger patient population. We currently prefer either midazolam (3–5 mg) or diazepam (5–8 mg) for sedation. Midazolam has the advantage of a more rapid and shorter action and better retrograde amnesia. In addition, its action can be reversed at the end of the procedure. It is also our current practice to use a secretion-drying agent in all patients under the age of forty. This is because younger patients tend to produce copius secretions during the procedure. These may be intolerable to the patient resulting in the procedure having to be aborted. Our current preference is to use intravenous glycopyrronium in an appropriate dose per kilogram to reduce dry secretions.

The patient is then asked to roll over onto his or her left side and to approximate chin to chest. An absorbent drape is put under the patients face and covering his shoulder and left arm. The bite guard is positioned over the shaft of the transesophageal probe. The operator holds the handle of the probe with his left hand and the right hand supports the probe at a distance of roughly 20 cm from the tip. During insertion the tip of the transducer is initially flexed anteriorly so as to gain contact with the tongue. The probe is then gradually advanced until the hypopharynx is reached. Thereafter the tip of the probe is slightly retroflexed so as to gain contact with the posterior aspect of the hypopharynx and to stay away from the epiglottis. With the probe in this position the patient will normally gag. The patient is then asked to swallow and following successful swallowing the probe is then rapidly advanced in the oesophagus to the level of the left atrium. Once the probe is inserted the patient is asked to breath normally and the biteguard is secured so as to prevent any damage of the transducer.

Certainly modifications of the above described technique of probe insertion exist, and individual operators will evolve their own methods of probe introduction with growing experience. However, despite the variations between individual techniques, several important aspects should be kept in mind. Firstly, the probe should always stay in a midline position during introduction in order to prevent passage into the (lateral) piriform recesses of the pharynx. Under no circumstances should the probe be advanced against resistance. Once the oesophagus has been entered, the probe should be advanced to a level well below the bifurcation of the trachea, where it causes the least discomfort to the patient. Both high esophageal and gastric positions are less well tolerated.

Paediatric patients

Transesophageal studies in children below the age of 10 years are normally carried out under general anaesthesia using endotracheal intubation. However, some investigators have performed studies in younger children using ketamine anaesthesia without endotracheal intubation (5–7 mg/kg) and have reported good results with this technique. In our experience, this latter technique has several disadvantages. The response to ketamine appears to be rather unpredictable. In addition, children frequently swallow excessive air into their stomachs. Nasogastric tubes must then be passed after the procedure to let the air escape. Furthermore, following ketamine administration, there is often a marked constriction of the entrance to the oesophagus which can make esophageal intubation difficult. In the older child transesophageal studies can be performed safely with heavy sedation (midazolam) together with appropriate local anaesthesia as described above. Such studies are best performed on a day care basis.

Although transesophageal studies in children of more than 20 kilograms of bodyweight have been reported to be safe using adult transesophageal probes (tip circumference >50 mm) (20,21), we feel that this should not be attempted routinely. Probe insertion and manipulation with such large probes can be difficult, and is potentially traumatic. Our preference is to use dedicated paediatric probes in all children up to 50 kilograms. Above that weight ultrasound attenuation is generally too great to allow full diagnostic studies to be obtained using a paediatric probe. The lower end of the patient weight spectrum for the current generation of paediatric probes appears to be somewhere around 3.0 kilograms. However, successful studies have been reported down to a bodyweight of 2 kilograms (21).

Intraoperative studies and studies carried out under general anaesthesia

Transesophageal studies performed in either the perioperative period or in the intensive care unit will normally be carried out with the patient under general anaesthesia using endotracheal intubation. With the patient in the supine position, it is best for the operator to introduce the probe and to perform the study standing at the patient's head. Nasogastric tubes should be removed prior to probe insertion. In our experience, it has proved easiest to place the probe and connecting cable around the operator's neck, and to introduce the distal portion of the probe into the hypopharynx with the right hand, while the left hand remains free for manipulation. During insertion, the left hand may be used to lift the patient's mandible and to slightly extend the patient's neck. In orally intubated patients, the partially flexed probe is then passed along the palate, above the endotracheal tube, and is advanced into the hypopharynx. In nasotracheally intubated patients in the intensive care unit, the probe should be inserted from a rather lateral position and is then passed behind the endotracheal tube into the oesophagus. In such cases the left index finger should be used for orientation and accurate probe guidance within the mouth. In cases in whom probe insertion fails or meets resistance a further attempt may be undertaken, and if this fails the probe should then be inserted under direct laryngoscopic vision.

Monitoring

A reliable venous access and continuous electrocardiographic monitoring are prerequisites for all transesophageal studies. In fact, such monitoring is sufficient for the majority of outpatient studies. In cyanotic patients the additional monitoring of oxygen saturations should be performed using a finger-tip oximeter. Blood pressure monitoring in our experience is of little value in the outpatient setting. However, during studies in patients undergoing surgical correction or in the intensive care unit the echocardiographer should take advantage of the abundance of concomitant monitoring information available in these two clinical settings.

Transesophageal studies in patients with congenital heart disease should only be performed in areas where there is equipment for cardiopulmonary resuscitation ready at hand. In particular, a reliable suction apparatus and oxygen supply are mandatory. A complete set of drugs for resuscitation should be prepared, and equipment for intubation and defibrillation should be available.

Endocarditis prophylaxis

In the past there has been evidence brought forward that bacteraemia is a frequent finding during transesophageal studies (22,23). Thus, several investigators have advocated giving antibiotic endocarditis prophylaxis as a routine measure. This is in contrast to the experience with thousands of transesophageal studies being performed without antibiotic prophylaxis with no case of associated endocarditis having been documented. Moreover, accepted guidelines on endocarditis prophylaxis (24) do not list upper gastrointestinal diagnostic procedures as an indication. Recently, two prospective studies have reported on the incidence of positive blood cultures both during and after transesophageal studies. These studies confirmed that the incidence of bacteraemia associated with gastroscopy is very low and may indeed be explained by contamination during blood sampling. We currently do not use antibiotic prophylaxis in any patient, and have not experienced a single case of endocarditis following a transesophageal study in our extensive study population with both congenital and acquired cardiac disease.

CONTRAINDICATIONS EXCLUSION CRITERIA

A list of absolute and relative contraindications to a transesophageal study has not yet been agreed upon by either the American Society of Echocardiography or by the Echocardiography Working Group of the European Society of Cardiology. Thus, every centre will develop and pursue its own policy. Currently we do not attempt transesophageal studies in patients with (a) severe upper spinal disease, (b) severe disorders of the upper gastrointestinal tract, and (c) severe coagulation disorders. In addition, studies in patients with severe pulmonary hypertension are carried out only under general anaesthesia with endotracheal intubation. Children of less than 4 kilograms bodyweight are not studied at our institution unless the information likely to be derived from the transesophageal study is crucial for patient management.

THE STANDARD EXAMINATION PROTOCOL

All transesophageal studies carried out to assess congenital heart disease should follow a standardised scheme. The investigator should observe the rules of sequential chamber analysis, the approach most widely used in the categorisation of congenital malformations of the heart. Firstly, the type of venous connections to the heart should be described. Thereafter the location and the morphology of the atrial chambers is assessed. Then the atrioventricular connection is defined and finally the form of the ventriculo-arterial connection is documented. Only thereafter are specific lesions more closely examined. This approach may appear time-consuming and complicated to the adult cardiologist, but it is only on the basis of this framework that the description of congenital cardiac malformations is meaningful.

The examination

The probe is initially advanced to image the transesophageal four chamber plane. The position of the cardiac apex should be noted. This can be on the left, midline or on the patient's right side (dextrocardia). Minor degrees of cardiac malposition will go undetected by transesophageal imaging. Patients with dextrocardia are as easily studied as normal patients. Probe manipulation in such cases just involves a 90 degree clockwise rotation of the probe from the normal esophageal imaging position (whereas in precordial ultrasound techniques this requires a mirror image examination technique). After establishing the position of the cardiac apex, the probe should then be slightly advanced together with clockwise rotation of the probe, so as to demonstrate the liver from a scan position near the esophageal hiatus. The infradiaphragmatic segment of the inferior caval vein is visualised by this manoeuvre, and by gradual probe withdrawal the pattern of drainage of the hepatic veins established. The distal portion of the inferior caval vein should then be followed to the (right) atrial chamber. Further probe withdrawal using right lateral scan positions will then demonstrate the connection of the superior caval vein to the atrial chamber. Immediately posterior to this the right upper pulmonary vein is visualised, and repeat probe insertion together with clockwise rotation will demonstrate the right lower pulmonary vein near its site

Table 2.4 *Summary of the sequence of imaging planes used during transesophageal echocardiographic investigations in the assessment of congenital heart disease*

Standard examination planes	Visualisation of cardiac structures	Examples of pathology visualised
Transgastric planes	Ventricular morphology	Ventricular dominance
	Ventricular relations	Supero/inferior ventricles
	Ventricular function	
	Chordal apparatus MV	Parachute MV
	Inferior atrioventricular vein	Interruption
	Hepatic veins	Individual drainage
	Atrioventricular valves	Common valve orifice
Lower oesophagus	Coronary sinus	Unroofed CS
		Dilated CS
	Muscular inlet septum	Muscular inlet VSD
	Tricuspid valve	Ebstein's malformation
		Tricuspid atresia
	4-chamber view	Offsetting atrioventricular valves
		Atrioventricular septal defects
		Perimembranous VSD
Left atrial views	Mitral valve	Valvar regurgitation
		Endocarditis
	Atrial septum	Patent oval foramen
		Deficiencies of the oval fossa
	Pulmonary veins	Anomalous connection
	Atrial chambers	Atrial arrangement
		Mustard baffles
		Cor triatriatum
	LV outflow tract	Membranes
		Arterial override
Mid oesophagus	Atrial septum	Sinus venosus defect
		Juxtaposition
	VA junction	Transposition/malposition
	Superior atrioventricular vein	Anomalous drainage
	Aortic valve	Valvar aortic stenosis
	RV outflow tract	Infundibular stenosis
	Pulmonary trunk	Patent ductus arteriosus
		Supratrioventricular alvar stenosis
	Pulmonary arteries	Palliative shunts
		Peripheral stenosis
Thoracic aorta	Aortic arch, descending aorta	Coarctation
		Collaterals

CS = coronary sinus; LV = left ventricle; MV = mitral valve; RV = right ventricle; VA = ventriculo-arterial; VSD = ventricular septal defect.
Note: In the sequential analysis of congenital heart disease atrial morphology has to be determined first, thereafter atrioventricular and ventriculoarterial connections should be defined and systemic and pulmonary venous drainage determined. Only thereafter the examination should focus on the relevant lesions.

of connection with the (left) atrial chamber. Ninety degree clockwise rotation of the probe will then allow visualisation of the left lower pulmonary vein, and, following gradual probe withdrawal, the left upper pulmonary vein and their site of drainage to the atria (see Chapter 3.1). Colour flow mapping studies will help the rapid identification of the site of connections of the four pulmonary veins. The left sided atrial appendage is normally visualised just anterior and medially to the left upper pulmonary vein. The right atrial appendage should then be imaged by a clockwise rotation of the probe from this scan position. The examination of the morphologic features of either atrial appendage will then allow the direct diagnosis of the atrial arrangement (see Chapter 3.2). Following this documentation of the cardiac position, and the definition of both the venous connections and the atrial arrangement, the next step should be to define the type of atrioventricular connection using a series of transesophageal four-chamber views (see Chapter 3.4). Finally the morphology of the ventriculo-arterial junction should be visualised by scanning high esophageal views (see Chapter 3.9) and the mode of ventriculo-arterial connection established. The relation of the great arteries to one another and to the underlying ventricular chambers is best defined using a series of slight probe manipulations.

Thus having defined the ventriculo-arterial connection and the spatial relations of the great vessels to one another, the process of sequential chamber localisation is complete and the transesophageal examination should then proceed to the assessment of the individual lesions.

This examination should also be performed in a standard sequential manner. The venous return to the heart should be assessed in more detail, as should be the atrial chambers, the atrial septum, the atrioventricular valves, the ventricular chambers and the ventricular septum and, finally, the great arteries. Colour flow mapping should be performed at all cardiac levels for the rapid identification of abnormal flow patterns, and pulsed and continuous wave Doppler interrogation should be performed at relevant areas of interest. The use of colour M-mode studies, in our experience, has proved to be particularly valuable in young children with rapid heart rates, since it allows a more precise temporal resolution of abnormal flow patterns. A synopsis of the standard transesophageal views which are used in the assessment of congenital cardiac malformations is listed in Table 2.4.

REFERENCES

1. FRAZIN L, TALANO JV, STEPHANIDES L, LOEB HS, KOPEL L, GUNNAR RM. Esophageal echocardiography. *Circulation* 1976; **54:** 102–8.
2. SOUQUET J, HANRATH P, ZITELLI L, et al. Transesophageal phased array for imaging the heart. *IEEE Trans Biomed Engineer* 1982; **29:** 707.
3. HANRATH P, KREMER P, LANGESTEIN BA, MATSUMOTO M, BLEIFELD W. Transoesophageale Eckokardiographie: Ein neues Verfahren zur dynamischen Ventrikelfunktionsanalyse. *Dtsch Med Wochenschr* 1981; **106:** 525–32.
4. HANRATH P, SCHLÜTER M, LANGENSTEIN BA, et al. Detection of ostium secundum atrial septal defects by transoesophageal cross-sectional echocardiography. *Br Heart J* 1983; **49:** 350–8.
5. OMOTO R, KYO S, MATSUMURA M, SHAH P, ADACHI H, MATSUNAKA T, TACHIKAWA K. Recent technological progress in transoesophageal colour Doppler flow imaging with special reference to newly developed biplane and paediatric probes. In Erbel R, et al. (eds), *Transoesophageal echocardiography.* Berlin: Springer-Verlag, 1989.
6. COHEN GI, CHAN KL. Biplane transoesophageal echocardiography: clinical applications of the long-axis plane. *J Am Soc Echo* 1991; **4:** 155–63.
7. COHEN GI, CHAN KL, VALLEY VM. Anatomic correlations of the long-axis views in biplane transoesophageal echocardiography. *Am J Cardiol* 1990; **66:** 1007–12.
8. PANDIAN N, HSU T, WEINTRAUB A, SCHWARTZ S, SIMONETTI J, GORDON G. Realtime multiplane transoesophageal echocardiography using a prototype phased array TEE probe with 180 dgree scan plane steering capability: Method, echo-anatomic correlations and early clinical experience. *J Am Coll Cardiol* 1992; **19:** no. 4 (suppl.).
9. OMOTO R, KYOS S, MATSUMURA M, ADACHI H, MARUYAMA M, MATSUNAKA T. New direction of biplane transoesophageal echocardiography with special emphasis on real-time biplane imaging and matrix phased-array biplane transducer. *Echocardiography* 1990; **7:** 691–8.
10. STÜMPER O, ELZENGA NJ, HESS J, SUTHERLAND GR. Transoesophageal echocardiography in children with congenital heart disease – an initial experience. *J Am Coll Cardiol* 1990; **16:** 433–41.
11. SEWARD JB, KHANDERIA BK, OH JK, et al. Transoesophageal echocardiography: technique, anatomic correlations, implementations and clinical applications. *May Clin Proc* 1988; **63:** 649–80.
12. MITCHELL M, SUTHERLAND GR, ROELANDT J. Transesophageal echocardiography – a state of the art review. *J Am Soc Echo* 1988; **1:** 363–77.

13. STÜMPER O, FRASER AG, HO SY, *et al.* Transoesophageal echocardiography in the longitudinal axis. Correlation between anatomy and images and its clinical implications. *Br Heart J* 1990; **64:** 282–8.

14. SEWARD JB, KHANDERIA BK, EDWARDS WD, *et al.* Biplane transoesophageal echocardiography; anatomic correlations, image orientation and clinical applications. *Mayo Clin Proc* 1990; **65:** 1193–213.

15. BANSAL RC, SHAKUDO M, SHAH PM, *et al.* Biplane transoesophageal echocardiography: technique, image orientation and preliminary experience in 131 patients. *J Am Soc Echo* 1990; **5:** 348–66.

16. NANDA NC, PINHEIRO L, SANYAL RS. Transoesophageal biplane echocardiographic imaging: technique, planes and clinical usefulness. *Echocardiography* 1990; **7:** 771–88.

17. RICHARDSON SG, WEINTRAUB AR, SCHWARTZ SL, *et al.* Biplane transesophageal echocardiography utilizing transverse and sagittal imaging planes. Technique, echo-anatomic correlations, and display approaches. *Echocardiography* 1991; **8:** 293.

18. SEWARD JB. 'Nonanatomic' correlations of transesophageal echocardiography. *Echocardiography* 1991; **8:** 669–70.

19. RICHARDSON SG, PANDIAN NG. Echo-anatomic correlations and image display approaches in transesophageal echocardiography. *Echocardiography* 1991; **8:** 671–4.

20. RITTER SB. Pediatric transesophageal color flow imaging 1990: the long and short of it. *Echocardiography* 1990; **7:** 713–25.

21. RITTER SB. Transesophageal real-time echocardiography in infants and children with congenital heart disease. *J Am Coll Cardiol* 1991; **18:** 569–80.

22. DENNIG K, SEDLMAYR V, SELING B, RUDOLPH W. Bacteremia with transesophageal echocardiography [abstract]. *Circulation* 1989; **80:** II-473.

23. GÖRGE G, ERBEL R, HENRICHS J, *et al.* Positive blood cultures during transesophageal echocardiography [abstract]. *J Am Coll Cardiol* 1990; **15:** 62a.

24. DELAYE J, ETIENNE J, FERUGLIO GA, *et al.* Prophylaxis of infective endocarditis for dental procedures. Report of a Working Party of the European Society of Cardiology. *Eur Heart J* 1985; **6:** 826–8.

TEE in the primary diagnosis of congenital heart disease

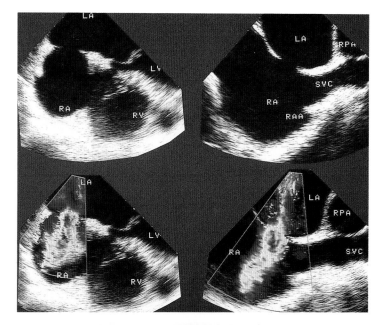

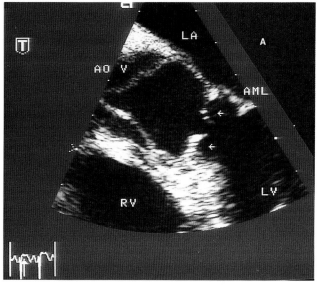

Normal and anomalous venous connections to the heart

O. Stümper

INTRODUCTION

Definition of the venous connections to the heart, both systemic and pulmonary, is among the initial steps in the assessment of patients with congenital heart disease. Anomalies of the venous connections are a frequent finding in patients with complex lesions, and their identification is especially important where a corrective surgical procedure is planned.

Precordial cross-sectional imaging is a good technique when used in the preoperative definition of anomalous venous connections in early childhood (1,2). The sensitivity with which total anomalous pulmonary venous connections can be documented in infancy is such that routine preoperative cardiac catheterisation is no longer considered essential (3). The more recent advent of both pulsed Doppler and colour flow mapping techniques further increased the diagnostic accuracy of precordial ultrasound in this respect (4). However, problems still persist in the definition of certain types of (partial) anomalous pulmonary venous connections or in the documentation of anomalies of the systemic venous drainage. Moreover, in patients with poor precordial ultrasound windows, for instance in adolescents or in children with thoracic or spinal cage anomalies, the transthoracic approach frequently cannot provide a definite diagnosis or the ultimate exclusion of such lesions.

Cardiac catheterisation techniques are considered to be the ultimate diagnostic test for the identification of systemic venous connections. Pulmonary venous connections, on the other hand, are frequently difficult to evaluate by cardiac catheterisation and angiocardiography. The major limitation of the technique would appear to be the poor definition of the sites of the venous connections relative to the atrial structures, in particular to the atrial septum.

Magnetic resonance imaging has been suggested by some investigators to be a valuable diagnostic technique in the preoperative assessment of this spectrum of lesions (5,6). However, the current limited availability and the high demands in operating time and manpower militate against its routine use.

Transesophageal echocardiography, which can provide a detailed insight into the cardiac chambers closest to the oesophagus, would appear to be a promising alternative diagnostic technique in cases where abnormalities of the venous connections cannot be definitively ruled out by precordial ultrasound techniques (7). An improved assessment of sinus venosus-type atrial septal defects, when compared with transthoracic ultrasound examinations, has been reported (8,9). However, little is known about its precise role in the assessment of the wide spectrum of these lesions. In this chapter the transesophageal assessment of normal systemic and pulmonary venous connections will be outlined first, before the methodology used to document the range of anomalous systemic and pulmonary venous connections is discussed in more detail.

NORMAL VENOUS CONNECTIONS

SYSTEMIC

With the transducer positioned at the junction of the oesophagus with the stomach, and by scanning towards the right side of the patient, a cross-sectional image of the liver is obtained. The hepatic veins are readily identified, and by decreasing the level of probe insertion, their confluence with the infradiaphragmatic segment of the inferior caval vein is documented. When the probe is withdrawn further and rotated slightly counterclockwise the connection of the inferior caval vein with the right atrium is documented. Anteriorly the Eustachian valve is visualised. Further counterclockwise rotation of the probe demonstrates the distal portion of the coronary sinus and its drainage into the right atrium (Fig. 2.6). Owing to the rapid movement of the base of the heart relative to the oesophagus, the coronary sinus can be visualised only during part of the cardiac cycle in the majority of cases. However, its site of drainage and the dimension of its distal portion can be assessed in every patient studied.

The superior caval vein is documented by scanning a high esophageal transverse axis view. It is seen anterior to the right pulmonary artery, and, when the probe is advanced further, just anterior to the right upper pulmonary vein. Following further probe advancement the connection of the superior caval vein with the right atrial cavity is delineated. Medially to the site of connection, the superior limbus of the atrial septum is well visualised. In addition, on transverse axis imaging of this area, a crest of atrial tissue will be seen laterally and extending anteriorly to the site of connection of the superior caval vein into the right atrium. This is the crista terminalis. Following gradual withdrawal of the probe a short segment of the mid section of the superior caval vein frequently can be visualised cranial of the right main bronchus. At this site the azygos vein joins the superior caval vein on its posterior aspect. This vessel is normally not visualised in children unless it is dilated, such as in patients with an interrupted inferior caval vein. Visualisation of the confluence of the right brachiocepalic vein and the innominate vein is unusual on transesophageal imaging, as the interposition of lung tissue normally precludes adequate image acquisition. With experience, a segment of the innominate vein can be visualised anterior to the aortic arch both on cross-sectional imaging and colour flow mapping

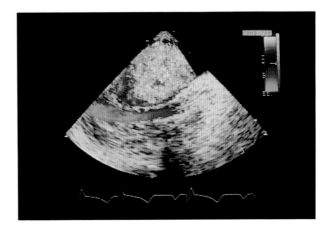

Figure 3.1 *Transverse axis colour flow mapping study used in the definition of the innominate vein (IV; encoded in blue), lying anterior to the transverse aortic arch.*

(Fig. 3.1). However, it should be remembered that transesophageal imaging and probe manipulation cranial to the pulmonary artery bifurcation is often poorly tolerated in the awake patient, and thus should be limited. It is best performed only at the end of the study.

When using longitudinal axis imaging longer segments of both the superior and inferior caval veins can be documented. This is certainly a definite advantage when compared with transverse axis imaging. In addition, visualisation of the azygos vein is facilitated. The imaging planes thus obtained are parallel to the orientation of both caval veins and the atrial septum. Thus, assessment of the degree of override of the caval veins over a sinus venosus atrial septum defect is enhanced when using longitudinal imaging planes. It is noteworthy that in most cases studied the superior caval vein drains into the right atrium more medially than the inferior caval vein. Thus, slight clockwise rotation has to be employed when the inferior caval vein is assessed from a scan position used for documentation of the superior caval vein.

PULMONARY

The left upper pulmonary vein is readily visualised when the probe is rotated counterclockwise from the position used to interrogate the aortic valve. It is separated from the left atrial appendage by a crest of atrial tissue (Fig. 3.2). The direction of the distal portion of the left upper pulmonary vein is such that it is directly parallel to the ultrasound beam.

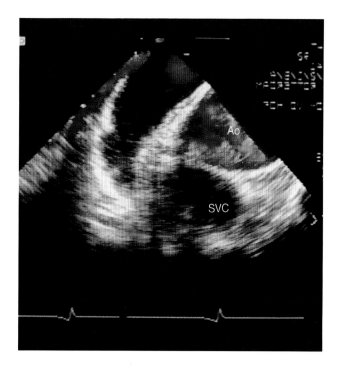
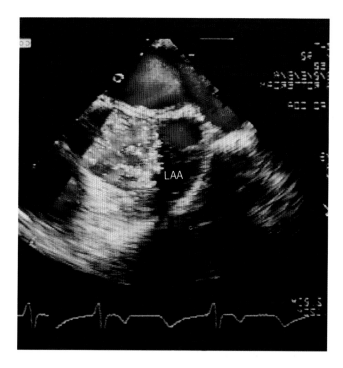

Figure 3.2 *Transesophageal definition of the normal connection of both the right upper and left upper pulmonary veins to the left atrium. The right upper pulmonary vein is visualised just posterior to the superior caval vein; and the left upper pulmonary vein is seen lying posterior to the left atrial appendage (LAA).*

Following slight probe advancement together with minimal counterclockwise rotation the left lower pulmonary vein is visualised. It enters the left atrium in a more frontal plane than the left upper pulmonary vein. Routinely a more proximal segment of the left lower pulmonary vein can be visualised lying anterior to the descending aorta. Repositioning of the probe to the position used for the assessment of the superior caval vein, will allow the right upper pulmonary vein to be visualised draining to the right atrium. Again its orientation is almost parallel to the ultrasound beam, allowing for high-quality pulsed wave Doppler interrogation of pulmonary venous flow patterns with an optimal angle of incidence. Frequently, the confluence of the right upper and the right middle lobe pulmonary vein can be demonstrated by transesophageal transverse axis imaging. The upper lobe pulmonary vein enters the left atrium in a rather oblique fashion and more cranially than the middle lobe pulmonary vein, which courses in a more frontal plane. This is noteworthy in the precise definition of the site of drainage of all four pulmonary veins; the middle lobe vein should not be mistaken for the right lower pulmonary vein. Documentation of the right lower pulmonary vein is the most difficult of the four pulmonary veins. It enters the left atrium inferiorly and in a rather postero-anterior fashion. Conclus-

ively, the probe has to be advanced further and has to be rotated even further clockwise. However, in some cases difficulties will be encountered in gaining good probe contact and thus adequate image quality from this scan position. Nevertheless, in our paediatric experience, the site of connection of the right lower pulmonary vein could be visualised in 92% of all cases (10).

Table 3.1 *Assessment of pulmonary venous connections by precordial (PE) and transesophageal (TEE) ultrasound studies*

Pulmonary vein	PE	TEE
LUPV	76%	100%
RUPV	84%	100%
LLPV	37%	97%
RLPV	18%	92%

When compared with transthoracic ultrasound techniques, transesophageal transverse axis imaging has proved to be a much more sensitive technique in the documentation of the site of connection of all four pulmonary veins (Table 3.1). In addition, the technique allows for high-quality pulsed wave Doppler studies of pulmonary venous flow patterns. This provides a most sensitive diagnostic technique for use in the detection of even minor pulmonary venous obstructions. Such obstructions are characterised by the finding of continuous turbulent flow within the veins or at their orifices throughout the cardiac cycle (Fig. 3.3).

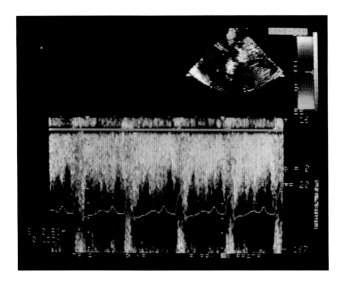

Figure 3.3 *Pulsed wave Doppler tracing diagnostic of mild pulmonary venous obstruction. There is continuous turbulent flow which does not reach baseline during the cardiac cycle.*

Pressure gradients can be calculated from pulsed wave Doppler recordings. In combination with high-quality cross-sectional imaging from the oesophagus the precise morphologic correlate of these lesions can be documented. This should be regarded an important contribution in the diagnosis and late postoperative follow-up of all patients with anomalous pulmonary venous connections.

Analysed in conjunction with the atrioventricular valve flow patterns, the documentation of pulmonary venous flow patterns potentially offers a new diagnostic modality in the assessment of diastolic ventricular function (11–13). Recently there has been much research performed in the interpretation of pulmonary venous flow patterns in patients with acquired cardiac disease. It appeared tempting to adopt some of these concepts for an improved assessment of subtle haemodynamic changes associated with congenital heart disease. Thus, in a pilot study carried out at our institutions, pulmonary venous flow patterns were evaluated in detail together with the patterns of atrioventricular inflow, and were then correlated with invasive pressure recordings obtained during simultaneous cardiac catheterisation. However, in our limited study population of some 60 patients, with a wide spectrum of congenital cardiac lesions, we were unable to detect any consistent patterns of changes which would predict abnormal diastolic function. In particular, there was no correlation between pulmonary venous flow patterns with either the magnitude of intracardiac shunting or the absolute volume of pulmonary blood flow. This perhaps is not surprising when one considers the intrinsic distensibility of the pulmonary venous bed. Furthermore, in all patients with an atrial septal defect, the pattern of pulmonary venous return appears to be largely related to the flow pattern across the communication rather than to reflect atrial and (left) ventricular chamber properties. Although the ratio between systolic and diastolic flow components of pulmonary venous flow patterns was found to change in patients with isolated left ventricular outflow obstruction, the study population was too small to detect any correlation with the severity of the obstruction or with the degree of impairment of left ventricular function. Until now, the routine pulsed wave Doppler evaluation of pulmonary venous flow patterns in patients with congenital heart disease would appear to be rewarding only in patients with a Mustard or Senning procedure for transposition of the great arteries (14) and in the pre- and postoperative evaluation and follow-up of patients undergoing a Fontan-type procedure (Chapter 5).

ANOMALOUS SYSTEMIC VENOUS CONNECTIONS

Anomalies of the systemic venous connections are a frequent finding in patients with even relatively simple forms of congenital heart disease. Many of these lesions do not have haemodynamic significance and will be recognised only incidentally. However, in patients with more complex congenital cardiac lesions, associated anomalies of the systemic venous connections may have clinical significance. The precise documentation or the definite exclusion of these lesions is essential prior to any planned surgical procedure, since they may significantly alter both the technique of venous cannulation and the operative approach (15,16).

The anatomy of systemic venous return is complex, and thus, not surprisingly, there are many variations of normal and numerous possibilities of abnormal connections. Four main systemic venous systems should be considered: (1) the superior vena cava system together with the coronary sinus, (2) the inferior vena cava system, (3) the azygos system, and (4) the hepatic venous system. In the majority of cases anomalies of the inferior vena cava system are associated with anomalies of the azygos and the hepatic venous system. Thus these systems will be considered together.

Anomalies of the superior vena cava system

PERSISTENT LEFT SUPERIOR CAVAL VEIN

Persistence of the left superior caval vein is found in up to 4.4% of all patients with congenital heart disease (17) and is thus the most frequent form of anomalous systemic venous connection. In the vast majority of cases the vein is connected to the systemic venous atrium via an enlarged coronary sinus. Other sites of drainage of the superior caval vein

include the roof of the left atrium or the pulmonary venous atrium via an unroofed coronary sinus. In some 60% of all cases there is a communication with the right sided superior caval vein via a bridging (innominate) vein.

Transthoracic, and in particular suprasternal echocardiography has been reported by Huhta and colleagues to be an extremely sensitive technique in the assessment of these lesions. They reported a success rate for the documentation of a left superior caval vein of 95%, and a success rate of 72% in the detection of bilateral superior caval veins in the presence of a bridging vein (1). However, in clinical practice, and in particular in the older child or adolescent with congenital heart disease, it remains frequently difficult either to define or to definitively exclude a left persistent superior caval vein. Cardiac catheterisation, together with hand injection of contrast into the innominate vein, is still considered the gold standard in the detection of these lesions. Alternatively transesophageal echocardiography now allows a detailed morphologic diagnosis.

On transverse axis imaging the presence of a left persistent superior caval vein is readily documented by visualisation of an echo-free space interposed be-

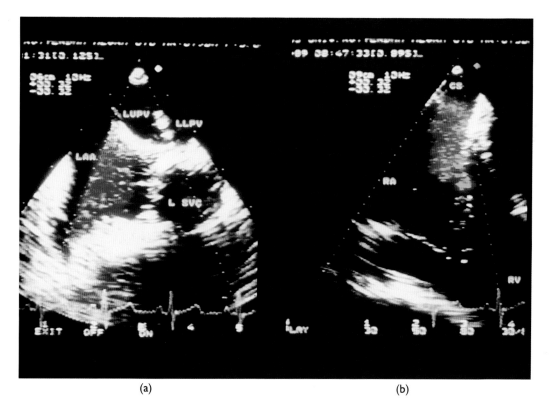

(a)　　　　　　　　　　　　　(b)

Figure 3.4 *Transesophageal colour flow mapping study in a child with a left superior caval vein draining to the coronary sinus.* **(a)** *The left persistent superior caval vein is seen as an echo-free space interposed between the left atrial appendage and the left sided pulmonary veins.* **(b)** *Probe advancement allows demonstration of the coronary sinus as being the site of connection.*

tween the left atrial appendage and the left upper pulmonary vein (Fig. 3.4). This location is constant and it is independent of the exact site of drainage or any form of cardiac malposition. In cases where the vessel is connected to the coronary sinus this can then be followed by slight probe advancement together with gradual clockwise rotation. Cranially a left persistent superior caval vein can be documented anterior to the left pulmonary artery. Interposition of the left main bronchus precludes the visualisation of the more proximal segment. Further probe withdrawal and scanning of the aortic arch allows assessment of the presence and size of the bridging (innominate) vein (Fig. 3.5).

Connection of the left persistent superior caval vein to the left sided atrium is found predominantly in cases with complex congenital heart disease, such as in patients with atrial isomerism. This entity is equally well documented by transesophageal cross-sectional imaging, whereas it frequently may go unrecognised by transthoracic imaging (7). Its mode of drainage can be assessed by slight variations in the depth of probe insertion after the visualisation of the vessel at its typical location interposed between the left sided atrial appendage and the left upper pulmonary vein.

Using transesophageal transverse axis imaging, problems persist in the definition of drainage of the left superior caval vein to the left atrium via an unroofed coronary sinus. In this situation, in our experience, the imaging planes that can be obtained do not allow adequate visualisation of the absence

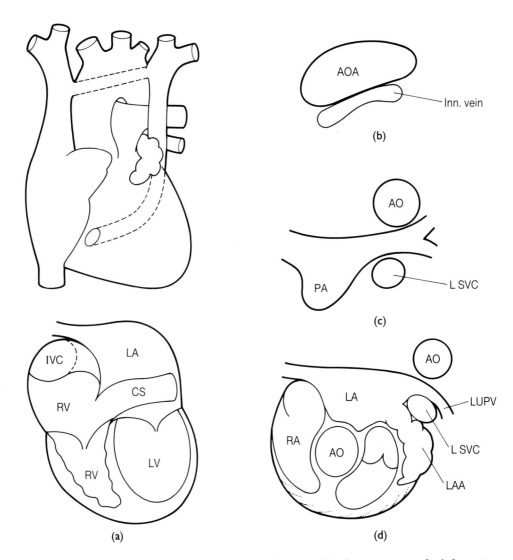

Figure 3.5 *Diagrammatic representation of transverse axis scan planes used in the assessment of a left persistent superior caval vein.* **(a)** *Level of the aortic arch.* **(b)** *Level of the left pulmonary artery.* **(c)** *Level of the arterial valves.* **(d)** *Level of the floor of the atrial chambers.*

of the roof of the coronary sinus. It is only the failure of documentation of the coronary sinus at its normal position, after having demonstrated a left superior caval vein, or the detection of an atrial septal defect at the site of its expected drainage into the right atrium, which may suggest the diagnosis.

It may be expected that the use of longitudinal transesophageal imaging planes will allow a better definition of this lesion. In addition these imaging planes should allow for an improved visualisation of the proximal portions of both superior caval

veins (18). More recent experience with this technique in the assessment of a persistent left superior caval vein, proved that the longitudinal imaging plane enhances the visualisation of the connection of this vessel to the coronary sinus, and allows for a better demonstration of the more cranial course (Fig. 3.6). However, in all of the cases studied so far the correct diagnosis could be obtained by transverse axis imaging on its own. Thus, it appears that biplane imaging is not a prerequisite in the transesophageal diagnosis of these lesions.

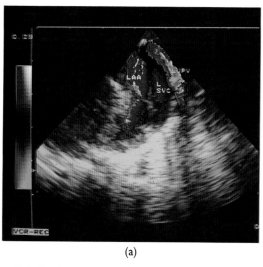

(a)

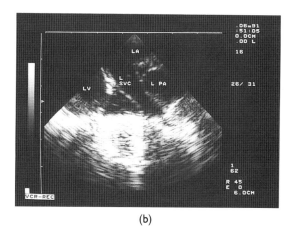

(b)

Figure 3.6 *Biplane transesophageal study in a patient with a left superior caval vein.* **(a)** *The transverse axis plane demonstrates the characteristic features.* **(b)** *The longitudinal axis plane allows the visualisation of a long segment of the vessel coursing anteriorly to the left pulmonary artery and then draining to the coronary sinus.*

ANOMALIES OF THE RIGHT SUPERIOR CAVAL VEIN

In the presence of a persistent left superior caval vein, the right superior caval vein may be absent. This rare anomaly is recognised by careful scanning of the roof of the right atrium and then scanning more cranially anterior to the right pulmonary artery. Anomalous drainage of the right superior caval vein to the left atrium is somewhat more frequent and has been reported to occur even as an isolated lesion (19). However, the two cases we have encountered so far have had an associated atrial septal defect. In both it was not possible to detect this anomaly by complete precordial ultrasound studies including subcostal and suprasternal examination, because of the generally poor definition of the cranial portion of the atrial chambers by these techniques. Angiography did not allow us to determine the site of drainage of the right superior caval vein relative to the atrial septum. Transesophageal

cross-sectional imaging, on the other hand, clearly defined the superior limbus of the atrial septum and the lateral crest of tissue of the junction of the right superior caval vein which was in direct continuation with the limbus (Fig. 3.7). The right upper pulmonary vein drained into the left atrium immediately posteriorly. However rare these examples may be, they document the superiority of transesophageal echocardiography in the detailed morphologic assessment of lesions involving the superior sinus venosus area.

It is unlikely that the addition of longitudinal axis imaging may significantly enhance the definition of this type of lesion. As pointed out above, transverse axis imaging always allows definition of the presence and the site of drainage of the superior caval vein relative to the atrial septum. Longitudinal axis imaging is only felt to allow for a better documentation of the degree of override of the superior caval vein above a sinus venosus atrial septal defect.

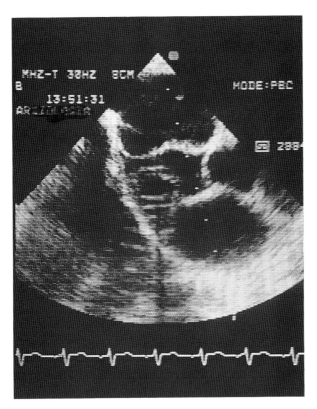

Figure 3.7 *Transverse axis imaging in a patient with connection of the right superior caval vein to the left sided atrium. By following the superior caval vein caudally the rim of atrial tissue that guards its orifice laterally was found to be in continuity with the superior limbus of the atrial septum. The site of drainage of the right upper pulmonary vein is seen directly posterior.*

Anomalies of the inferior vena cava system

Interruption of the inferior caval vein with azygos continuation to the superior caval vein is the most frequently encountered anomaly of this systemic venous system. The underlying deficiency is an absence of the infradiaphragmatic segment of the inferior caval vein. Systemic venous blood from the lower body half is rerouted via a dilated azygos system to drain via the superior caval vein into the right atrium. Hepatic venous return is directly into the atrial chambers, usually the right sided one. The majority of patients in whom this lesion is encountered will have complex congenital heart disease, and there is a strong association with left atrial isomerism. In fact, interruption of the inferior caval vein is used in precordial ultrasound techniques to infer left atrial isomerism (20). However, it is well established that interruption of the inferior caval vein can be present in patients with a normal atrial arrangement (atrial situs solitus) [see Chapter 3.2].

On transesophageal examination of the liver, absence of the infradiaphragmatic segment of the inferior caval vein is readily appreciated. The hepatic veins are visualised, and slight probe withdrawal will document their mode of drainage into the atrial chambers. In particular in patients with left atrial isomerism there may be several sites of drainage. Rotation of the probe to the patient's right will normally demonstrate a dilated venous channel to the right of the spine, which is the azygos vein. By following this channel further cranially, its connection with the superior caval vein can be demonstrated. The site of connection is to the posterior aspect of the distal superior caval vein, just above the right main bronchus. Interposition of the bronchus may preclude the adequate visualisation on transverse axis imaging planes. More recent experience with longitudinal axis imaging confirmed that the assessment of these lesions is largely enhanced by the latter technique.

Other anomalies of the inferior vena cava system include bilaterally inferior caval veins, a rare congenital anomaly, which we have not encountered so far.

When compared with transthoracic ultrasound techniques in the assessment of inferior caval vein anomalies, transesophageal echocardiography, in the majority of cases, has little to offer in the way of new insights. However, in some patients hepatic venous connections may be better demonstrated, and the supradiaphragmatic portion of a dilated azygos vein is frequently better visualised. It is felt that the transesophageal documentation of the pattern of both hepatic and azygos venous abnormalities is further enhanced by the routine use of biplane imaging equipment.

ANOMALOUS PULMONARY VENOUS CONNECTIONS

Anomalous connections of the pulmonary veins to either the right atrium or to a systemic vein are a relatively uncommon finding in congenital heart disease. However, the definite exclusion or the detailed documentation of such abnormalities is of crucial importance in all patients who are being considered for surgical correction. The wide spectrum of these lesions can be divided into two groups: 1. partial anomalous pulmonary venous connections and 2. total anomalous pulmonary venous connections. Whereas patients with the first condition may remain clinically asymptomatic, patients with total anomalous pulmonary venous connections in the vast majority of cases will present in cardiac failure in early infancy. However, rarely some patients with total anomalous pulmonary venous connections may not present until early adulthood (21).

Partial anomalous pulmonary venous connections

In these conditions one or more (but not all) pulmonary veins connect to the right atrium, the coronary sinus or to a systemic vein. It is of interest that 9% of patients with atrial septal defects were reported to have partial anomalous pulmonary venous connections (22). Although any one of the four pulmonary veins may be connected to any systemic venous structure, anomalous connection of the right upper pulmonary vein to either the superior caval vein or directly to the right atrium is by far the most common lesion encountered. Anomalous connection of the left upper pulmonary vein to either the innominate vein or a persistent left superior caval vein ranks second in frequency. Anomalous connections of the lower pulmonary veins is far less frequent and may be either to the right atrium, the coronary sinus or to the inferior vena cava system.

ANOMALOUS CONNECTION OF THE RIGHT UPPER PULMONARY VEIN

Transesophageal transverse axis imaging of the superior aspect of the atrial chambers readily identifies this lesion. On such scans the right upper pulmonary vein will not be documented at its normal site just posterior to the position where the superior caval vein enters the right atrium (Fig. 3.8(a)). In our experience this feature is diagnostic (7). Slight withdrawal of the probe, so as to image the distal portion of the superior caval vein, will allow documentation of the site of connection in cases where the vein drains to the right superior caval vein at the level of the right pulmonary artery. However, the interposition of the right main bronchus may preclude identification of the site of connection to the superior caval vein where it is more cranial. This, however, is encountered in the minority of cases. In cases where the right upper pulmonary vein is connected directly to the right atrium slight probe advancement will readily identify the connection (Figs 3.8(b) and (c)).

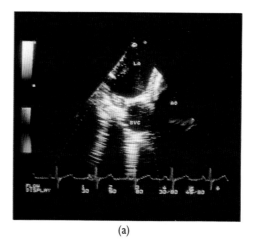

(a)

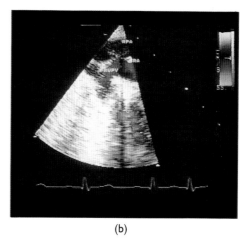

(b)

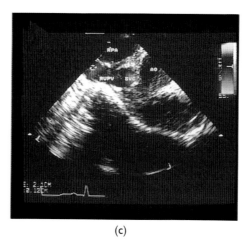

(c)

Figure 3.8 *Anomalous connection of the right upper pulmonary vein.* **(a)** *The failure to demonstrate the vessel at its normal site just posterior to the superior caval vein is diagnostic.* **(b)** *Drainage of the right upper pulmonary vein to the high right atrium.* **(c)** *Drainage to the low superior caval vein.*

Potential pitfalls for transesophageal evaluation of these lesions include the presence of individual drainage of the right upper lobe and right middle lobe pulmonary vein to different sites within the right atrium or to the superior caval vein. This then may result in mistaking the (normally connected) middle lobe vein for the right upper pulmonary vein, and thus missing anomalous connection of the upper lobe pulmonary vein. Although we have not encountered such a problem so far, the right middle lobe pulmonary vein is orientated in a much more frontal plane than the right upper lobe pulmonary vein; a feature which may be helpful in distinguishing them. Longitudinal axis imaging may be expected to be helpful in the definition of such lesions, since it allows a better visualisation of a long segment of the superior caval vein. Using adequate clockwise rotation of the probe it should be feasible to document the exact number of anomalous pulmonary veins to the superior caval vein, and to provide the surgeon with quantitative data about the distances between the sites of drainage and the atrial chambers.

ANOMALOUS CONNECTION OF THE LEFT UPPER PULMONARY VEIN

In patients with this lesion the left upper pulmonary vein is not visualised at its normal position just posterior and to the left of the left atrial appendage, when scanning mid-esophageal transverse axis planes. The abnormal course of the vessel and its site of connection then have to be carefully sought for. Using clockwise rotation of the probe the descending aorta is visualised and a more proximal segment of the left upper pulmonary vein can normally be detected lying anterior to the aorta. The use of colour flow mapping is essential for the rapid identification of the vessel. Alternatively the vessel should be sought for anterior to the left pulmonary artery. The pulmonary arteries are normally dilated in this condition, and thus there are fewer difficulties in adequate visualisation of this vessel anterior to the left main bronchus. Finally the innominate vein should be scanned anterior to the aortic arch (see above), since this vessel is the most frequent site of drainage. In patients in whom a left

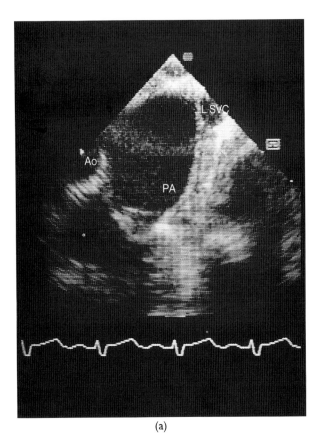

(a)

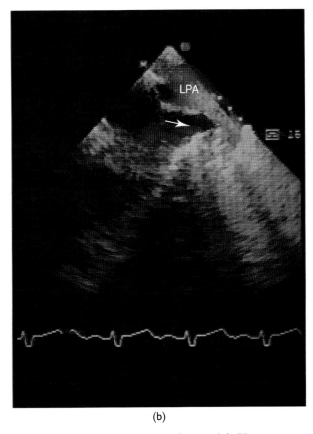

(b)

Figure 3.9 *Anomalous connection of the left upper pulmonary vein to a left persistent superior caval vein.* **(a)** *Transverse axis imaging of the pulmonary artery bifurcation identifies the left superior caval vein lying anterior to the left pulmonary artery.* **(b)** *Subsequent scanning of the course of this vessel, using colour flow mapping, readily identifies the site of connection of the left upper pulmonary vein (encoded in red).*

persistent superior caval vein is documented, the entire course of this vessel has to be examined, as abnormal connection of the left upper pulmonary vein to it is a definite possibility (Fig. 3.9). Using the above examination techniques it is possible to diagnose the presence of these lesions reliably, and in the majority of cases it should also be possible to define the exact site of connection.

ANOMALOUS CONNECTIONS OF THE LOWER PULMONARY VEINS

Connection of the right lower pulmonary vein to the right atrium is readily diagnosed on transesophageal colour flow mapping studies of the inferior aspect of the atrial chambers, obtained from scan positions near the esophageal hiatus (Fig. 3.10). The same applies for anomalous connection of the right lower pulmonary vein to the immediate infradiaphragmatic portion of the inferior caval vein, and to the coronary sinus. Other sites of anomalous connection of this vessel are difficult to assess by transesophageal imaging. In addition, failure to document the normal connection of the right lower pulmonary vein at the inferior aspect of the left atrium is not a diagnostic sign for anomalous connection of this vessel (unlike for the upper pulmonary veins). So far we have not encountered a patient with partial anomalous connection of the left lower pulmonary vein. However, anomalous connection to the right atrium or to the coronary sinus may be expected to be documented with ease. In the latter condition, the finding of a dilated coronary sinus in the absence of a persistent left superior caval vein may be indicative and should lead to detailed colour flow mapping studies which will make the diagnosis.

In summary, when compared with precordial ultrasound studies in the assessment of partial anomalous pulmonary venous connections, the advantages of transesophageal echocardiography are manifold. Firstly, the technique allows the definitive identification of the site of connection of all four pulmonary veins in the vast majority of normal individuals (Table 3.1). This is independent of the patient's size, the presence of associated lesions, or the presence of cardiac malposition. In turn, this routinely allows the definite exclusion of partial anomalous pulmonary venous connection, a contribution which cannot be overemphasised in the diag-

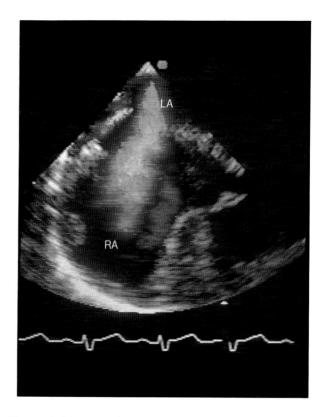

Figure 3.10 *Anomalous connection of both the right middle and the right lower pulmonary vein draining to the right atrium.*

nosis of congenital heart disease. In the majority of patients thus identified of having partial anomalous pulmonary venous connection, the technique allows for the definition of the exact site of connection. Finally, in comparison with angiocardiography, the technique allows for a much more detailed assessment of the exact morphology of this spectrum of lesions. Thus, at our institutions, transesophageal echocardiography has become the diagnostic technique of first choice in the evaluation of patients with suspected anomalous pulmonary venous connections.

Total anomalous pulmonary venous connection

The majority of patients with a total anomalous pulmonary venous connection present during early infancy. The diagnosis is routinely made by precordial ultrasound techniques and subsequent surgical correction is in general performed on this basis alone (3,4). Thus, there is only limited need for transesophageal echocardiography in the preoperative evaluation. However, some cases who have unobstructed pulmonary venous return and a wide interatrial communication, may not present until later childhood or as adolescents. The sites of total anomalous venous connections as assessed by several large autopsy series are summarised in Table 3.2.

In the few cases with total anomalous venous connection we have studied so far, transesophageal echocardiography was of value in several instances. The major contribution was found to be in the improved exclusion of mixed patterns of anomalous connections when compared with precordial ultrasound. The pulmonary venous confluence (collector) was consistently visualised at the posterior aspect of the left atrium. Close examination of the confluence could define the number and the exact

site of connection of each of the four pulmonary veins and the proximal portion of its communication with the systemic venous system. Cardiac types of total anomalous pulmonary venous connection could be documented over their entire course (Fig. 3.11). However this may prove difficult in particular for infradiaphragmatic types of total anomalous connections.

Table 3.2 *Sites of total anomalous pulmonary venous connections*

Left innominate vein	32%
Coronary sinus	17%
Right atrium	10%
Right superior caval vein	13%
Portal venous system	19%
Multiple sites	7%
Unknown	2%

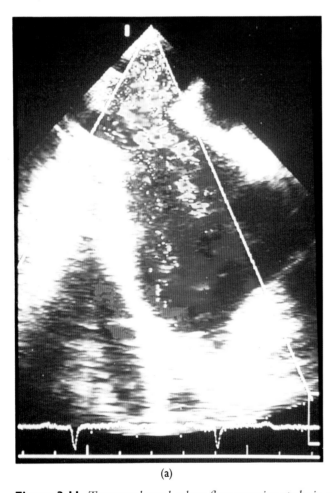

(a)

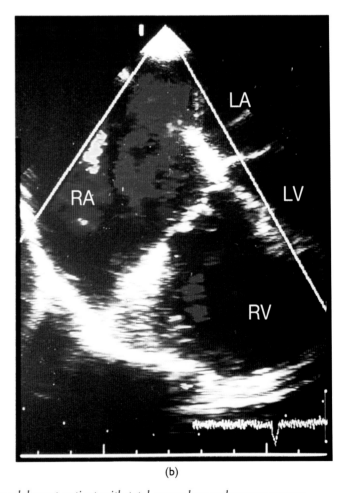

(b)

Figure 3.11 *Transesophageal colour flow mapping study in an adolescent patient with total anomalous pulmonary venous connection at cardiac level.* **(a)** *Scanning at the level of the atrial chambers allowed rapid identification of the common collector, which drained posteriorly to the right atrium. In addition, the individual sites of connection of the four pulmonary veins were defined.* **(b)** *Associated atrial septal defect with right-to-left shunting.*

REFERENCES

1. HUHTA JC, SMALLHORN JF, MACARTNEY FJ, ANDERSON RH, DELEVAL M. Cross-sectional echocardiographic diagnosis of systemic venous return. *Br Heart J* 1982; **48:** 388–403.

2. SMALLHORN JF, SUTHERLAND GR, TOMMASINI G, HUNTER S, ANDERSON RH, MACARTNEY FJ. Assessment of total anomalous pulmonary venous connection by two-dimensional echocardiography. *Br Heart J* 1981; **46:** 613–23.

3. HUHTA JC, GUTGESELL HP, NIHILL MR. Cross-sectional echocardiographic diagnosis of total anomalous pulmonary venous connection. *Br Heart J* 1985; **53:** 525–34.

4. SMALLHORN JF, FREEDOM RM. Pulsed Doppler echocardiography in the preoperative evaluation of total anomalous pulmonary venous connection. *J Am Coll Cardiol* 1986; **8:** 1413–20.

5. JULSRUD PR, EHMAN RL. The 'Broken ring' sign in magnetic resonance imaging of partial anomalous pulmonary venous connection to the superior vena cava. *Mayo Clin Proc* 1985; **60:** 874–9.

6. DIETHELM L, DERY R, LIPTON MJ, HIGGINS CB. Atrial-level shunts: sensitivity and specificity of MR in diagnosis. *Radiology* 1987; **162:** 181–6.

7. STÜMPER O, VARGAS-BARRON J, RIJLAARSDAM M, et al. The assessment of anomalous systemic and pulmonary venous connections by pediatric transesophageal echocardiography. *Br Heart J* 1991; **66:** 411–19.

8. WEIGEL TJ, SEWARD JB, HAGLER DJ. Transesophageal echocardiography in anomalous pulmonary and systemic venous connections. *Circulation* 1990; **812V** (suppl): 339 (abstract).

9. KRONZON I, TUNICK PA, FREEDBERG RS, SCHWINGER ME. Sinus venosus type atrial septal defect is frequently missed by conventional echocardiography and is better detected by transesophageal echocardiography. *J Am Coll Cardiol* 1990; **15:** 1174A (abstract).

10. STÜMPER O, HESS J, SUTHERLAND GR. Paediatric transesophageal echocardiography – the value of a new diagnostic technique. *Int J Card Imag* 1990; **5:** 19.

11. RAJAGOPALAN B, FRIEND JA, STALLARD, LEE GJ. Blood flow in pulmonary veins. II: The influence of events transmitted from the right and left sides of the heart. *Cardiovasc Res* 1979; **13:** 677–83.

12. KEREN G, SHEREZ J, MEGIDISH R, LEVITT B, LANIADO . Pulmonary venous flow patterns – its relationship to cardiac dynamics: A pulsed Doppler echocardiographic study. *Circulation* 1985; **71:** 1105–12.

13. KEREN G, SONNENBLICK EH, LEJEMTEL TH. Mitral anulus motion: relation to pulmonary vnous and transmitral flows in normal subjects and in patients with dilated cardiomyopathy. *Circulation* 1988; **78:** 621–9.

14. KAULITZ R, STÜMPER O, FRASER AG, KREIS A, TUCILLO B, SUTHERLAND GR. The potential value of transoesophageal evaluation of individual pulmonary vein flow after an atrial baffle procedure. *Int J Cardiol* 1990; **28:** 299–308.

15. BOSHER LH. Problems in extracorporeal circulation relating to venous cannulation and drainage. *Ann Surg* 1959; **149:** 652–63.

16. DELEVAL MR, RITTER DG, MCGOON DC, DANIELSON GK. Anomalous systemic venous connection. Surgical considerations. *Mayo Clin Proc* 1975; **50:** 599–610.

17. WINTER FS. Persistent left superior vena cava; survey of world literature and report of thirty additional cases. *Angiology* 1954; **5:** 90–132.

18. STÜMPER O, FRASER AG, HO SY, et al. Transoesophageal echocardiography in the longitudinal axis: correlation between anatomy and images and its clinical implications. *Br Heart J* 1990; **64:** 282–8.

19. EZEKOWITZ MD, ALDERSON PO, BULKLEY BH, et al. Isolated drainage of the superior vena cava into the left atrium in a 52-year-old man. *Circulation* 1978; **58:** 751–6.

20. HUHTA JC, SMALLHORN JF, MACARTNEY FJ. Two dimensional echocardiographic diagnosis of situs. *Br Heart J* 1982; **48:** 97–108.

21. ENGLE MA. Total anomalous pulmonary venous drainage. *Circulation* 1972; **46:** 209–16.

22. GOTSMAN MS, ASTLEY R, PARSONS C. Partial anomalous pulmonary venous drainage in association with atrial septal defect. *Br Heart J* 1965; **27:** 566–73.

Morphology and pathology of the atrial chambers

O. Stümper

INTRODUCTION

The anatomy of the atrial chambers is complex and is frequently not fully appreciated by precordial ultrasound techniques. Both atrial chambers consist of a venous component and an atrial appendage. The venous component serves as a compliant filling chamber. The atrial appendages on the other hand do not have a specific function. However, they are the determinants of the morphology of the corresponding atrial chamber, and thus the atrial arrangement (1). Abnormalities of the atrial arrangement (atrial situs) are relatively rare, but are of significance in complex congenital heart disease. They are associated *inter alia* with anomalies of the site and course of the conduction tissue (2). Thus, knowledge of the atrial arrangement is important prior to any surgical correction.

A further abnormality frequently associated with complex congenital heart disease is juxtaposition of the atrial appendages (3). In this condition both atrial appendages lie side by side rather than on opposite sides of the arterial trunk. The abnormal location of the atrial appendages is associated with an abnormal orientation of the atrial septum. Again the presence of this lesion has important implications on selected surgical procedures.

Whereas the venous components of the right and left sided atrial chambers can be adequately visualised from either subcostal or parasternal ultrasound windows, the atrial appendages are not. In contrast, both atrial appendages are routinely visualised by transesophageal imaging. Thus, the transesophageal approach can contribute the preoperative assessment of congenital lesions involving these structures. In this chapter the definition of atrial appendage morphology by transesophageal imaging will be described, as well as the characteristic features of juxtaposition of the atrial appendages and the appearances of the range of obstructive lesions within the atria.

ATRIAL ARRANGEMENT

Determination of the atrial arrangement (atrial situs) is the fundamental diagnostic step required for sequential chamber localisation in the diagnosis of congenital heart disease (4,5). The normal atrial arrangement is described as atrial situs solitus – a condition where the morphologically right atrial appendage is located on the right side, with the morphologically left atrial appendage on the left of the arterial pedicle. The mirror image arrangement is described as atrial situs inversus. The presence of bilateral morphologically right or left atrial appendages is described as either right or left atrial isomerism (6). In the majority of cases the atrial arrangement is concordant with both the visceral and the bronchial arrangement. This in turn has led to the clinical practice which infers the atrial arrangement from the presence, the morphology and the location of the thoracic and abdominal organs. For instance, the strong association of bilaterally left atrial appendages with the presence of multiple spleens has resulted in the term 'polys-plenia' being used to describe this entity (7). Similarly, absence of the spleen is frequently found in patients with bilaterally right atrial appendages. Such cases are also described by the term 'asplenia syndrome'.

With transthoracic ultrasound techniques, documentation of the presence and the relative location of the infradiaphragmatic great vessels to one another is used to assess anomalies of the atrial arrangement (8). In addition, radiographic documentation of the bronchial anatomy has been found to be a useful indicator of atrial arrangement (9). However, it is well documented that cases of discord between both the abdominal and bronchial arrangement and the atrial arrangement exist (10,11). Thus, only direct visualisation of both atrial appendages can provide the definitive diagnosis of atrial arrangement. In newborns, precordial echocardiography can sometimes allow the demonstration of both atrial appendages by using a series of parasternal short axis views. However, with increasing patient size and the naturally occurring reduction in the precordial ultrasound window, direct visualisation of both atrial appendages from the precordium becomes a virtual impossibility.

Atrial appendage morphology

The right atrial appendage is characterised by a short triangular shape with a blunt ending. The junction of the appendage with the venous cavity of the atrial chamber is broad. The left atrial appendage is characterised by a long, narrow lumen with marked crenellations. The tip of the left atrial appendage is pointed. The junction with the venous component of the atrial chamber is characteristically narrow (Fig. 3.12).

These morphologic features are readily appreciated when scanning high transesophageal transverse axis views of the atrial chambers. In particular the morphology of the junctions of both atrial appendages with their respective venous chambers can be clearly visualised. This latter morphologic feature is the most constant, and thus most important criterion for the definition of atrial appendage morphology. Both the dimension of the lumen of the appendage cavity as well as the extent of crenellations may be altered by the underlying haemodynamic lesion. Transesophageal echocardiographic visualisation and definition of the morphology of both atrial appendages thus offers for the first time the direct diagnosis of atrial situs in all patients studied (12). It may prove to be the most reliable technique in the preoperative diagnosis.

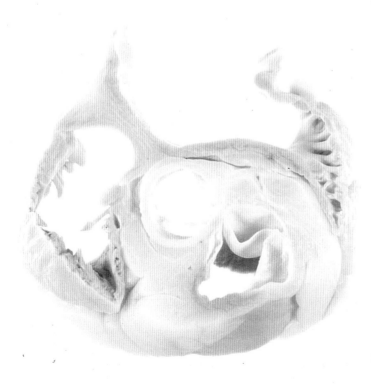

Figure 3.12 *Transverse anatomic section of a normal heart obtained at the level of the atrial appendages.*

Atrial situs solitus

The right sided atrial appendage is characterised by having a broad junction with the venous component of the atrial chamber and having a short, triangular lumen and a blunt ending (Fig. 3.12). Frequently, the tip of the right atrial appendage cannot adequately be visualised on transverse axis imaging, because of its anterior and superior location. Moreover, in some cases a more cranial position of the right atrial appendage can result in a crest of tissue seen on transverse axis cross-sectional imaging. However, in most cases, with anterior transducer tip angulation, it will be possible to scan the entire appendage lumen. The broad junction of the right sided atrial appendage with the venous component of the atrial chamber can be visualised in all cases. Visualisation of the crista terminalis (the strand of atrial tissue separating the smooth atrial free wall from the trabeculated wall of the atrial appendage itself) also will be documented in the majority of cases.

The left sided atrial appendage will then be visual-ised by using counterclockwise rotation of the probe. It is located just inferior and to the left of the pulmonary trunk. Inferiorly the left ventricular free wall and both the left main and circumflex coronary artery will be seen. Posteriorly and to the left, the left atrial appendage is separated by a crest of tissue from the site of drainage of the left upper pulmonary vein into the atrial chamber. The junction of the left atrial appendage with the venous component of the atrial chamber is characteristically narrow; its lumen is rather long, narrow and crenelated.

Documentation of the arrangement of the atrial appendages should be among the initial steps during transesophageal studies carried out in the assessment of congenital heart disease. It is of major importance where precordial and abdominal ultrasound studies have suggested an abnormal atrial arrangement, such as with an interruption of the inferior caval vein. This may be found both in cases with atrial situs solitus or in those with left atrial isomerism (Fig. 3.13). Transverse axis imaging, in our experience, will provide the definite diagnosis in virtually every patient studied. The additional use of longi-

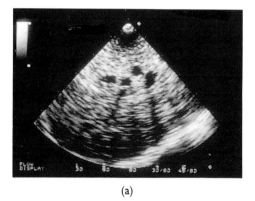

(a)

(c)

Figure 3.13 *Sequence of transesophageal images in a patient with an interrupted inferior caval vein.* **(a)** *The hepatic scan confirms absence of the infradiaphragmatic section of the inferior caval vein. The hepatic veins have a common confluence. Subsequent scanning of the right (b) and (c) atrial appendages documents atrial situs solitus. Arrow = right atrial appendage; asterisk = left atrial appendage.*

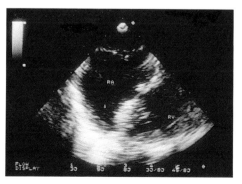

(b)

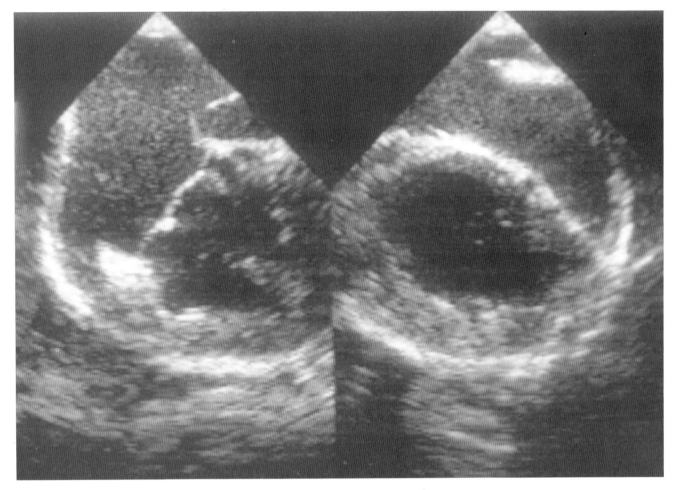

Figure 3.14 *Transverse transesophageal sections of the atrial appendages in a patient with atrial situs inversus. The left-sided right atrial appendage is seen having a broad junction and a triangular shape. The right-sided, morphologically left atrial appendage is seen having a very narrow junction produced by a prominent crenellation and a pointed ending.*

tudinal axis imaging sometimes allows a more rapid diagnosis to be obtained.

Atrial situs inversus

This condition is often referred to as the 'mirror image atrial arrangement'. Using transesophageal imaging, the morphologically right sided atrial appendage will be visualised on the patient's left side, the morphologically left atrial appendage on the patient's right (Fig. 3.14). Again, it is the junction of the atrial appendages with the venous component of the atrial chamber which is the most consistent diagnostic feature in the determination of append-

age morphology. The range of commonly associated lesions may lead to a distention of the atrial appendage lumen, which in turn may distort the morphology of the lumen of the atrial appendage. In contrast, the dimensions of the junctions of the atrial appendages remain unaffected.

Atrial isomerism

These conditions are characterised by the presence of bilateral morphologically right or left atrial appendages. Atrial isomerism is thus subdivided into right or left atrial isomerism. In the majority of such cases, the range of associated severe cardiac lesions will suggest the diagnosis in early infancy. In right atrial isomerism the most common associated cardiac lesions include dextrocardia, anomalous pulmonary venous connections, univentricular atrioventricular connections and transposition of the great arteries with either pulmonary stenosis or atresia. In left atrial isomerism there is a high incidence of biventricular atrioventricular connections, with double outlet of the right ventricle (1,6,13,14). In right atrial isomerism, there is a high incidence of bilateral superior caval veins and total anomalous pulmonary venous connections, whereas in left atrial isomerism there is characteristically interruption of the inferior caval vein with azygos continuation. Partial anomalous pulmonary venous connections are frequently encountered. A careful assessment of the venous connections therefore has to be carried out in all cases where the initial diagnosis suggests atrial isomerism.

In patients with right atrial isomerism, the transesophageal study will document the presence of identical atrial appendages, having a broad junction with the venous component of the atrial chamber (Fig. 3.15). In addition, the lumen of either atrial

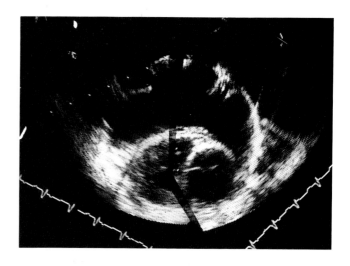

Figure 3.15 *Composite transesophageal image in a patient with right atrial isomerism. Both the right and the left sided atrial appendage are seen having a broad junction with the venous components. In addition there is virtual absence of the atrial septum (common atrium) and transposition of the great arteries.*

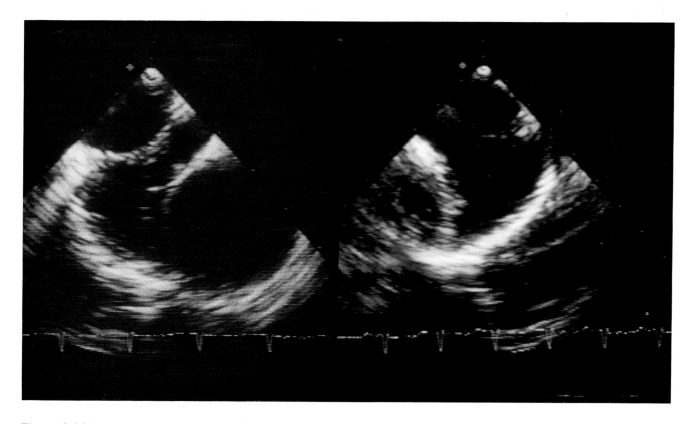

Figure 3.16 *Transverse axis scans in a child with right atrial isomerism. Both atrial appendages have a broad Lumen and a triangular shape. The junction of the left sided, morphologically right appendage is compressed by a largely dilated persistent left superior caval vein (asterisk).*

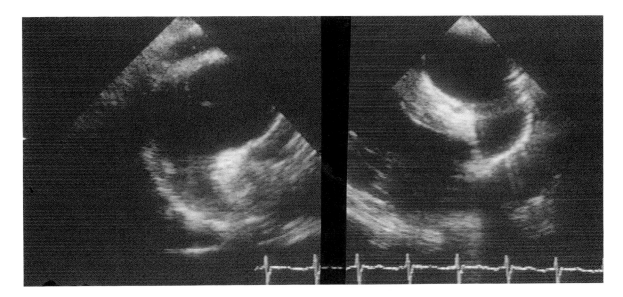

Figure 3.17 *Transesophageal documentation of left atrial isomerism. Both atrial appendages have a narrow junction with the venous component of the atrial chambers. The lumen of the left sided, morphologically left atrial appendage is markedly distended because of high left atrial pressures.*

appendage is wide, has a triangular shape and characteristically a blunt ending. A left superior caval vein is encountered in about half the cases, and is then visualised lying interposed between the left upper pulmonary vein and the left sided, morphologically right atrial appendage. This in turn may lead to a compression of the junction of the left sided appendage, with the morphology of the appendage cavity becoming the most important feature for the determination of appendage morphology (Fig. 3.16).

In patients with left atrial isomerism, both atrial appendages will be found to demonstrate a narrow junction with the venous component of the atrial chamber (Fig. 3.17). Interruption of the inferior caval vein with azygos continuation is encountered in only 60% of these cases (14), and accounts for some of the limitations of transthoracic ultrasound techniques in the unequivocal definition of atrial arrangement.

JUXTAPOSITION OF THE ATRIAL APPENDAGES

Juxtaposition of the atrial appendages is a rare anomaly and one which is normally associated with complex congenital heart disease, in particular with complete transposition of the great arteries or tricuspid atresia (3). This condition may be associated with all of the above described types of atrial arrangement. Left juxtaposition, a condition in which both atrial appendages lie side-by-side on the left side of the arterial trunk (Fig. 3.18), is the most commonly encountered form and occurs about six times more often than right juxtaposition (3,15). Knowledge of the presence of this malformation is important to the surgeon when considering either a Mustard or Senning procedure for complete trans-

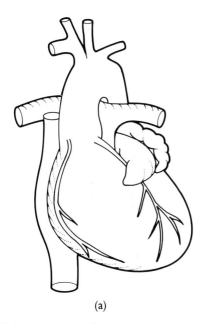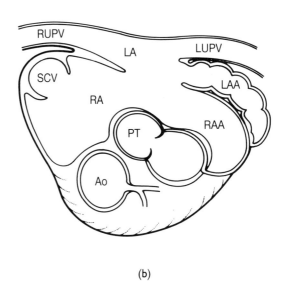

Figure 3.18 (a) *Diagram of a heart with left juxtaposition of the atrial appendages and transposition of the great arteries.* **(b)** *The transverse axis transesophageal image obtained at the level of the atrial appendages is characteristic for this entity.*

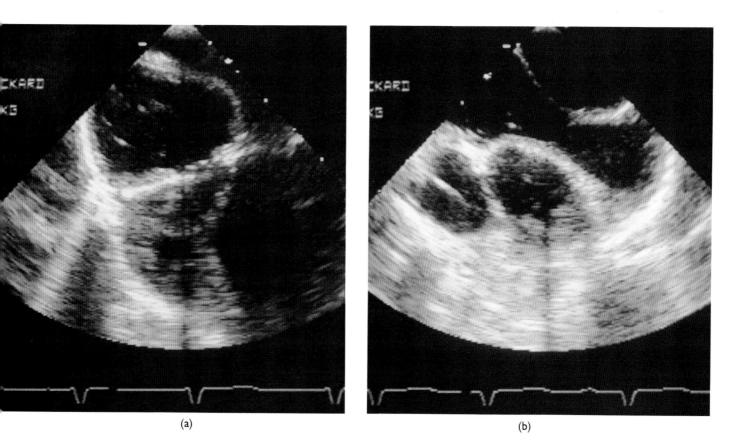

(a)   (b)

Figure 3.19 *Transverse axis sections in a patient with left juxtaposition of the atrial appendages.* **(a)** *The atrial septum is seen in a more frontal plane than in a heart with normal appendage arrangement.* **(b)** *The right atrial appendage is seen to the left of the arterial pedicle. Compare with Fig. 3.18.*

position of the great arteries or a Fontan-type procedure (16). In addition, a Rashkind septostomy may be difficult in this malformation because of the resultant abnormal orientation of the atrial septum (17). The diagnosis of juxtaposed atrial appendages can be made by angiocardiography, but only when special emphasis is placed on identifying this anomaly (18). In infants and young children, precordial cross-sectional imaging was reported to be a valuable investigative technique in the preoperative diagnosis (19,20). However, difficulties may persist in the older child with a limited precordial ultrasound window. In contrast, this anomaly is readily recognised on transesophageal cross-sectional imaging of the atrial chambers (21). In fact, the technique may be considered to be the definitive preoperative diagnostic technique for the identification or exclusion of juxtaposition of the atrial appendages.

In left juxtaposition characteristically there is a malorientation of the atrial septum when scanning transesophageal four-chamber views. The midportion of the atrial septum is found in a more frontal plane and its superior portion is found to form the floor and the posterior wall of the juxtaposed right atrial appendage when the probe is slightly withdrawn (Fig. 3.19). In our experience, neither the transesophageal definition of atrial appendage morphology, nor documentation of the systemic and pulmonary venous connections, is compromised by the presence of this abnormality. In the majority of cases an associated secundum-type atrial septal defect will be present. Such defects are readily identified on transesophageal imaging studies, whereas they may go unrecognised during prior precordial ultrasound studies. The defect is typically found to be located rather superiorly and close to the junction of either atrial appendage with the atrial chambers. This may account for some of the difficulties encountered during diagnostic and therapeutic cardiac catheterisations in these patients. The use of transesophageal ultrasound studies should be considered a valuable adjunct to catheter guidance during these procedures (see Chapter 4.2).

In patients with right juxtaposition of the atrial appendages both atrial appendages are positioned to the right of the arterial pedicle. Although we have not encountered this lesion in any of our patients studied so far, it may be anticipated that right juxtaposition would be equally well diagnosed by transesophageal imaging. The orientation of the atrial septum may be expected to be rather from left posterior to right anterior, with the superior aspect forming the floor and the posterior wall of the atrial appendage of the left sided atrial chamber.

Cor triatriatum sinister and supramitral membrane

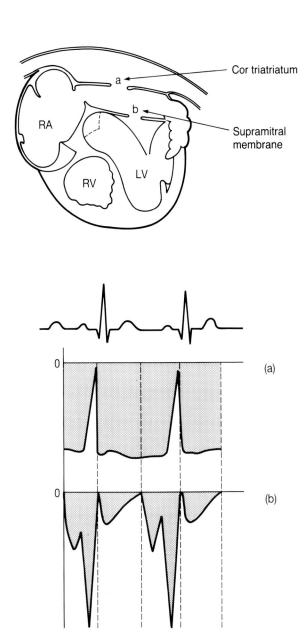

Figure 3.20 *Diagram of cor triatriatum and supramitral membrane with the corresponding pulsed wave Doppler tracings when sampling at the site of connection.*

This section will briefly discuss the transesophageal appearances of this rare range of congenital lesions. Partitioning of the left atrial chamber (cor triatriatum sinister) will usually result in the patient presenting during infancy with severe pulmonary venous congestion. Characteristically a fibromuscular membrane septates the left atrial chamber into a proximal compartment, which receives the pulmonary veins, and a distal compartment which is in communication with the mitral valve and the left atrial appendage. About half of the cases show an associated atrial septal defect, which classically communicates with the distal chamber. The presence of an atrial septal defect that communicates with the proximal chamber should lead to consideration whether the encountered lesion represents a supramitral membrane rather than a cor triatriatum sinister (Fig. 3.20). Documentation of the lateral attachment of the membrane relative to the orifice of the left atrial appendage may give the final clue in this differentiation.

In cor triatriatum sinister the size of the communication between the proximal and distal chambers determines the clinical picture. In cases with a wide unobstructive communication, recognition may be delayed until adolescence. The diagnosis in most cases can be made by transthoracic cross-sectional imaging studies (22). Pulsed wave Doppler interrogation across a restrictive communication will demonstrate a continuous turbulent flow pattern. The contribution of transesophageal echocardiographic studies in these patients lies in the improved definition of the attachments of the fibromuscular membrane relative to the left atrial appendage and the atrial septum (Fig. 3.21). In addition, the technique allows for a more detailed demonstration of the site and the number of communications between the two chambers, and the ultimate definition of the sites of pulmonary venous return (23,24).

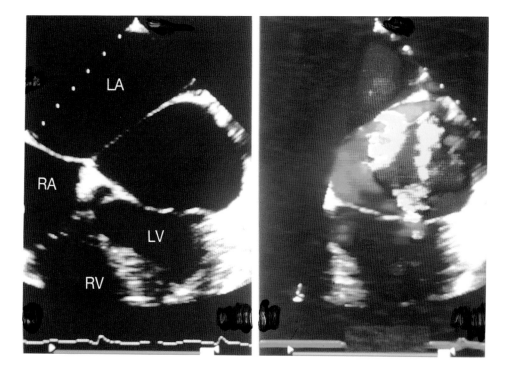

Figure 3.21 *Transverse axis transesophageal study in an adult patient with cor triatriatum and intact atrial septum. The dividing membrane is clearly seen within the left atrial chamber (arrows). (Courtesy P. Hanrath, RWTH Aachen, Germany)*

In patients with supramitral membrane the obstructive lesion is characteristically located a short distance above the mitral valve annulus. The left atrial appendage is incorporated into the proximal chamber. An atrial septal defect, if present, establishes a communication between the proximal chamber and the right atrium, resulting usually in a continuous non-restrictive left-to right shunt. Pulsed wave Doppler interrogation will document a high-velocity diastolic flow pattern across the communication of the proximal chamber with the supramitral chamber. When compared with transthoracic ultrasound studies, the transesophageal approach offers an improved assessment of the precise morphology of the lesion and its relation to the mitral valve apparatus, the left atrial appendage and the pulmonary veins. This is particularly true in older patients with poor precordial ultrasound windows. Although the addition of longitudinal axis imaging can provide additional imaging information, in particular with respect to the definition of the inferior and the superior attachments of these membranes, the diagnosis will be obtained readily by transverse axis imaging on its own.

VENOUS VALVES

With transesophageal imaging studies the Eustachian valve can be visualised in every patient studied. This valve guards the orifice of the inferior caval vein at its connection with the right atrium. Anteriorly it is attached to the inferior portion of the atrial septum posterior to the site of drainage of the coronary sinus. The orifice of the coronary sinus is guarded by the Thebesian valve. However, this thin structure is rarely appreciated during transesophageal imaging studies. In fetal life the function of these venous valves is to direct the oxygenated

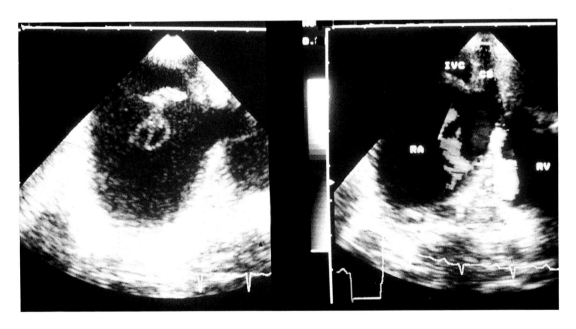

Figure 3.22 *Transesophageal study in a child with pulmonary atresia and intact ventricular septum. The Eustachian valve forms a redundant tissue aneurysm, that was thought to represent an atrial mass lesion on precordial imaging. The coronary sinus drains normally.*

inferior caval blood to the left atrium. Routinely they regress in late fetal life and early childhood. However, in some cases they persist in their original dimensions. A grossly enlarged Eustachian valve may be found in particular in patients with stenosis or atresia of the tricuspid or pulmonary valve (Fig. 3.22). Persistence of these valves in other patients may result in an aneurysmal enlargement with protrusion into the right ventricle in diastole. In other cases apparent localised or generalised thickening of the Eustachian valve may be encountered and may be interpreted on transthoracic studies to represent a right atrial mass lesion. The use of transesophageal studies in these patients is rewarding, since such studies will allow an improved definition of the underlying morphology.

The extreme end of the spectrum of persistence of the venous valves is represented by a complete partitioning of the right atrial chamber (cor triatriatum dexter), an exceedingly rare lesion (25). Transesophageal imaging would appear to be the diagnostic technique of choice in the preoperative diagnosis of these lesions, since it provides a much better insight into the right atrial chamber than does precordial ultrasound. Attachments of the valves should be demonstrated clearly and it may be expected that the site and the number of communications between the proximal and the distal chambers can be demonstrated with ease. In two cases in our series, where precordial ultrasound studies suggested a cor triatriatum dexter, the transesophageal study defined wide communications at the superior portion of the atrial chamber without any obstruction to blood flow.

ATRIAL MASS LESIONS

Cardiac tumors are a rare finding in the paediatric patient population (26). The majority of these tumors involve the ventricular chambers, but both primary and secondary tumors may involve the atrial chambers. Although precordial ultrasound techniques allow for the detailed diagnosis of intracardiac tumors and mass lesions in infants and young children (27), the technique is frequently limited in the older age group (28). Transesophageal imaging in such cases may be of additional value in particular in defining tumor infiltration of the atrial and atrioventricular levels of the heart. In addition, involvement of the pulmonary venous return can be readily diagnosed on transverse axis imaging,

while involvement of the caval venous system is better defined on longitudinal plane imaging. In patients with atrial myxoma, transesophageal imaging has been reported to allow a more comprehensive assessment of the morphology and the extent of the disease (29). Similarly, atrial thrombus formation is better demonstrated on transesophageal than on transthoracic ultrasound studies (30). However, in our experience, mural thrombi which adhere to either the roof or the floor of the atrial chambers may go unrecognised on transverse axis imaging. Longitudinal axis imaging is largely superior in this respect. Finally, endocarditis jet lesions of the atrial chambers due to long venous lines, pacemaker lead infection (31) or thrombosis are better assessed by transesophageal than by transthoracic imaging. Thus, transesophageal ultrasound studies should be considered to be the diagnostic technique of first choice in patients with suspected atrial mass lesions.

REFERENCES

1. SHARMA S, DEVINE W, ANDERSON RH, ZUBERBUHLER JR. The determination of atrial arrangement by examination of appendage morphology in 1842 heart specimens. *Br Heart J* 1988; **60:** 227–31.
2. DICKINSON DF, WILKINSON JL, ANDERSON KR, SMITH A, HO SY, ANDERSON RH. The cardiac conduction system in situs ambiguus. *Circulation* 1979; **59:** 879–84.
3. CHARUZI Y, SPANOS PK, AMPLATZ K, EDWARDS JE. Juxtaposition of the atrial appendages. *Circulation* 1973; **47:** 620–7.
4. LEV M. Pathologic diagnosis of positional variations in cardiac chambers in congenital heart disease. *Labor Invest* 1954; **3:** 71–82.
5. TYNAN MJ, BECKER AE, MACARTNEY FJ, QUERO-JIMINEZ M, SHINEBOURNE EA, ANDERSON RH. Nomenclature and classification of congenital heart disease. *Br Heart J* 1979; **41:** 544–53.
6. MACARTNEY FJ, ZUBERBUHLER JR, ANDERSON RH. Morphological considerations pertaining to recognition of atrial isomerism. *Br Heart J* 1980; **44:** 657–67.
7. VAN PRAAGH R. Terminology of congenital heart disease. Glossary and comments. *Circulation* 1977; **56:** 139–43.
8. HUHTA JC, SMALLHORN JF, MACARTNEY JF. Two dimensional echocardiographic diagnosis of situs. *Br Heart J* 1982; **48:** 97–108.
9. DEANFIELD JE, LEANAGE R, STROOBANT J, CHRISPIN AR, TAYLOR JFN, MACARTNEY FJ. Use of high kilovoltage filtered beam radiographs for detection of bronchial situs in infants and young children. *Br Heart J* 1980; **44:** 577–83.

10. STANGER P, RUDOLPH AM, EDWARDS JE. Cardiac malpositions. An overview based on study of sixty-five necropsy specimens. *Circulation* 1977; **56:** 159–72.

11. CARUSO G, BECKER AE. How to determine atrial situs? Considerations initiated by three cases of absent spleen with a discordant anatomy between bronchi and atria. *Br Heart J* 1979; **41:** 559–67.

12. STÜMPER O, SREERAM N, ELZENGA NJ, SUTHERLAND GR. The diagnosis of atrial situs by transesophageal echocardiography. *J Am Coll Cardiol* 1990; **16:** 442–6.

13. ROSE V, IZUKAWA I, MOSES CAF. Syndromes of asplenia and polysplenia: A review of cardiac and non-cardiac malformations in 60 cases with special reference to diagnosis and prognosis. *Br Heart J* 1975; **37:** 840–52.

14. CHIU IS, HOW SW, WANGG JK, et al. Clinical implications of atrial isomerism. *Br Heart J* 1988; **60:** 72–7.

15. BECKER AE, BECKER MJ. Juxtaposition of atrial appendages with normally orientated ventricles and great arteries. *Circulation* 1970; **41:** 685–92.

16. URBAN AE, STARK J, WATERSTON DJ. Mustard's operation for transposition of the great arteries complicated by juxtaposition of the atrial appendages. *Ann Thorac Surg* 1976; **21:** 304–10.

17. TYRELL MJ, MOES CAF. Congenital Levoposition of the right atrial appendage: its relevance to balloon septostomy. *Am J Dis Child* 1971; **121:** 508–10.

18. HUNTER AS, HENDERSON CB, URQUHART W, FARMER MB. Left-sided juxtaposition of the atrial appendages: report of four cases diagnosed by cardiac catheterization and angiocardiography. *Br Heart J* 1973; **35:** 1184–9.

19. CHIN AJ, BIERMAN FZ, WILLIAMS RG, SANDERS SP, LANG P. Two-dimensional echocardiographic appearance of complete left-sided juxtaposition of the atrial appendages. *Am J Cardiol* 1983; **52:** 346–8.

20. RICE MJ, SEWARD JB, HAGLER DJ, EDWARDS WD, JULSRUD PR, TAJIK AJ. Left juxtaposted atrial appendages: diagnostic two-dimensional echocardiographic features. *J Am Coll Cardiol* 1983; **5:** 1330–6.

21. STÜMPER O, RIJLAARSDAM M, VARGAS-BARRON J, ROMERO A, HESS J, SUTHERLAND GR. The assessment of juxtaposed atrial appendages by transoesophageal echocardiography. *Int J Cardiol* 1990; **29:** 365–71.

22. OSTMAN-SMITH I, SILVERMAN NH, OLDERSHAW P, LINCOLN C, SHINEBOURNE EA. Cor triatriatum sinistrum. Diagnostic features on cross-sectional echocardiography. *Br Heart J* 1984; **51:** 211–19.

23. SCHLÜTER M, LANGENSTEIN BA, THIER W, et al. Transesophageal two-dimensional echocardiography in the diagnosis of cor triatriatum in the adult. *J Am Coll Cardiol* 1983; **2:** 1011–15.

24. TUCILLO B, STÜMPER O, HESS J, et al. Transesophageal echocardiographic evaluation of atrial morphology in children with congenital heart disease. *Eur Heart J* 1992; **13:** 223–31.

25. HANSING CE, YOUNG WP, ROWE CC. Cor triatriatum dexter. Persistent right sinus venosus valve. *Am J Cardiol* 1972; **30:** 559–64.

26. CHAN HSL, SONLEY MJ, MOES CAF, et al. Primary and secondary tumors of childhood involving the heart, pericardium and great vessels. *Cancer* 1985; **56:** 825–36.

27. MARX GR, BIERMAN FZ, MATTHEWS E, WILLIAMS R. Two-dimensional echocardiographic diagnosis of intracardiac masses in infancy. *J Am Coll Cardiol* 1984; **3:** 827–32.

28. COME PC, RILEY MF, MARKIS JE, MALAGOLD M. Limitations of echocardiographic techniques in evaluation of left atrial masses. *Am J Cardiol* 1981; **48:** 947–53.

29. OBEID AI, MARVASTI M, PARKER F, et al. Comparison of transthoracic and transeosophageal echocardiography in diagnosis of left atrial myxoma. *Am J Cardiol* 1989; **63:** 1006–8.

30. ASCHENBERG W, SCHLÜTER M, KREMER P, SCHRÖDER E, SIGLOV V, BLEIFELD W. Transesophageal two-dimensional echocardiography for the detection of left atrial appendiage thrombus. *J Am Coll Cardiol* 1986; **7:** 163–6.

31. VAN CAMP G, VANDENBOSSCHE JL. Recognition of pacemaker lead infection by transesophageal echocardiography. *Br Heart J* 1991; **65:** 229–30.

Atrial septal defects

G. R. Sutherland

INTRODUCTION

Ultrasound has a major role to play in the management of atrial septal defects both in their diagnosis and in subsequent clinical decision-making. Some of the earliest M-mode echocardiographic descriptions of congenital heart disease were studies that identified a number of M-mode and contrast M-mode echocardiographic features which were frequently associated with a defect in the atrial septum. However, the classification of atrial septal defects into their various morphologic forms only became possible with the introduction of high-resolution two-dimensional imaging. Using a combination of precordial and subxiphoid scanning, the site of a defect in the atrial septum could be visualised as could associated lesions such as: (1) the atrioventricular valve abnormalities associated with a partial atrioventricular septal defect, (2) the presence of a left superior vena cava and (3) the direct visualisation of anomalies of pulmonary venous drainage. However, transthoracic ultrasound imaging (even when using high-frequency transducers in infants) may be a sub-optimal technique as in some patients false positive areas of 'echo dropout' can occur within the normal atrial septum. It was the subsequent introduction of colour flow mapping which could confirm transseptal flow that led to an increase in diagnostic accuracy in the identification of the presence of an atrial septal defect. However, the initial enthusiasm for the accuracy of the colour flow mapping technique in correctly identifying transseptal flow has waned with experience. It has

only been with the introduction of transesophageal imaging (initially only single transverse plane imaging and latterly in the bi- or multiplane mode) that the range of anomalies and defects of the atrial septum and their associated morphologic abnormalities can be identified and classified with certainty (1,2). For example, the combination of biplane transesophageal imaging and colour flow mapping can allow the identification of the site of drainage of all four pulmonary veins in virtually every patient. Thus entities such as isolated partial anomalous pulmonary venous drainage or obstructed drainage of the pulmonary veins (following re-routing of these at cardiac surgery by an interatrial baffle) can all accurately be diagnosed using the transesophageal technique. The introduction of umbrella device closure for secundum atrial septal defects has led to a re-evaluation of the imaging techniques available to monitor the placement of such devices (3). Bi- or multiplane transesophageal imaging would appear to be the technique of choice (see Chapter 4.3) for use both in appropriate patient selection and in the real-time monitoring of device closure.

This chapter will review the anatomy and function of the normal atrial septum. It will describe commonly occurring abnormalities of that septum. It will discuss the morphology of the varying types of atrial septal defect and will indicate how these can best be diagnosed using the transesophageal technique. The role of transesophageal monitoring in the closure of defects within the atrial septum is discussed in Chapter 4.3.

THE MORPHOLOGY AND TRANSESOPHAGEAL ECHOCARDIOGRAPHIC APPEARANCES OF THE NORMAL ATRIAL SEPTUM AND PULMONARY VEINS

The normal atrial septum

The true interatrial septum is the relatively small area of fusion of the atrial walls which surrounds the oval fossa. The oval fossa itself is closed by a flap valve which takes origin from the limbus of the oval fossa. Superiorly and posterior to the true interatrial septum, the two medial atrial walls are separated to a variable extent by an interatrial fat pad. Inferiorly, the secundum atrial septum is contiguous with the primum atrial septum. These morphologic components of the atrial septum are all well recognised by transesophageal echocardiography as are the two cavae, the venous valves within the right atrium and the site of drainage of the coronary sinus.

To demonstrate these features, the transverse plane transesophageal probe should be inserted to the level at which the superior vena cava/right atrial junction is visualised. Then by slight further advancement of the probe, a postero-superior portion of the true interatrial septum will be visualised lying between the two atrial chambers. As the probe is advanced slightly further, the relatively thick area of fusion of the atrial walls will be seen to thin and the flap valve of the oval fossa will come into view. This is normally visualised as an appreciably thinner structure than the surrounding true atrial septum. In the majority of patients, the flap valve is a static structure which appears to have only one layer. In some patients, however, this may be correctly appreciated as a structure with two layers in which flow (visualised by colour flow mapping) may be present between the layers. Anteriorly and inferiorly, the flap valve of the oval fossa will be seen to be fused with the thicker echo of the anterior portion of the true interatrial septum. The transducer then can be slowly advanced in order to scan the whole of the flap valve of the foramen ovale and the true interatrial septum in the transverse plane. The inferior rim of the true interatrial septum is often poorly visualised in this scanning plane. However, the coronary sinus, the orifice of the in-

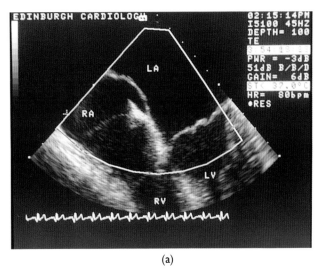

(a)

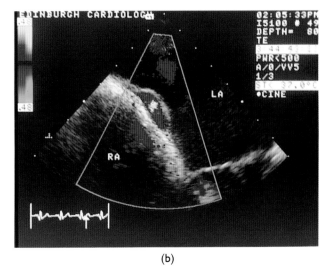

(b)

Figure 3.23 (a) *A transesophageal four-chamber transverse plane image of the atrial septum. In this image, the components of the atrial septum are well visualised. Posteriorly, the thin interatrial septum fuses with the flap valve of the foramen ovale which, during the inspiratory phase of a valsalva manoeuvre, is seen to bulge towards the left atrium. Inferiorly, the lower rim of the flap valve is contiguous with the anterior portion of the atrial septum. This thicker structure is seen to fuse anteriorly with the primum atrial septum which is visualised immediately posterior to the septal insertion of the mitral valve anterior leaflet.* **(b)** *A colour flow map taken from the above imaging sequence. In this transesophageal cut, the imaging plane is slightly anterior to that in (a). The combination of (a) and (b) illustrate the tunnel-like morphology which is frequently associated with the flap valve of the foramen ovale. In this image, we see flow occurring between the flap valve of the foramen and the true interatrial septum. It has been our experience that where such colour appears between layers of the foramen, normally there is probe patency of the foramen.*

ferior vena cava and the venous valves which guard it are normally well visualised in this transverse plane scan.

Longitudinal plane transesophageal imaging of the atrial septum will frequently better demonstrate the morphology of the atrial septum than transverse plane scanning. The superior fat pad separating the two medial atrial walls is better demonstrated using this plane. The morphology of the rim of the fossa ovalis and the flap valve are also better appreciated. The longitudinal plane has a further advantage in that it allows an excellent visualisation of the lower margin of the fossa ovalis and its relationship to the inferior caval orifice. The transesophageal imaging features associated with both normal and abnormal interatrial septae are illustrated in Figs 3.23–3.25.

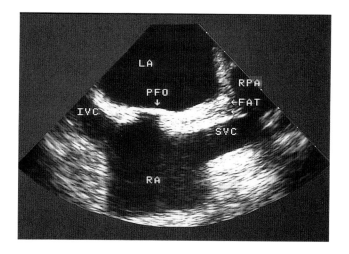

Figure 3.24 *A transesophageal long axis image of the atrial septum acquired from a normal adult patient. In this imaging plane, the anatomy of the atrial septum is well visualised. Superiorly, the two atrial walls are well seen separated by an interatrial fat pad. The flap valve of the foramen ovale is seen as a much thinner structure which fuses inferiorly with the thickened true interatrial septum. The true interatrial septum is seen as a small area surrounding the flap valve of the foramen ovale.*

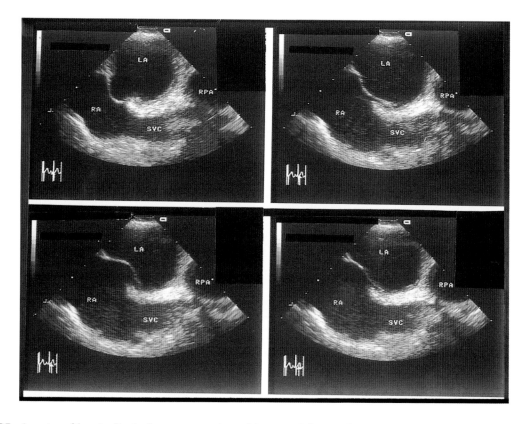

Figure 3.25 *A series of longitudinal plane transesophageal images of the atrial septum from a patient with a true aneurysm of the atrial septum. The four images are sequential images from one cardiac cycle. Note the freely mobile flap valve of the foramen moves alternatively right-to-left and then left-to-right dependent on the presence of either atrial or ventricular systole. Such an abnormally mobile atrial septum may be found in up to 5% of normal patients.*

Normal pulmonary venous drainage

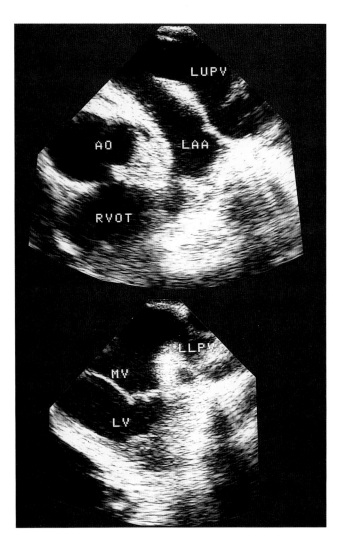

Figure 3.26 *A transverse plane transesophageal study of the left pulmonary veins. The left upper pulmonary vein (LUPV) is seen to drain to the left atrium posterior to the orifice of the left atrial appendage (LAA). Where drainage of the left upper pulmonary vein is normal, this will be seen in 100% of patients using this imaging plane. With slight probe insertion and a leftwards tip angulation a short segment of the lower pulmonary vein will normally be seen below the left atrial appendage. The drainage of this vein can be confirmed by the use of colour flow mapping. The left lower pulmonary vein will normally be visualised in some 90% of patients using the transverse plane alone.*

Transesophageal imaging in the transverse plane can allow identification of the site of drainage of all four pulmonary veins in the majority of patients with congenital heart disease. Both the left upper and right upper pulmonary veins should be visualised in 100% of patients where drainage is normal. Only the left lower and more specifically the right lower pulmonary vein may be difficult to visualise in transverse plane imaging. Using a transverse plane scanning technique, the right upper pulmonary vein can be visualised to drain to the left atrium with the course of the vein running posterior to the right atrium just below the right pulmonary artery. Slight probe insertion from this imaging plane and directing the transducer tip slightly to the patient's right will allow visualisation of the right lower pulmonary vein. Then by rotating the transducer towards the patient's left, it is possible to scan across the left atrium to visualise the left upper pulmonary vein (Fig. 3.26). This will be seen to drain to the left atrium at a position immediately posterior to the mouth of the left atrial appendage. To attempt to identify the left lower pulmonary vein, the probe should then be inserted slightly further with the probe tip imaging towards the postero-lateral aspect of the mitral valve ring. Using this scan plane, a short segment of the left lower pulmonary vein will be seen to drain to the left atrium. Direct two-dimensional imaging of the pulmonary veins may prove difficult. Colour flow mapping is a great adjunct in their identification. Where imaging is of poor quality, then by simply turning on the colour map the presence of flow from a vein into the atrium can often be confirmed. Subsequent interrogation of the jet visualised on the colour map by pulsed Doppler will confirm that this flow is pulmonary venous in origin.

Although the majority of patients with congenital heart disease will have four individual pulmonary veins, slight variations in this morphology may occur (4). Anatomic variations in the veno-atrial connections occur in approximately 10% of the normal population. The most frequent anomaly is the presence of a common right or left pulmonary vein. In this entity, the common confluence may be formed outside or within the pericardial cavity. (The latter situation is the more common.) Bilateral common trunks may occur as may a single common trunk into which all four veins drain prior to entering the left atrium. In a proportion of patients, pulmonary venous return from the right lung will be by three veins, that is, a right upper, a right middle and a right lower (Fig. 3.27). This morphology can be well appreciated by either transverse or longitudinal plane scanning. Longitudinal plane imaging is a definite advantage in the identification of normal or abnormal pulmonary venous return. It has been our experience at Edinburgh that the normal drainage pattern of all four pulmonary veins can be more easily identified by longitudinal plane scanning (Fig. 3.28). The main advantage is that the longitudinal plane allows a better visualisation of drainage of the lower pulmonary veins on either side. The technique used to visualise the pulmonary veins using longitudinal scanning is as follows: the probe should be inserted to a level in which the flap valve of the foramen ovale is seen centrally placed within the atrial septum and the vena cavae are imaged in their long axes. The probe then should be rotated to the patient's right. Gradual rotation will bring the right upper pulmonary vein into view as it drains to the left atrium directly below the right pulmonary artery. This vein is usually easily visualised and the presence of flow to the atrium can

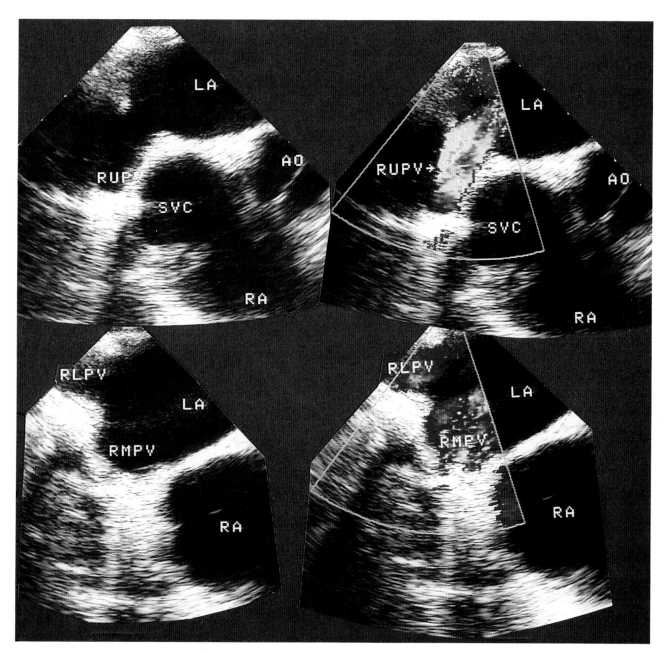

Figure 3.27 *A composite montage to illustrate the technique used to identify normal drainage of the right pulmonary veins. This imaging study is carried out in the transverse plane. In the upper left panel, the right upper pulmonary vein is seen to drain to the left atrium posterior to the superior vena cava. In normal patients, this pattern of venous drainage will be identified in 100% of cases. In the right upper panel, colour flow mapping is used to confirm the presence of flow from this vein into the left atrium. With probe insertion to a lower level, the right lower pulmonary vein will be seen to drain posteriorly to the left atrium. In many cases, there will be a separate drainage of the right middle pulmonary vein to the left atrium. This is seen in both left panels. The colour flow map in the right lower panel confirms the presence of flow from both the right lower and right middle pulmonary vein to the left atrium. Drainage of the right lower pulmonary vein is the most difficult to image of all four veins using the transverse plane. This may be visualised in only some 85% of cases.*

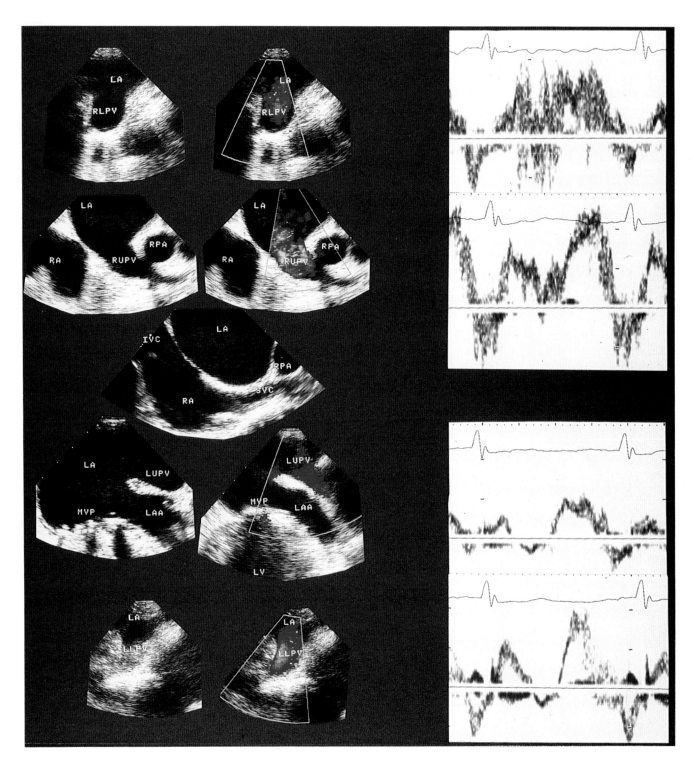

Figure 3.28 *A composite longitudinal plane transesophageal study demonstrating the drainage of all four pulmonary veins. Longitudinal plane imaging is a great advantage in the study of normal and abnormal pulmonary venous drainage. In our experience, it is easier to identify the normal drainage of all four veins using the longitudinal plane approach. With a combination of transverse and longitudinal plane imaging, it is our experience that all four veins can be shown to drain normally in patients with normal pulmonary venous drainage. Where a vein is not visualised, it should be presumed that there is partial anomalous pulmonary venous drainage.*

be confirmed by colour flow mapping and pulsed Doppler examination. Once the site of drainage of this vein has been verified, the probe should be slightly advanced and the transducer tip turned further to the patient's right. This will normally bring a short segment of the right lower pulmonary vein into view as it drains into the right atrium. Once again, colour flow mapping and pulsed Doppler will confirm the presence of pulmonary venous flow. If a right middle pulmonary vein is present, this will be visualised between these two veins as the scan towards the patient's right side takes place. The probe should then be rotated to the patient's left to visualise the left atrial appendage. The left upper pulmonary vein should be easily visualised draining superior to the orifice of the left atrial appendage. Once this vein has been visualised, then the probe should be rotated slightly further to the patient's left and advanced. This will normally bring the left lower pulmonary vein into view. This vein may prove most difficult of the four to visualise using long axis scanning. Only a short segment may be seen and the presence of pulmonary venous flow should be confirmed by the use of colour flow mapping.

It has been our experience that by using biplane transesophageal scanning, we can identify normal pulmonary venous drainage in virtually all patients in whom this is present. The addition of the longitudinal imaging plane has been a definite benefit in this respect.

THE MORPHOLOGY OF ATRIAL SEPTAL DEFECTS

Defects in the atrial septum may be of four main morphologic types. These are (1) secundum atrial septal defects (2), sinus venosus atrial septal defects (3), coronary sinus atrial septal defects and (4) partial atrioventricular septal defects. Each of the four types of atrial septal defect has unique morphologic features which are readily recognised by transesophageal echocardiography. The incidence of each defect in our own consecutive prospective series at Edinburgh is given in Table 3.3. Each defect will now be described in turn.

Table 3.3 *The sites and incidence of each type of atrial septal defect*

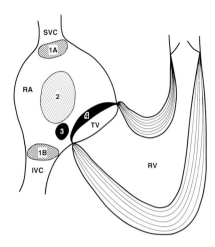

IA = superior sinus venosus (11)
IB = inferior sinus venosus (0)
2 = secundum (52)
3 = coronary sinus (1)
4 = primum (17)

Series: 81 consecutive prospective cases at Edinburgh, Nov. 1990 to June 1992.

SECUNDUM ATRIAL SEPTAL DEFECTS

These are centrally placed defects within the atrial septum which involve in part or in whole the flap valve of the fossa ovalis. The fossa ovalis itself is normally placed centrally with the right atrial aspect of the atrial wall, but this structure may be abnormal in both position and shape and may have marked deficiencies in its muscular rims. Ferreira *et al.*(5) in a pathologic study of 100 hearts with defects within the oval fossa showed the fossa to be centrally placed in 43, placed slightly toward the inferior vena cava in 51, to be displaced to the mouth of the inferior vena cava in four and displaced to the mouth of the superior vena cava in two. Such defects of the oval fossa may be single or multiple. They may be associated with an aneurysm of the atrial septum. They may also be associated with any of the other forms of atrial septal defect and with anomalies of pulmonary venous return. They may occur as isolated lesions or be associated with other complex cardiac anomalies. Transesophageal imaging is an excellent technique for use in the identification of the morphology of such defects (Figs 3.29–3.34), with biplane imaging being essential for the assessment of defect size and morphology when consideration is being given to possible device closure (6).

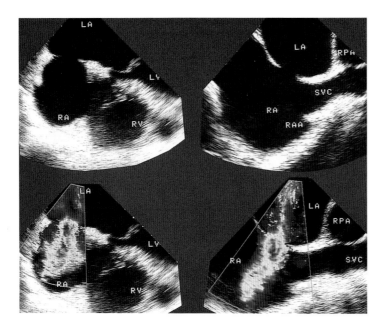

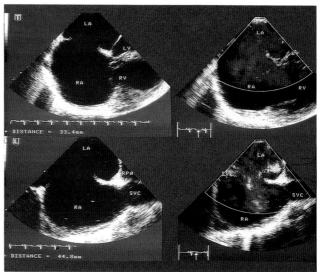

Figure 3.29 *A composite illustration of the morphology and flow associated with a central secundum atrial septal defect. In the left-hand panels (upper and lower), the defect is imaged in the transverse transesophageal plane. The defect is seen to lie centrally within the atrial septum with flow visualised across the defect (left lower panel) on colour flow mapping. In the right-hand panels (upper and lower), the defect is well visualised in the longitudinal plane. Again, the defect is seen to lie centrally within the atrial septum. Colour flow mapping again confirms trans-defect flow in the longitudinal plane.*

Figure 3.30 *A composite biplane transesophageal study of a patient with a large secundum atrial septal defect in whom there is little inferior rim. The upper two panels show the transesophageal transverse plane study, the lower two panels the longitudinal plane transesophageal study. In the transverse plane image, the defect measures some 3.3 cm with apparently good posterior and anterior rims. In the longitudinal plane study, the defect measures some 4.5 cm but in this imaging plane there is clearly little inferior rim. This study demonstrates the need for biplane imaging when considering the suitability of a defect for transcatheter closure. The deficiency in the inferior rim could only be seen in the longitudinal plane study.*

The size of such defects, the degree of displacement of the oval fossa and the structures contiguous to the defect margins vary considerably from defect to defect. Chen *et al.*(7), in a correlative clinical study in which 106 consecutive patients undergoing secundum atrial septal defect closure had a detailed examination of the atrial septal defect morphology at surgery, found that 66% of such defects were restricted to the central portion of the fossa ovalis, 3.7% had a superior displacement, 7.6% had an inferior displacement, 1.9% had in part no posterior rim, 2.8% had subtotal absence of the atrial septum, with 9.4% having a completely fenestrated and 8.5% a partially fenestrated secundum septum. They found the shape of the secundum defects to be oval with the major diameter (i.e. antero-posterior) ranging from 10 to 50 mm in size with a mean of 28 mm. The minor diameter (i.e. infero-superior) ranged from 4 to 30 mm with a mean of 15 mm. Based on a combination of defect size in both axis and the presence (or absence) of an adequate defect rim, Chen *et al.* suggested that defect closure by an umbrella device should have been feasible in approximately 50% of these patients.

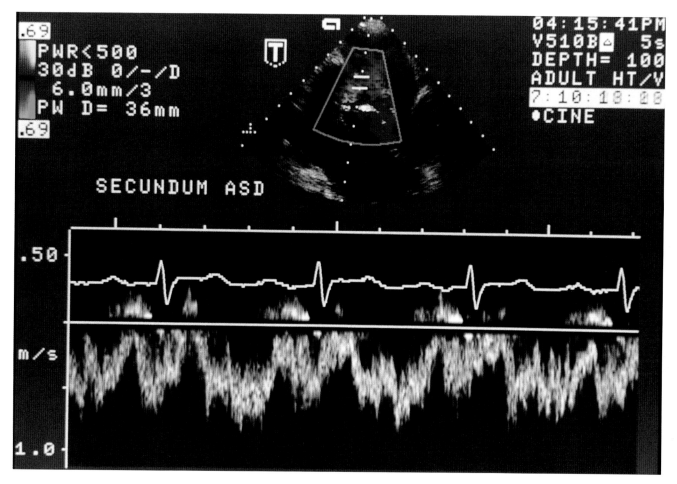

Figure 3.31 *A pulsed-Doppler transesophageal transverse axis study of the flow velocity profile across a large secundum atrial septal defect. This demonstrates predominantly left-to-right shunting with a minor degree of right-to-left shunting during atrial systole. This would be the normal flow pattern for a moderate to large size atrial septal defect. This velocity profile will vary from atrial septal defect to atrial septal defect, and will depend on the defect size, the degree of shunting, and atrial and ventricular compliance.*

To determine if a defect is present in the flap valve or in the surrounding true interatrial septum, a careful transesophageal study using both imaging and colour flow mapping is required (Fig. 3.29). To test the potential patency of the atrial septum, a peripheral venous contrast echocardiographic study during the release of a Valsalva manoeuvre is necessary (Fig. 3.34). In addition, pulsed Doppler (Fig. 3.33) and colour M-mode studies can be carried out to determine the characteristics of flow across any defect found in the secundum septum.

Transverse plane imaging of the atrial septum was one of the first diagnostic uses described for transesophageal echocardiography (8). To identify the flap valve of the foramen, the transducer tip should be directed towards the thin portion of the atrial septum. The probe tip should then be advanced and withdrawn to scan the whole length of the interatrial septum visible in the transverse plane.

Any defect greater than 2–3 mm in transverse dimension should readily be imaged. The position of the defect, the largest dimension of the defect in this plane (the major axis) and the structures contiguous to the defect should all be noted. Multiple defects should be excluded. Where there is doubt about the presence of a defect on imaging alone, a colour flow mapping study (with appropriate low velocity settings) should be carried out. Where the defect haemodynamics are non-restrictive, this may give additional confirmation of the presence of multiple defects. However, the colour flow mapping technique is of more value in the identification of multiple restrictive defects in the atrial septum (Fig. 3.33). In this situation, the use of the velocity variance map will readily identify multiple sites of turbulent flow exiting from the septum into the right atrium.

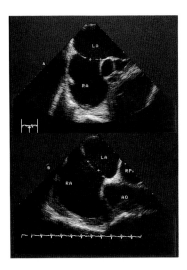

Figure 3.32 *A composite image from a patient with two defects in the secundum septum demonstrating in the upper panel a transverse plane study of the atrial septum and in the lower panel a longitudinal plane study. In the transverse plane transesophageal image one central atrial septal defect is seen (central arrow) and a possible second defect in the retro-aortic position is imaged. It was uncertain on the transverse plane study whether a second defect was indeed present. In the lower panel (the longitudinal plane study), the two atrial septal defects are clearly visualised. The more anterior defect in the retro-aortic position is the defect which was poorly imaged in the transverse plane study. This in fact is the larger defect. These two images again make it clear that a biplane study of the atrial septum is essential to rule out defects in the retro-aortic position. This area is not well seen on transverse plane scanning.*

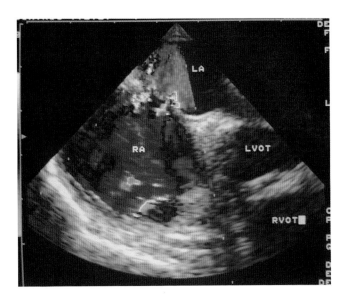

Figure 3.33 *A transverse plane transesophageal colour flow map study from a patient with multiple atrial septal defects. In this patient, the transverse plane imaging study suggested the foramen ovale to be intact. However, on colour flow mapping, two areas of turbulent transseptal flow are visualised across the foramen ovale. These are two small restrictive atrial septal defects.*

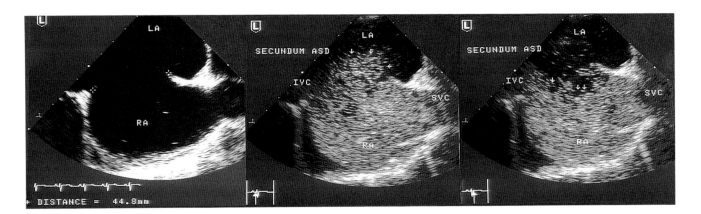

Figure 3.34 *A longitudinal plane transesophageal study demonstrating the value of peripheral venous contrast echocardiography and confirming the presence of transatrial flow. The contrast agent (Echovist) was injected into an anticubital vein. Right-to-left contrast flow is seen in the bottom left panel with left-to-right flow later during the cardiac cycle in the bottom right panel.*

Longitudinal plane transesophageal scanning is a valuable adjunct to transverse plane imaging. Experience with the new imaging planes available from longitudinal scanning has shown that not all the atrial septum can be scanned in the transverse plane. Transverse plane scanning may fail to or poorly image portions of the atrial septum which lie either in a retro-aortic root position (i.e. antero-inferiorly) or inferiorly towards the orifice of the inferior vena cava. These septal areas are normally well seen by longitudinal scanning (Fig. 3.32). A complete longitudinal plane scan of the flap valve of the foramen and the secundum atrial septum is commenced by imaging the atrial septum in the plane of the long axis of the caval veins (Fig. 3.24). As with transverse plane scanning, a full imaging and colour Doppler study should be carried out to determine if any defects are present. If a defect is present, its maximal dimension should be measured (the minor axis dimension of the defect). The probe may have to be advanced and withdrawn slightly to image the whole length of the interatrial septum. The imaging plane should then be rotated to the patient's right to sweep across the lateral portion of the septum until the drainage of both right pulmonary veins to left atrium has been seen. The probe tip should then be rotated to the patient's left to scan across the atrial septum until this structure drops out of view and the ascending aorta is visualised in its long axis. It is just before the aortic root is visualised that the retro-aortic portion of the atrial septum, not often visualised by transverse plane scanning, is seen. Again, the presence and size of any defect and its relationship to contiguous structures (i.e. the caval orifices, the coronary sinus, etc.) should be carefully noted. The long axis study should then be completed by defining the drainage pattern of both left pulmonary veins.

SINUS VENOUS ATRIAL SEPTAL DEFECTS

Transesophageal imaging would appear to be the best diagnostic technique to confirm the presence and the morphology of these defects. Subcostal echocardiography can image such defects in infants and small children but with increasing age this becomes increasingly difficult. Angiography is a less than optimal technique for defining both the morphology of the atrial defect and the co-existence of partial anomalous pulmonary venous drainage. We have no experience of the use of either computed tomography or MRI scanning in the assessment of these defects.

Sinus venosus defects may be sited either superiorly at the site of drainage of the superior vena cava to the atria or inferiorly at the site of drainage of the inferior vena cava. The former is by far the more common type. Both types are associated with partial anomalous pulmonary venous return. For the superior type the most common associated anomaly is abnormal drainage of the right upper pulmonary vein to the superior vena cava. However, a wide range of anomalies of drainage of the right pulmonary veins may co-exist.

Transesophageal imaging will readily confirm the morphology of both the superior and inferior types of sinus venosus defect and their associated anomalies of pulmonary venous return (1). Transverse plane imaging would appear to be the best imaging plane to select in investigating such defects. The probe should initially be advanced to image the lower portion of the superior vena cava in its transverse axis. With gradual probe advancement, the caval–right atrial junction will be brought into view. It is at this point that the postero-superior defect characteristic of a superior sinus venosus defect will be seen in the atrial septum, with the defect roofed by the orifice of the superior vena cava and the free atrial wall (Fig. 3.35(a)). The superior vena cava may often be seen in part to 'override' the defect. The remaining rim of the defect is part of the interatrial septum. In the majority of cases, further probe introduction will demonstrate that the foramen ovale (closed by its flap valve) is entirely discrete from the defect, thus confirming this is not a secundum defect. The probe then should be advanced to scan the orifice of the inferior vena cava to exclude the presence of a co-existing inferior sinus venosus defect. Having confirmed the morphology of the superior sinus venosus defect, the presence of anomalous pulmonary venous return should then be confirmed or excluded (as should the absence of a co-existing left superior vena cava). To do this, the probe should be withdrawn to image the area of the superior vena cava–right atrial junction and a subsequent careful transverse plane scan of the lower superior vena cava then made. This will normally reveal the presence of the right upper pulmonary vein draining directly to the lateral wall of the superior vena cava (Fig. 3.36). Colour flow mapping is useful to confirm this diagnosis. Care must be taken in such cases not to mistake the drainage of a hemiazygos systemic vein to the superior vena cava in this position as anomalous right upper pulmonary vein drainage. Thus in every case an additional scan should be made to confirm that there is no right upper pulmonary vein draining normally to the left atrium. As this structure should be visualised in 100% of cases where right upper pulmonary vein return is normal, absence of this structure is further evidence of partial anomalous venous return.

Longitudinal plane scanning has been suggested by some to be a better technique to demonstrate the morphology of superior sinus venosus defects. This has not been our experience. Indeed, the defect may be missed or its size much underestimated by scan-ning in the longitudinal plane. However, the defect will normally be imaged in this plane (Fig. 3.35(b)). The main problem with longitudinal plane imaging is that it may be difficult to confirm the anomalous drainage of the right upper pulmonary vein to the superior vena cava. However, we would imagine that longitudinal plane scanning might provide more information on the inferior form of sinus venosus defect than transverse plane scanning as the transverse approach often foreshortens the inferior portion of the atrial septum.

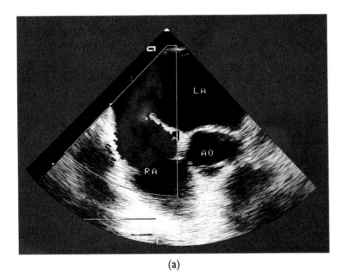

(a)

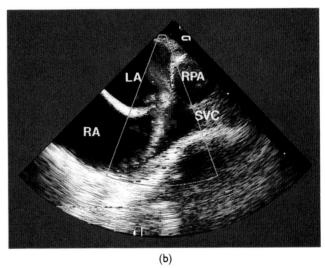

(b)

Figure 3.35 (a) *A transverse plane transesophageal image of a superior sinus venosus atrial septal defect. The morphologic features of the defect are well illustrated. The defect is roofed posteriorly by the atrial wall. Non-obstructive flow is seen to cross the defect.* **(b)** *The long axis transesophageal image from the same patient. The defect is not so well visualised in this plane but still the presence of the defect can be recognised. Left-to-right shunting is seen across the defect. The anomaly of drainage of the right upper pulmonary vein is not seen in either image. This can be identified by slight withdrawal of the probe using transverse plane scanning. In this plane, the right upper pulmonary vein will normally be seen to drain at the junction of the superior vena cava to the right atrium.*

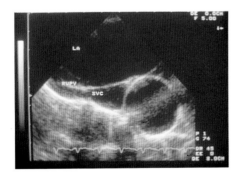

Figure 3.36 *Transverse plane transesophageal image of anomalous right upper pulmonary venous drainage to the superior vena cava in a case of a superior sinus venosus atrial septal defect.*

CORONARY SINUS DEFECTS

Of all the various types of atrial septal defect, the morphology of a coronary sinus atrial septal defect can be the most difficult to define from the precordial or subcostal imaging windows. These atrial septal defects are sited around the orifice of an un-roofed coronary sinus and have as part of the morphology a persistent superior vena cava of varying size. Normally the clue to the diagnosis is the precordial echocardiographic identification of the presence of a persistent left superior vena cava in a patient with clinical and echocardiographic evidence of right heart volume overload. The presence of a defect and its relationship to the orifice to the coronary sinus should then be sought using a variety of precordial and subcostal imaging positions which image the area of the coronary sinus. Colour flow mapping is a valuable adjunct in making this diagnosis as it can be used to confirm the presence of trans-defect flow. In addition, a left arm antecubital vein contrast echocardiographic study can be used to confirm both the presence of a left superior vena cava and (more importantly) its site of drainage.

As yet, there are no case reports of these relatively rare defects in the literature. In a consecutive series of 81 patients with clinical evidence of an atrial septal defect studied by ourselves (Table 3.3) only one had a coronary sinus defect. In this patient, the defect had been missed on prior precordial imaging. At a transverse plane transesophageal study, the secundum septum appeared intact. It was only with probe tip angulation to scan the atrial septum posteriorly around the coronary sinus that a small defect (1.2 cm in diameter) was seen immediately superior to the orifice of a dilated superior vena cava. The presence of the associated persistent superior vena cava was confirmed in the manner described in Chapter 3.1. We have no experience at Edinburgh of longitudinal or multiplane scanning in the diagnosis of such defects but we would speculate that the addition of other than transverse imaging planes should both enhance the definition of the site of drainage of the persistent left superior vena cava and should facilitate the imaging of the atrial septal defect.

PRIMUM ATRIAL SEPTAL DEFECTS PARTIAL ATRIOVENTRICULAR DEFECTS

MORPHOLOGIC FEATURES

These are common defects occurring with an incidence of 1–2% of all congenital heart defects. They are characterised by an absence in part or in total of the atrioventricular septum between the inferior limbic band of the atrial septum and the inlet portion of the ventricular septum, and are sited adjacent to the atrioventricular valve annuli. Most defects in the primum septum are large and non-restrictive but occasionally there is only minimal deficiency in the septum primum and the defect is restrictive. The atrioventricular valves are also abnormal. They share a common inlet with the attachments of the valves to the crest of the ventricular septum separating the outlets of the valves and thus obliterating any interventricular communication. The left atrioventricular valve normally has three leaflets (the normal anterior leaflet being divided into a superior and inferior portion by a 'cleft'). The right atrioventricular valve also has three leaflets.

PRECORDIAL AND SUBCOSTAL ECHOCARDIOGRAPHIC FEATURES

The diagnosis of a partial atrioventricular defect is normally very easily made by precordial or subcostal ultrasound imaging (9–11). The defect in the primum septum lying immediately above the plane of the atrioventricular valves is readily visualised. The apical four-chamber plane will demonstrate the common inlet to the atrioventricular valves and their divided outlet. In many patients, the appearance of an 'aneurysm' of the ventricular septum will be seen lying below the atrioventricular valves. This is caused by the insertion of the atrioventricular valve sub-valve apparatus inserting into the crest of the ventricular septum and thus closing off any potential interventricular communication. Subcostal and parasternal short axis scans will normally best demonstrate the detailed morphology of the atrioventricular valve leaflets (including the 'cleft') and chordal arrangements (12). A combination of colour flow mapping, continuous wave and pulsed Doppler will allow an accurate assessment of the intracardiac shunt, the presence (or absence) and severity of atrioventricular valve regurgitation, the pulmonary artery systolic pressure and the site and severity of any co-existing lesions such as left ventricular outflow tract obstruction (13).

In our experience, it is rare not to acquire the above information in its entirety even in adult patients. What role therefore does transesophageal imaging play in this patient group?

TRANSVERSE PLANE SCANNING

The atrioventricular junction is well visualised by transverse plane scanning from the oesophagus. Deficiencies in the primum atrial septum are well seen (Fig. 3.37). The common inlet of the atrioventricular valve is well characterised as are abnormalities in the valve leaflets. However, except in cases where precordial imaging is poor, these morphologic details are as well or often better imaged from the precordium. This is also true of related colour flow mapping and spectral Doppler studies. The real advantage of a diagnostic transesophageal study

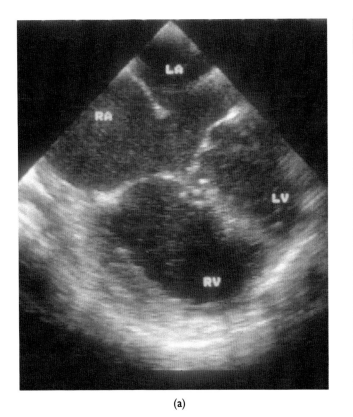

(a)

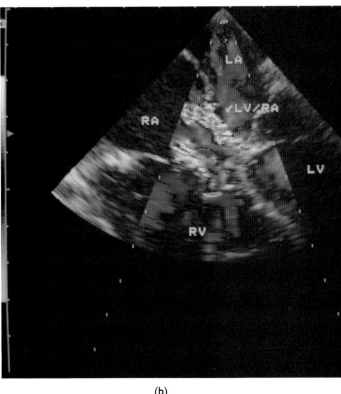

(b)

Figure 3.37 *A composite transverse plane transesophageal image from a patient with a partial atrioventricular septal defect.* **(a)** *The primum atrial septal defect is well seen as is the morphology of the atrioventricular valve and the presence of close-packed chordae closing the ventricular component.* **(b)** *In the colour flow mapping image, two jets of valve regurgitation are imaged, (1) a direct left ventricular right atrial jet and (2) the jet of tricuspid incompetence.*

most commonly lies in the definition of finer details of the morphology. These include (1) the identification of an associated double orifice mitral valve, (2) the better definition of obstruction within the left ventricular outflow tract and (3) the recognition of co-existing lesions such as partial anomalous pulmonary venous drainage, cor triatriatum or obstructive lesions within the right ventricle (biplane imaging). However, the real clinical role of transesophageal imaging in either partial or complete atrioventricular defects lies in intraoperative and immediate postoperative studies in patients undergoing surgical repair (14). Although for the majority of intraoperative studies in congenital heart disease we consider epicardial imaging to be superior to the transesophageal approach (see Chapter 4) in patients undergoing atrioventricular valve surgery (either replacement or repair) the transesophageal approach to monitoring may be preferred. In addition, during the early postoperative period precordial echocardiography may be of limited value in the ventilated patient. In this situ-

ation, transesophageal imaging (with the concomitant use of a right heart contrast agent) is often invaluable in confirming the adequacy of a surgical repair or in identifying the cause and determining the severity of a residual lesion (Fig. 3.38).

LONGITUDINAL PLANE IMAGING

Longitudinal plane imaging is a poor substitute for transverse plane imaging in the study of atrioventricular septal defects. The primum defect itself is poorly characterised and the morphology of the atrioventricular valves not so well defined as by transverse plane imaging (Fig. 3.39). However, the addition of a longitudinal plane study is often of value in better defining the morphology of the pulmonary venous drainage, the morphology and severity of the valve regurgitation, the site and nature of any associated left ventricular outflow tract obstruction and the morphology of the right ventricular outflow tract. Specific associated lesions poorly characterised by longitudinal plane scanning include the presence of left ventricular to right atrial shunting and the presence of a double-orifice mitral valve. Both these latter lesions are well characterised by transverse plane scanning (see Chapter 3.5).

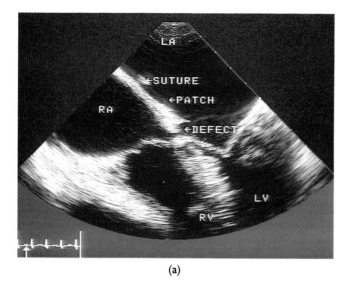

(a)

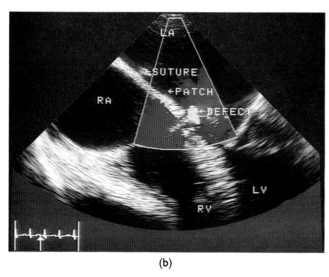

(b)

Figure 3.38 (a) *A transverse plane transesophageal image in a patient with a partial atrioventricular septal defect. The primum defect is well imaged in this imaging plane as is the morphology of the atrioventricular valve.* **(b)** *A longitudinal plane study from the same patient. The primum atrial septum defect is imaged in this plane. It is unusual, however, to see the defect so well. Transverse plane imaging is the optimal technique for identification of such defects.*

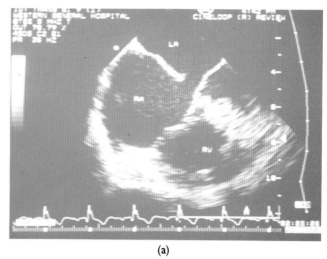

(a)

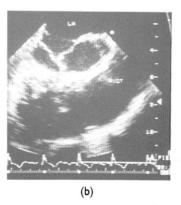

(b)

Figure 3.39 *A transverse plane transesophageal image taken in the four-chamber plane for a patient who had prior surgical closure of her partial atrioventricular septal defect. The imaging study suggested the presence of a small residual defect immediately above the atrioventricular valves. Colour flow mapping confirms the presence of a small left-to-right shunt at the bottom end of the atrial patch. This residual shunt had been missed at prior precordial echocardiography.*

TRANSGASTRIC IMAGING

Imaging the heart in the transverse plane from the fundus or lesser curvature of the stomach will produce a series of images essentially the same as those produced by subcostal imaging. The transgastric approach will often allow visualisation of the whole anterior bridging leaflet of a complete atrioventricular septal defect. (This structure is often poorly imaged during an intraesophageal study whereas the morphology of the posterior bridging leaflet is best imaged from within the oesophagus). In addition, transgastric transverse plane imaging may prove to be the optimal transesophageal approach to visualising and determining the haemodynamic importance of the cleft in the anterior leaflet of a primum defect.

COMPLETE AND INTERMEDIATE FORMS OF ATRIOVENTRICULAR DEFECTS

MORPHOLOGY

Complete and intermediate forms of atrioventricular septal defects have in common a complete deficiency of the atrioventricular septum and a ventricular component to the defect. The common atrioventricular valve has five leaflets, with an anterior and posterior bridging leaflet and three lateral leaflets. The bridging leaflets have connections in both ventricles while the lateral leaflets have attachments to only the ventricle in which they are sited. The common form of the defect (in which the associated ventricular septal defect is unrestrictive) can be subdivided into three morphologic types (the Rastelli classification) according to the morphology of the anterior bridging leaflet. This surgically derived classification is probably less clinically important than the need to determine the chordal or papillary muscle arrangement in the left ventricle or the alignment of the common valve with respect to the ventricles. Normally the common atrioventricular valve is aligned with its mid-point over the ventricular septum with equal amounts of valve tissue related to each ventricle. Rarely, the common valve is 'unbalanced' and is predominately related to one ventricle. Extreme degrees of 'unbalance' will result in hypoplasia of the ventricle which has little of the atrioventricular valve orifice related to it.

There is a spectrum of morphology between such a common defect and a partial atrioventricular defect. The 'intermediate' forms have a ventricular component to the defect which is partially closed by the atrioventricular valve septal attachments.

PRECORDIAL AND SUBCOSTAL ECHOCARDIOGRAPHIC FEATURES

As with partial atrioventricular defects, the major morphologic features which characterise the complete or intermediate forms are well defined by a combination of precordial and subcostal imaging. The deficiencies in the atrial and ventricular septa are well seen using either apical four-chamber or subcostal views. The valve leaflet morphology is best imaged using sub-xiphoid or parasternal short axis views. These latter two views also allow an excellent appreciation of the morphology and spatial relationships of the common atrioventricular valve and papillary muscles to the ventricular chambers. The combination of colour flow mapping studies integrated with spectral Doppler interrogation will define whether the ventricular component is restrictive or non-restrictive and the associated patterns of valve regurgitation.

TRANSOESOPHAGEAL IMAGING

Little needs to be added to the discussion of the role of transesophageal imaging in partial defects. For a complete atrioventricular defect, transverse plane transesophageal imaging will define the presence of a ventricular component and can better define the morphology and chordal and papillary muscle arrangement of the posterior bridging leaflet. Using the transesophageal approach, the anterior bridging leaflet and the arrangement of its sub-valve apparatus are best imaged from the transgastric position. However, these morphologic features are normally well defined by a combination of precordial and subcostal scanning. Transesophageal echocadiography in this defect group should be used diagnostically only where precordial imaging is poor, where there is a need for better definition of either the papillary muscle arrangement or the substrate for any co-existing left ventricular outflow tract obstruction. As stated earlier, the main role of transesophageal imaging in this defect group is in the monitoring of surgical repair.

REFERENCES

1. TUCILLO B, STÜMPER O, HESS J, et al. Transesophageal echocardiographic evaluation of atrial morphology in children with congenital heart disease. *Eur Heart J* 1992; **13:** 223–31.

2. STÜMPER O, VARGAS-BARRON J, RIJLAARSDAM M, ROMERO A, ROELANDT JRTC, HESS J, SUTHERLAND GR. Assessment of anomalous systemic and pulmonary venous connections by transoesophageal echocardiography in infants and children. *Br Heart J* 1991; **66:** 411–18.

3. HELLENBRAND WE, FAHEY JT, McGOWEN FX, WELTIN GE, KLEINMAN CS. Transoesophageal echocardiographic guidance of transcatheter closure of atrial septal defect. *Am J Cardiol* 1990; **66:** 207–13.

4. PINHEIRO L, NANDA NC, JAIN H, SANYAL R. Transesophageal echocardiographic imaging of the pulmonary veins. *Echocardiography* 1991; **8:** 841–8.

5. FERREIRA SMAG, YEN HO S, ANDERSON RH. Morphologic study of defects of the atrial septum within the oval fossa: implications for transcatheter closure of left-to-right shunt. *Br Heart J* 1992; **67:** 316–20.

6. MORIMOTO K, MATSUZAKI M, TACHMA Y, ONO S, TANAKA N, MICHISHIGE H, MURATA K, ANNO Y, KUSUKAWAR. Diagnosis and quantitative evaluation of secundum-type atrial septal defect by transoesophageal Doppler echocardiography. *Am J Cardiol* 1990; **66:** 85–91.

7. CHEN KC, GODMAN MJ. Morphological variations of fossa ovalis atrial septal defects (secundum). The feasibility for transcutaneous closure using the 'Clam-Shell' device. *Br Heart J* 1993; **69:** 52–6.

8. HANRATH P, SCHLUTTER M, LANGENSTEIN BA, et al. Detection of ostium secundum atrial septal defects by transoesophageal cross-sectional echocardiography. *Br Heart J* 1983; **49:** 350–8.

9. SMALLHORN JF, TOMMASINI G, ANDERSON RH, MACARTNEY FJ. Assessment of atrioventricular septal defects by two dimensional echocardiography. *Br Heart J* 1982; **47:** 109–21.

10. SILVERMAN NH, ZUBERBUHLER JR, ANDERSON RH. Atrioventricular septal defects: cross-sectional echocardiographic and morphologic comparisons. *Int J Cardiol* 1986; **13:** 309–31.

11. CARBERA A, PASTOR E, GALDANO JM, MODESTO C, CABRERA JA, ALCIBAR J, PENA R. Cross-sectional echocardiography in the diagnosis of atrioventricular septal defect. *Int J Cardiol* 1990; **28:** 19–23.

12. CHIN AJ, BIERMAN FZ, SANDERS SP, WILLIAMS RG, NORWOOD WI, CASTANEDA AR. Subxyphoid 2-dimensional echocardiographic identification of left ventricular papillary muscle anomalies in complete common atrioventricular canal. *Am J Cardiol* 1983; **51:** 1695–9.

13. HEYDARIAN M, GRIFFITH BP, ZUBERBUHLER JR. Partial atrioventricular canal associated with discrete subaortic stenosis. *Am Heart J* 1985; **109:** 915–17.

14. ROBERTSON DA, MUHIUDEEN IA, SILVERMAN NH, TURLEY K, HAAS GS, CAHALAN MK. Intraoperative transoesophageal echocardiography of atrioventricular septal defect. *J Am Coll Cardiol* 1991; **18:** 537–45.

Atrioventricular junction anomalies

O. Stümper

INTRODUCTION

Anomalies of the atrioventricular junction are a frequent finding in complex congenital heart disease. Whereas the paediatric cardiologist is familiar with the terminology to describe such lesions, the adult cardiologist will sometimes experience difficulties in adequately describing the wide range of lesions encountered. Thus, a reappraisal of the terminology will precede the description of the transesophageal findings (Fig. 3.40).

Atrioventricular connections can be either biventricular (each atrium is connected to one of the two ventricles) or univentricular (both atrial chambers are connected to a single ventricle). In hearts with biventricular atrioventricular connections there can exist either concordant, discordant or ambiguous connections (1). Concordance of the atrioventricular connection describes a state where the morphologically right atrium is connected to a morphologically right ventricle, and the morphologically left atrium to a morphologically left ventricle. The use of the term concordance is not influenced by the morphology of the atrioventricular valves: there can be either two perforate valves, a common valve or one imperforate valve. Discordance of the atrioventricular connection describes a state where the morphologically right atrium connects to a morphologically left ventricle and vice versa. The term ambiguous biventricular atrioventricular connection finally describes the fact that either two morphologically right or left atrial chambers exist (atrial isomerism) and are connected to two ventricles (independent of atrioventricular valve morphology). The spectrum of lesions that have in the past been grouped under the term 'univentricular' hearts are strictly speaking all those hearts in which the two atrial chambers (irrespective of their morphology) are connected to one ventricular chamber of varying morphology. Most often both atrial chambers will be connected to a morphologically left ventricle (double-inlet left ventricle) or to a ventricular chamber of indeterminate morphology. Sometimes hearts with absence of the right or the left atrioventricular connection ('single inlet') are included in this group, but the terms tricuspid or mitral atresia are more widely used in clinical practice.

The various forms of the mode of biventricular atrioventricular connections describe the morphology and the relation of the atrioventricular valves and their subvalvar apparatus to the ventricular chambers. There can be two perforate valves, one imperforate valve or a common atrioventricular valve. Finally the atrioventricular valves can be overriding or straddling.

After having defined the morphology and the position of the atrial chambers (Chapter 3.2), the crucial step in the determination of the atrioventricular connection is to document the relation of the atrial chambers to the individual ventricular chambers. A morphologically right ventricle is characterised by, firstly, coarse trabeculations of its apical trabecular component; secondly, by chordal attachments of the corresponding atrioventricular valve to the septal surface; and thirdly, by a complete muscular outlet, which characteristically results in a fibrous discontinuity between the

BIVENTRICULAR CONNECTIONS

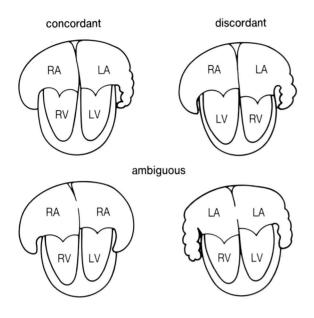

concordant   discordant

ambiguous

UNIVENTRICULAR CONNECTIONS

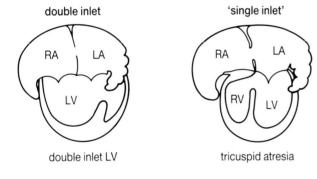

double inlet   'single inlet'

double inlet LV   tricuspid atresia

Figure 3.40 *Diagram summarising the different types of atrioventricular connections.*

atrioventricular and arterial valve of the right ventricle. A morphologically left ventricle is characterised, firstly, by fine trabeculations of the apical trabecular septum; secondly, by the absence of chordal attachments of the corresponding atrioventricular (mitral) valve to the septal surface; and thirdly, by a fibrous continuity of the atrioven-

tricular valve with the arterial valve. In hearts with an intact inlet portion of the ventricular septum, the morphologically right atrioventricular valve is typically attached more apically relative to the septal attachment of the morphologically left atrioventricular valve; a sign which is most often used in the rapid identification of ventricular topology.

Precordial ultrasound techniques have been shown to provide an accurate diagnosis of the atrioventricular junction in the vast majority of children with congenital heart disease (2–4). However, in the adolescent or adult patient population with relatively poor precordial ultrasound windows diagnostic difficulties may arise. Furthermore, in patients with an inlet ventricular septal defect, resulting in an attachment of both atrioventricular valves at the same level, diagnostic ambiguities may be encountered.

Magnetic resonance imaging has been used in several institutions in the assessment of atrioventricular junction anomalies (5–7). These studies suggested that the technique is at its best in the definition of the relation of the atrial and the ventricular chambers to one another. However, detailed pictures of the subvalvar apparatus of the atrioventricular valves are frequently difficult to obtain (8). This is mainly related to the fact that magnetic resonance imaging is a gated technique with long acquisition times. Thus, the technique is of little value in the exclusion of chordal straddling.

Transesophageal echocardiography, in our experience, is a most appropriate and useful technique for the assessment of this range of lesions. It is a real-time imaging technique that allows a detailed evaluation of the precise morphology of the subvalvar apparatus of both atrioventricular valves (9). However, an accurate assessment of certain aspects of ventricular chamber morphology and the definition of the relation of the ventricular chambers to one another is limited using single-plane imaging techniques. Although the introduction of biplane imaging technology has enhanced the transesophageal evaluation of the relationship of the atrioventricular junction to the ventricular chambers and their outflow tracts, current experience is still too limited to allow judgments on its exact diagnostic value. Transthoracic and subcostal echocardiographic studies, which combine high-resolution cross-sectional imaging together with unlimited imaging planes, remain the first-line diagnostic techniques. We currently consider transesophageal imaging a second-line imaging technique and perform studies in all patients in whom diagnostic ambiguities on the morphology of the atrioventricular junction persist.

CONCORDANT ATRIOVENTRICULAR CONNECTIONS

The definition of concordant atrioventricular connections is based on the documentation of, firstly, the atrial chamber morphology (Chapter 3.2) and, secondly, the demonstration of appropriate ventricular chamber morphology. Offsetting of the atrioventricular valves in patients with an intact inlet portion of the ventricular septum is best documented using low four-chamber views. In patients with an inlet ventricular septal defect, transesophageal cross-sectional imaging rapidly identifies the characteristic pattern of chordal insertion of both atrioventricular valves. Thus, the technique allows unequivocal chamber definition in the vast majority of cases. In contrast, the various patterns of ventricular trabeculation are difficult to assess by transesophageal imaging. This is mainly related to the large distances between the apical portions of the ventricular chambers and the oesophagus. Instead, demonstration of fibrous continuity between the atrioventricular valve and the arterial valve should be used as an additional marker in the definition of left ventricular morphology in cases where ambiguity persists. This can be performed best by the use of longitudinal axis imaging planes.

DISCORDANT ATRIOVENTRICULAR CONNECTIONS

Typically, discordance of the atrioventricular connection is found together with discordance of the ventriculo-arterial junction. This combination is usually referred to as congenitally corrected transposition of the great arteries. However, double outlet of the right ventricle or single outlet with pulmonary atresia are other types of abnormal ventriculo-arterial connections that may coexist with atrioventricular discordance. Having defined the location and the morphology of the atrial chambers (normal or mirror-image arrangement), transverse axis cross-sectional imaging of the atrioventricular junction will rapidly identify the ventricular inver-

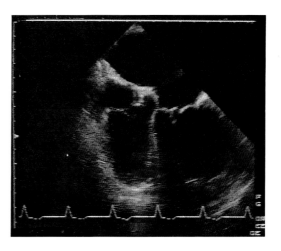

Figure 3.41 *Transesophageal four-chamber view in a patient with dextrocardia, atrial situs solitus and congenitally corrected transposition. Note the reversed offsetting of the atrioventricular valves and the malalignment between the atrial and the ventricular septum. Definition of the intracardiac anatomy is not impaired by the cardiac malposition.*

sion. It is the definition of the chordal insertions of both atrioventricular valves which is of most value in the assessment of these lesions (Fig. 3.41). Frequently, particularly in the older patient population, this is better performed by transesophageal than by precordial cross-sectional imaging. In approximately 80% of patients with congenitally corrected transposition there will be an associated ventricular septal defect, typically located in the inlet portion (10). In such cases the classical pattern of reversed offsetting of the atrioventricular valves is not present. The definition of ventricular morphology therefore depends on, firstly, documentation of the chordal implantation of the atrioventricular valves, and, secondly, definition of the relation of the atrioventricular valves to the arterial valves. Fibrous continuity between the right sided atrioventricular valve and the pulmonic valve can be demonstrated best using either a sequence of transverse axis planes or a single longitudinal axis cut.

Abnormalities of the atrioventricular valves, and in particular the left sided valve, are frequently encountered in patients with congenitally corrected transposition. An Ebstein-like malformation of the

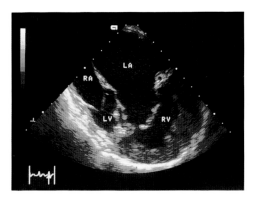

Figure 3.42 *Ebstein's malformation of the tricuspid valve in a patient with congenitally corrected transposition. There is displacement and tethering of both the septal and the anterior leaflet of the left sided, morphologically right atrioventricular valve.*

left sided, morphologically tricuspid valve, is recognised by apical displacement of in particular the septal and the anterior leaflet (Fig. 3.42). Tethering of the individual leaflets and the degree of displacement, however, in most cases will be better demonstrated on transthoracic apical four-chamber views. The great distances between the oesophagus and the area of interest frequently preclude an adequate assessment from within the oesophagus (see Chapter 3.5). Furthermore, straddling of the chordal apparatus of either the right or the left atrioventricular valve through a ventricular septal defect is encountered in a proportion of cases. The precise description of such an anomaly is of crucial importance prior to any attempted surgical repair. This, in our experience, can best be performed using transesophageal imaging (Fig. 3.43). Finally, incompetence of the left sided atrioventricular valve is an almost universal finding in the older patient with congenitally corrected transposition of the great arteries. Transesophageal studies should be carried out in patients with severe valvar regurgitation, in order to assess the potential for reconstructive surgery.

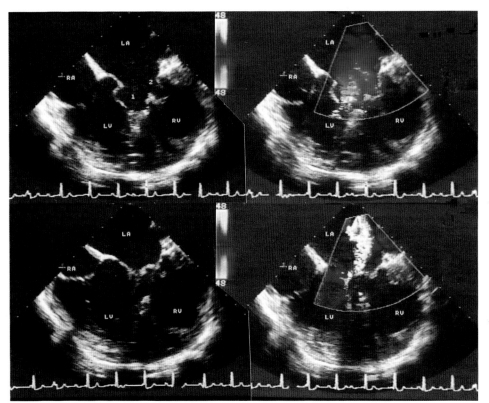

Figure 3.43 *Transesophageal ultrasound study in a patient with congenitally corrected transposition and ventricular septal defect. On precordial imaging the left sided atrioventricular valve was judged to be normal. Transesophageal four-chamber views demonstrate double orifice of the left sided atrioventricular valve (top left). The chordal attachment of the medial component is straddling the ventricular septal defect (bottom left). Colour flow mapping documents unobstructed diastolic ventricular inflow through both valve components (top right) and mild to moderate regurgitation of the medial component during systole (bottom right).*

Subpulmonary obstruction is another lesion commonly present in atrioventricular discordance. This is usually better assessed by transesophageal imaging than by precordial imaging. Poor definition of the subpulmonary area by transthoracic ultrasound techniques has been previously reported (11), and is the most problematic area in the precordial echocardiographic evaluation of atrioventricular discordance. Abnormal atrioventricular valve architecture, such as reduplication of the anterior leaflet of the mitral valve, is readily identified from the oesophagus, as is the presence of abnormal chordal attachments or tissue tags and aneurysm formation of the membranous ventricular septum (Fig. 3.44). Less frequently, the subpulmonary obstruction will be found to be caused by the presence of a fibromuscular membrane.

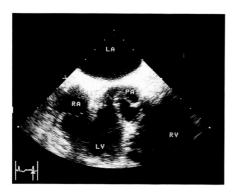

Figure 3.44 *Transverse axis image of a subpulmonary obstruction in a patient with congenitally corrected transposition. Aneurysm formation of the membranous ventricular septum as the cause of obstruction is clearly identified. Involvement of either atrioventricular valve apparatus could be excluded.*

AMBIGUOUS ATRIOVENTRICULAR CONNECTIONS

In patients with atrial isomerism a biventricular atrioventricular connection is defined to be ambiguous, as the criteria for concordance or discordance no longer apply. Following the transesophageal definition of isomeric atrial chamber morphology (Chapter 3.2), the atrioventricular junction should be assessed using a series of four-chamber views which will readily identify a biventricular connection where this is present. In patients with left atrial isomerism this will be so in some 70% of cases, whereas only one-third of patients with right atrial isomerism have a biventricular atrioventricular connection (12). The remaining patients with atrial isomerism will be found to have a univentricular atrioventricular connection, typically a double-inlet left ventricle.

In patients with a biventricular atrioventricular connection only about one-quarter have two separate atrioventricular valves, the remainder having a common atrioventricular valve. In rare cases either the right or the left atrioventricular connection may be an imperforate atrioventricular valve. These entities should be easily recognisable on transesophageal cross-sectional imaging. The major contributions of the technique to this rare spectrum of lesions lie in the unequivocal definition of the atrial situs, and in the superior image quality that can be obtained particularly in the adolescent and adult group when compared with transthoracic ultrasound techniques. The latter undoubtedly is of major relevance in the re-evaluation of previously assigned inoperable patients.

TRICUSPID ATRESIA

Strictly speaking the term tricuspid atresia does not classify a type of atrioventricular connection, but rather describes hearts which have in common that the only return of systemic venous blood to the ventricular chamber(s) is via an interatrial communication. The morphologic correlate is either an absent atrioventricular connection or (much more rarely) an imperforate atrioventricular valve. In hearts with an absent atrioventricular connection there is complete discontinuity between the right atrial and ventricular myocardium. The underlying ventricle has no inlet component – it consists of only a trabecular and an outlet portion. In contrast, in hearts with an imperforate tricuspid valve, there is atresia of a severely hypoplastic valve. The underlying ventricular chamber has an inlet portion and there is evidence of a subvalvar apparatus (Fig. 3.45). Although distinguishing between these two entities is of little, if any, clinical significance, their differentiation is desirable as it allows a more accurate morphologic description of the underlying pathology. Whereas this occasionally is difficult to establish by precordial ultrasound techniques, transesophageal imaging allows for a better understanding of these lesions. In fact it may be expected that the technique should prove comparable to magnetic resonance imaging in the definition of these malformations (13).

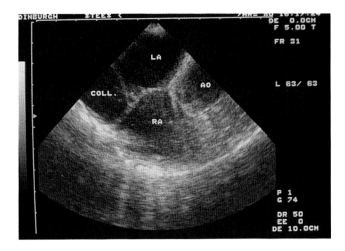

Figure 3.46 *Transeosophageal view of the common collector of pulmonay venous blood in a child with total anomalous pulmonary venous drainage and tricuspid atresia. Using combined imaging and colour flow mapping studies the site of connection of all four pulmonary veins and the unobstructed communication of the collector (COLL.) with the left atrium could be documented.*

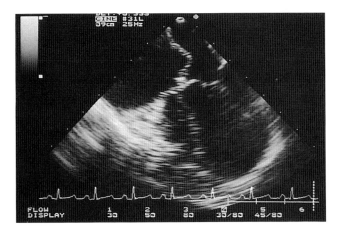

Figure 3.45 *Transesophageal four-chamber view in a child with tricuspid atresia. A small imperforate membrane is clearly visualised on cross-sectional imaging. Note the characteristic appearance of the atrial septum with a rather redundant flap valve of the oval fossa.*

Definition of the type of the ventriculo-arterial connection in hearts with tricuspid atresia should follow the guidelines set out above. In the most common form the ventriculo-arterial connection will be concordant, with the aorta posterior and to the right of the pulmonary artery. There will be a restrictive muscular interventricular communication to a rudimentary anterior outlet chamber

(14). Neither the size of the ventricular septal defect nor the morphology of the outlet chamber are well assessed by transesophageal imaging. In fact, in our experience, the technique has nothing to offer in the assessment of these aspects of the lesion when compared with transthoracic imaging. In about one-quarter of patients with tricuspid atresia, the ventriculo-arterial connection will be discordant. In such cases there is a high incidence of additional cardiovascular anomalies, which should be ruled out during the transesophageal study.

Transesophageal studies in the preoperative assessment of patients with tricuspid atresia should focus on a detailed definition of both the systemic and pulmonary venous return (Chapter 3.1), and on evaluation of the atrial chamber and atrial septal morphology (Chapters 3.2, 3.3). The presence of anomalous venous connections greatly influences the operative technique and outcome (15). A left superior caval vein is frequently encountered in patients with tricuspid atresia, and will be identified on high esophageal views of the left atrium. Partial or total anomalous pulmonary venous connections should be ruled out in all patients studied (Fig. 3.46). With respect to the atrial septum, the transesophageal study should be tailored to exclude multiple defects. Coexisting coronary sinus atrial septal defects, which occur in about 2.5% of patients with tricuspid atresia (16), should be specifically excluded. Using transverse axis imaging, this requires detailed imaging and colour flow mapping studies of the distal portion and the site of drainage of the coronary sinus. However, such defects can be missed on transverse axis plane scanning. Longitudinal plane imaging would appear to be the technique of choice in identifying such defects. A further anomaly which is frequently encountered in patients with tricuspid atresia and transposition of the great arteries is juxtaposition of the atrial appendages. The preoperative definition of this lesion may be of considerable value in planning a Fontan procedure.

The majority of patients with tricuspid atresia will undergo a number of palliative procedures, such as pulmonary artery banding or pulmonary artery shunting, before they are considered for a Fontan-type repair. In all such patients transesophageal ultrasound studies should also be used for a detailed assessment of the central pulmonary artery system. It is especially in the exclusion of discrete obstructions of the branch pulmonary arteries (which may preclude a subsequent Fontan procedure), that transesophageal imaging has been shown to be superior to transthoracic imaging.

Based on our current experience, the use of transesophageal ultrasound to study patients with tri-cuspid atresia is highly rewarding both in the preoperative definition of the underlying morphology and in the exclusion of associated anomalies. The information thus obtained can then be used to plan the subsequent catheterisation and surgical procedure.

MITRAL ATRESIA

In hearts with mitral atresia the tissue between the floor of the left atrium and the left ventricle always consists of dense fibrous tissue. This can take the form either of a thin fibrous cord or of a compact membrane (17). The underlying ventricle is typically severely hypoplastic. Most commonly the ventricular septum is intact and there is atresia of the aortic valve. Such hearts are grouped under the term 'hypoplastic left heart syndrome'. Because of the severity of these lesions patients present in the neonatal period and the definitive diagnosis is made by precordial cross-sectional imaging (18).

Patients who have a ventricular septal defect and a normal aorta may survive and present only later. In such cases a Fontan-type procedure (total cavopulmonary anastomosis) may be a surgical option. Thus, in the rare cases to be investigated with these

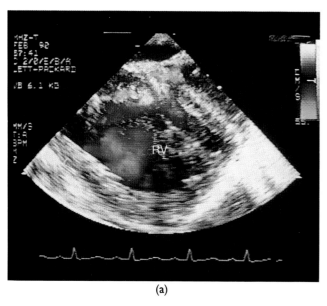

(a)

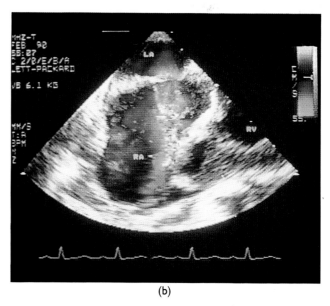

(b)

Figure 3.47 *Transesophageal imaging study in a child with mitral atresia and double-outlet right ventricle.* **(a)** *The imperforate mitral valve and the ventricular septal defect are documented on four-chamber views.* **(b)** *There is a restrictive central atrial septal defect with left-to-right shunting. The transesophageal study was performed for guidance and monitoring of blade septostomy.*

lesions, the transesophageal study should focus on an assessment of the systemic and the pulmonary venous connections, and the morphology of the atrial septum (Fig. 3.47). The information to be derived from such studies may lead to a more accurate planning of subsequent cardiac catheterisation or an interim interventional procedure such as blade septostomy to establish unobstructed pulmonary venous return.

DOUBLE-INLET VENTRICLES

In these hearts both atrial chambers are connected to the same ventricle. The ventricular chamber may be of left or right ventricular morphology and there may be two separate atrioventricular valves, a common atrioventricular valve orifice, or atresia of one of the atrioventricular valves. The most common form within this range of lesions is a double-inlet left ventricle. This is associated in about 90% with transposition of the great arteries. Thus, the aorta in such hearts arises from an anterior outlet chamber of right morphology. However, concordant ventriculo-arterial and double-outlet connections can also exist. Abnormalities of the atrioventricular valves frequently coexist, and should be ruled out by a transesophageal study.

It is particularly in the detailed definition of the insertion of the subvalvar apparatus of both atrioventricular valves that transesophageal imaging has proved to be of additional value to precordial imaging in the preoperative evaluation. In some cases surgical septation, thus establishing a biventricular repair, may be an option. We would consider preoperative transesophageal studies in such patients essential for the accurate definition of the chordal attachments of either atrioventricular valve to the ventricular chambers, and for planning of the potential plane of the patch used to septate the ventricle (Fig. 3.48). In hearts which cannot be septated, a Fontan-type procedure represents the only surgical option. A large proportion of such patients will be found to have transposition of the great arteries with subaortic obstruction. Transesophageal studies should be performed in these patients in order to rule out any chordal straddling through the restrictive ventricular septal defect, which may preclude surgical enlargement of the defect.

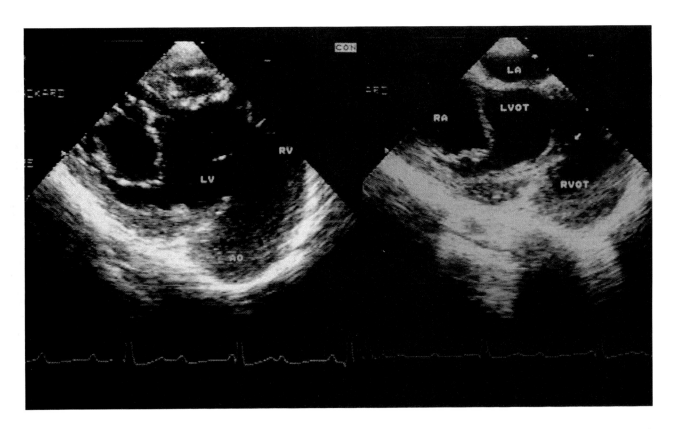

Figure 3.48 *Transverse axis imaging in a patient with a double-inlet left ventricle, defining the relation of the atrioventricular valves and subvalvar apparatus to one another and to the ventricular chambers.*

CRISS-CROSS HEARTS AND SUPERO-INFERIOR VENTRICLES

The terms 'criss-cross heart' and 'supero-inferior ventricles' describe complex spatial ventricular relations rather than abnormalities of the atrioventricular junction. In criss-cross hearts the systemic and the pulmonary venous returns cross at the level of the atrioventricular valves. The atrioventricular connection itself may be concordant or discordant. There is always a large perimembranous ventricular septal defect. In hearts with supero-inferior relation of the ventricular chambers, the atrioventricular connection may again be either concordant or discordant. The plane of the ventricular septum is almost horizontal, with one ventricle lying on top

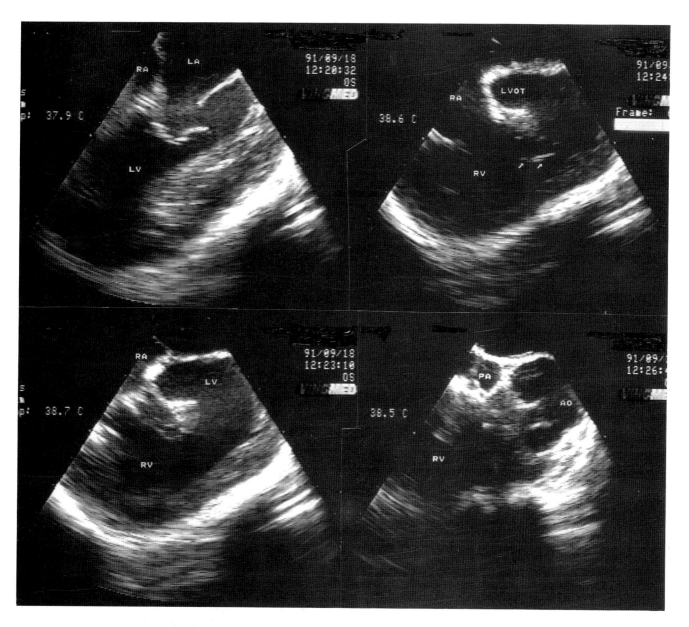

Figure 3.49 *Transesophageal transverse axis imaging in a child with atrial situs solitus, concordant atrioventricular and discordant ventriculo-arterial connections. The ventricular chambers are arranged in a superior-inferior fashion. Scanning low esophageal views, the relationship of the mitral valve apparatus to the inferior, morphologically left, ventricle is defined (top left). Gradual withdrawal of the probe visualises the ventricular septal defect (bottom left), and documents the attachments of the tricuspid valve to the outlet septum and the anterior free wall of the superior, morphologically right, ventricle (top right). Finally the relationship of the great arteries to one another and to the right ventricular outflow tract are demonstrated (bottom right).*

of the other. Typically there is a ventricular septal defect. The ventriculo-arterial junction in such hearts is in most cases discordant, but may also be concordant, or double-outlet. Again abnormalities of the atrioventricular valves are a frequent finding.

Transthoracic and subcostal cross-sectional imaging is the diagnostic technique of choice in the initial diagnosis and preoperative evaluation (19). In patients in whom these techniques remain ambiguous, particularly in the definition of atrioventricular valve morphology and subvalve apparatus, transesophageal ultrasound studies may be of additional value. Using a strict sequence of esophageal short axis views, detailed tomographic images of the heart can be obtained (Fig. 3.49). This allows a comprehensive assessment of the intracardiac morphology, and in particular of the atrioventricular valve apparatus relative to the ventricular chambers and to any coexisting ventricular septal defect. Transgastric views are best in defining the relation of the ventricular chambers to one another. It is felt that the addition of biplane transesophageal imaging will further enhance the transesophageal assessment of such complex hearts.

SUMMARY

The majority of patients with abnormal atrioventricular connections have complex intracardiac anatomies and a wide range of associated cardiovascular anomalies. In a high proportion of these patients a Fontan-type procedure is the only form of surgical treatment, making a detailed preoperative assessment mandatory. Transesophageal ultrasound studies should be considered an integral part of any such pre-surgical evaluation. In our experience, the technique frequently provides invaluable information for subsequent patient management and allows for a detailed planning of further diagnostic tests. Areas of particular strength of the technique include the definition of venous connections, atrial chamber morphology and abnormalities of the atrioventricular valves. With respect to definition of the ventricular chambers, their morphology and spatial relation to one another, transthoracic ultrasound techniques and magnetic resonance imaging remain superior diagnostic techniques. However, in the adolescent and adult patient population transesophageal imaging should be considered the diagnostic technique of first choice.

REFERENCES

1. TYNAN MJ, BECKER AE, MACARTNEY FJ, QUERO-JIMINEZ M, SHINEBOURNE EA, ANDERSON RH. Nomenclature and classification of congenital heart disease. *Br Heart J* 1979; **41:** 544–53.
2. HAGLER DJ, TAJIK AJ, SEWARD JB, EDWARDS WD, MAIR DD, RITTER DG. Atrioventricular and ventriculoarterial discordance (corrected transposition of the great arteries): wide-angle two-dimensional echocardiographic assessment of ventricular morphology. *Mayo Clin Proc* 1981; **56:** 591–600.
3. FOALE R, STEFANINI L, RICKARDS A, SOMERVILLE J. Left and right ventricular morphology in complex congenital heart disease defined by two dimensional echocardiography. *Am J Cardiol* 1982; **49:** 93–9.
4. SMALLHORN JF, SUTHERLAND GR, ANDERSON RH, MACARTNEY FJ. Cross-sectional echocardiographic assessment of conditions with atrioventricular value leaflets attached to the atrial septum at the same level. *Br Heart J* 1982; **48:** 331–41.
5. BOXER RA, SINGH S, LACORTE MA, GOLDMAN M, STEIN HL. Cardiac magnetic resonance imaging in children with congenital heart disease. *J Pediatr* 1986; **109:** 460–4.
6. DIDIER D, HIGGINS CB, FISHER MR, OSAKI L, SILVERMAN NH, CHEITLIN MD. Congenital heart disease: gated MR imaging in 72 patients. *Radiology* 1986; **158:** 227–35.
7. GUIT GL, BLUEMM R, ROHMER J, et al. Levotransposition of the aorta: identification of segmental cardiac anatomy using MR imaging. *Radiology* 1986; **131:** 673–9.
8. BAKER EJ, AYTON V, SMITH MA, et al. Magnetic resonance imaging at a high field strength of ventricular septal defects in infants. *Br Heart J* 1989; **62:** 305–10.
9. SREERAM N, STÜMPER O, KAULITZ R, et al. The comparative value of surfac and transoesophageal ultrasound in the assessment of congenital abnormalities of the atrioventricular junction. *J Am Coll Cardiol* 1990; **16:** 1205–14.
10. EGLOFF M, ROTHLIN J, SCHNEIDER G, ARBENZ V, SCHÖNBECK M, SENNING O, TURINA M. Congenitally corrected transposition of the great arteries: a clinical and surgical study. *J Thorac Cardiovasc Surg* 1980; **28:** 228–32.
11. SUTHERLAND GR, SMALLHORN JF, ANDERSON RH, RIGBY ML, HUNTER S. Atrioventricular discordance: cross-sectional echocardiographic-morphological correlative study. *Br Heart J* 1983; **50:** 8–20.
12. SAPIRE DW, HO SY, ANDERSON RH, RIGBY ML. Diagnosis and significance of atrial isomerism. *Am J Cardiol* 1986; **58:** 342–6.
13. FLETCHER BD, JACOBSTEIN MD, ABRAMOWSKY CR, ANDERSON RH. Right atrioventricular valve atresia – anatomic evaluation with MR imaging. *Am J Radiol* 1987; **148:** 671–4.
14. ANDERSON Rh, WILKINSON JL, GERLIS LM, SMITH A,

BECKER AE. Atresia of the right atrioventricular orifice. *Br Heart J* 1977; **39:** 414–28.

15. VARGAS FJ, MAYER JE, JONAS RA, CASTANEDA AR. Anomalous systemic and pulmonary venous connections in conjunction with atriopulmnary anastomosis – technical considerations. *J Thorac Cardiovasc Surg* 1987; **93:** 523–32.

16. RUMISEK JD, PIGOTT JD, WEINBERG PM, NORWOOD WI. Coronary sinus septal defect associated with tricuspid atresia. *J Thorac Cardiovasc Surg* 1986; **92:** 142–5.

17. GITTENBERGER-DE GROOT AC, WENINK ACG. Mitral atresia – morphological details. *Br Heart J* 1984; **51:** 252–8.

18. BASH SE, HUHTA JC, VICK GW III, GUTGESELL HP, OTT DA. Hypoplastic left heart syndrome: is echocardiography accurate enough to guide surgical palliation? *J Am Coll Cardiol* 1986; **7:** 610–16.

19. CARMINATI M, VALSECCHI O, BORGHI A, *et al.* Cross-sectional echocardiographic study of criss-cross hearts and superinferior ventricles. *Am J Cardiol* 1987; **59:** 114–18.

Congenital anomalies of the atrioventricular valves

G. R. Sutherland and N. Sreeram

INTRODUCTION

Transthoracic ultrasound studies of congenital anomalies of the atrioventricular valves normally provide reliable diagnostic information on both valve morphology and functional status. This applies to both children and adults (although image quality may be reduced in the latter age group). However, one area of diagnostic difficulty which may arise is in the definition of the morphology of the sub-valve apparatus and in the exclusion of chordal straddling. Transesophageal echocardiography (especially in its biplane or multiplane formats) potentially offers higher resolution imaging of valve morphology and should have advantages over precordial imaging in the assessment of valve regurgitation. This chapter will attempt to compare and contrast the values of each imaging approach in the detailed assessment of congenital lesions of the atrioventricular valves.

Using a combination of parasternal, apical and subcostal views to image multiple sectioning planes, transthoracic echocardiography can identify all aspects of native atrioventricular valve morphology and function. This ability to scan the valve is related to the multiplicity of imaging planes available from this approach. Transesophageal imaging (even with the addition of transgastric imaging) is limited in the imaging planes available. One of the most important views used to scan an atrioventricular valve is the short axis cut at the level of the commissures. This view is never available from an intraesophageal position and is only feasible using transverse plane transgastric scanning. However, using appropriate transducer manipulation, a short axis transgastric view which visualises the commissures of both the mitral and tricuspid valves can be obtained in a proportion of patients. This can allow the evaluation of the effective valve orifice area, the leaflet morphology, the site of regurgitation (central orifice or commissural), the presence of a leaflet cleft and the presence of a leaflet perforation. In addition, neither transverse nor longitudinal plane scanning can correctly evaluate valve leaflet prolapse. Longitudinal plane scanning is more reliable than transverse plane scanning in this respect, but both planes may fail to identify minor or moderate degrees of leaflet prolapse which are readily identified using transthoracic imaging. Thus while transesophageal imaging is second best to transthoracic imaging in the evaluation of valve leaflet morphology and valve orifice area for either atrioventricular valve, it has major benefits in the assessment of the morphology and severity of valve regurgitation and in the assessment of the sub-valve apparatus. The whole question of the transesophageal evaluation of atrioventricular valve regurgitation is covered in Chapters 5.1 and 5.2 and will not be discussed further here. To determine the morphology of the sub-valve apparatus of the mitral valve from the oesophagus, a series of views must be used. The transverse plane transesophageal view images the sub-valve chordae in a foreshortened oblique view in which one papillary muscle lies behind the other. It is rarely possible to separate the papillary muscles out and to identify their primary and secondary chordae. It certainly is not possible to differentiate reliably between the normal papillary muscle architecture and a single papillary muscle using transverse plane imaging alone. This problem is normally easily resolved by switching to the longitudinal plane which separates out the two papillary muscles and can allow the identification of the attachments of both the primary and secondary chordae. Perhaps even a better view of these structures is that obtained from a transgastric long axis plane with the imaging array sited near the gastroesophageal junction. This view may be obtainable in only 40–50% of patients but where obtained gives the best images of the mitral valve sub-valve apparatus. Where doubts exist about the presence of a single papillary muscle, this can be further evaluated using a series of transgastric short axis views to follow the papillary muscles down into the ventricle to their site(s) of origin from the ventricular walls. The morphology of the tricuspid valve sub-valve apparatus is much more difficult to evaluate from the oesophagus as these structures are more complex and less-well organised and (when compared to the mitral valve) lie in the far imaging field. A combination of transesophageal and transgastric imaging should also be used to define these structures with transgastric longitudinal imaging often giving the most information on chordal and papillary muscle morphology. Transesophageal imaging is also of value in determining the presence or absence of valve override or chordal straddling (see later).

In summary, transesophageal imaging is an adjunct to transthoracic imaging in the preoperative evaluation of native atrioventricular valve morphology and function. Both approaches have their respective strengths and weaknesses as indicated above. They should be used in an integrated manner to study congenital atrioventricular valve anomalies. Transesophageal imaging, however, is the technique of choice for the evaluation of suspected prosthetic valve malfunction (see Chapter 5.2).

Ebstein's anomaly of the tricuspid valve

TRANSTHORACIC ECHOCARDIOGRAPHIC FEATURES

Ebstein's anomaly is characterised by displacement of part of the origin of the tricuspid valve leaflets from the atrioventricular junction into the cavity of the right ventricle (1). The septal and posterior leaflets are most commonly involved in the displacement. There is usually associated dysplasia of the leaflet tissue, and anomalous distal attachments of the leaflets. Such apical displacement results in 'atrialisation' of part of the inlet portion of the right ventricle. The anterosuperior leaflet may be normally attached at the atrioventricular junction, but the leaflet is usually enlarged and malformed, and may have focal or linear distal attachments (2). These anomalous attachments, and the abnormal leaflet morphology, may produce a tricuspid valve that is regurgitant, stenotic or both. The functional right ventricular cavity is frequently reduced, with dysplasia of its walls. Diminished pulmonary blood flow may result from a combination of obstruction at tricuspid valve level due to the anomalous distal attachments of the leaflets, to reduced volume of the functional right ventricle, to severe tricuspid regurgitation, or anatomic malformations of the pulmonary valve and outflow tract. There is an associated atrial septal defect in the majority of patients, the direction of the shunt through the defect being determined by the presence and degree of obstruction to pulmonary blood flow.

The diagnosis of Ebstein's anomaly can be conclusively made by transthoracic cross-sectional echocardiography (3–6). The apical four-chamber view enables appreciation of the inferior displacement of the junctional origin of the septal leaflet. There is normally some apical displacement (offsetting) of the septal leaflet of the tricuspid valve when compared with the proximal attachment of the anterior leaflet of the mitral valve. There may also be an overlap between patients with Ebstein's anomaly and normals when absolute displacement of the septal leaflet is considered. However, on indexing the displacement to the body surface area, Shiina et al.(3) found that apical displacement exceeding 8 mm/m^2 of body surface area appeared to be a sensitive predictor for Ebstein's anomaly. The displacement of the septal tricuspid leaflet was measured in the four-chamber view as the distance from the atrioventricular junction to the distal point of the septal leaflet attachment in systole. The point of maximal displacement may sometimes vary from the midpoint of the septal leaflet to a point between the septal and posterior leaflets (2). The insertion of all three tricuspid valve leaflets cannot be simultaneously visualised from the four-chamber view. The anterior and posterior leaflets may however be optimally imaged from the right ventricular inlet view, with the transducer rotated anti-clockwise through almost 90° from the four-chamber view, and angled upwards and medially (7–9). Occasionally, leaflet displacement may be appreciated only in this view. Subcostal views are also valuable in visualising the posterior leaflet if it cannot be seen from the precordial approach (7).

The anterior leaflet is typically elongated, and has a sail-like redundant motion which may be seen in both the apical four-chamber and parasternal long axis views. This redundant motion is responsible for the delayed closure of the tricuspid valve, which is the most characteristic M-mode echocardiographic feature of Ebstein's anomaly (10,11). With increasing severity of dysplasia of the septal leaflet the anterior leaflet exhibits an increasingly exaggerated motion, and the coaptation point of the two leaflets in the four-chamber view is displaced towards the ventricular septum. In extreme cases, the septal leaflet may be absent, and the anterior leaflet appears to function as a monocusp valve apparatus.

Various additional features may be appreciated in the four-chamber view. The relative sizes of the right atrium, atrialised portion of the right ventricle and the functional right ventricle may be assessed. The true right atrium is measured from the atrioventricular junction to the posterosuperior wall of the atrium. The right ventricle is measured from the atrioventricular junction to the ventricular apex. The atrialised portion is then the distance from the atrioventricular junction to the functional annulus at the leading edge of the tricuspid valve leaflets, and the functional right ventricle the difference between the total right ventricle and the atrialised portion (3). A comparable angiographic correlate to these measurements was proposed by Leung et al.(2), who calculated the displacement index of the tricuspid valve leaflets. This was the extent of maximal distal displacement of the tricuspid valve attachment from the atrioventricular junction in diastole, expressed as a proportion of the measured length of the inlet of the right ventricle (from atrioventricular junction to ventricular apex).

Depending on the degree of leaflet displacement, the functional right ventricle may be considerably diminished and dysplastic. The thickness of the right ventricular walls may be reduced, and the ventricular septum may bow towards the left, producing a crescentic left ventricular cavity. Extreme degrees of leftward septal displacement may produce left ventricular outlet obstruction. The left ventricle itself is intrinsically normal, but may appear small when compared to the dilated right-sided chambers. Some investigators have noted angiographic left ventricular abnormalities including mitral valve prolapse and ventricular dyskinesia (12,13), although these findings may be explained in part by leftward bowing of the septum and compression of the left ventricular cavity.

TRANSOESOPHAGEAL ECHOCARDIOGRAPHIC EVALUATION

Both transverse and longitudinal plane imaging can identify the morphologic and haemodynamic features associated with this lesion. The transverse plane approach (Fig. 3.50) can identify (1) the degree of inferior displacement of the origin of the septal leaflet from the atrioventricular junction; (2) the level of leaflet coaptation within the right ventricular cavity; (3) the morphology of the chordae and papillary muscles; and (4) the severity of the tricuspid regurgitation. Secondary features such as the degree of right atrial and right ventricular dilatation, the presence or absence of a secundum atrial septal defect or any shunting across a patent oval foramen will also be well defined using transverse plane imaging. Longitudinal plane imaging is of value in determining the degree of anterior leaflet displacement, the morphology of the posterior leaflet, the ventricular volume, the morphology of the sub-valve apparatus and in defining the presence and morphology of any obstructive lesions within the right ventricular outflow tract and at pulmonary valve level. Used in combination, the transverse and longitudinal planes can characterise Ebstein's anomaly of the tricuspid valve in great detail. However, this is not always the case. It is our impression that precordial imaging using a combination of parasternal long axis and apical four-chamber scans may better define the leaflet morphology and degree of displacement of the valve leaflets from the valve ring when compared with the often foreshortened imaging planes available from the oesophagus. In addition, none of the imaging techniques may give adequate information on the structure and function of the sub-valve apparatus. This may be better defined by epicardial imaging at the time of attempted surgical repair, but even this technique may be inadequate with surgical inspection being the only certain method of defining the morphology of the chordae and papillary muscles. A further advantage of the combined precordial and subcostal approach is the better Doppler alignment to the direction of right heart blood flow when compared with transesophageal imaging. Thus a complete and accurate Doppler haemodynamic assessment is only possible using the transthoracic approach.

While the diagnosis of Ebstein's anomaly may thus be established with certainty, there is a poor correlation between the morphologic findings and the resultant clinical severity of the lesion. In the largest series of patients studied using echocardiography, Shiina et al.(3) found that a lower functional class (based on the New York Heart

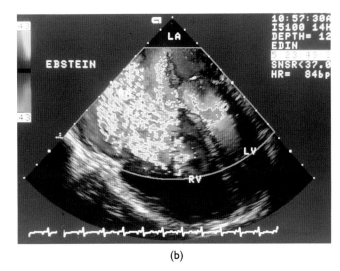

(a)

(b)

Figure 3.50 (a) *A transverse plane transesophageal image of the atrioventricular junction from a patient with Ebstein's anomaly of the tricuspid valve. The right ventricle is severely dilated and the tricuspid valve ring normally positioned but enlarged. The septal leaflet of the tricuspid valve (arrowed) is seen to be abnormally adherent to the right ventricular surface of the septum over one-third of its length.* **(b)** *A transverse plane colour Doppler study from the above patient. Note the gross tricuspid regurgitation with the valve orifice lying far within the right ventricular cavity. The 'atrialised' portion of the right ventricle is well appreciated.*

Association classification) was associated with: (1) a small functional right ventricle and a large atrialised portion; (2) extreme displacement or absence of the septal leaflet; (3) displacement of the anterior leaflet and tethering of its distal attachments; (4) aneurysmal dilatation of the right ventricular outflow tract with compression of the left ventricle. Aneurysmal dilatation was defined as a right ventricular outflow tract dimension in the parasternal short axis view greater than twice the diameter of the aortic root. Of these, absence of the septal leaflet and pronounced tethering and restricted mobility of the anterior leaflet were best related to diminished functional capacity. While no single feature adequately reflected functional disability, patients in NYHA classes III and IV appeared to have more of these structural abnormalities.

SURGICAL CONSIDERATIONS

Surgery for Ebstein's anomaly has taken the form of tricuspid valve repair (15–17) or replacement (18,19), together with repair of all associated defects. Although clinical severity is often associated with adverse morphologic features, none of the adverse morphologic features described previously enabled classification of patients into those who might benefit maximally from medical treatment and those in whom surgery would be required. Corrective surgery is therefore reserved for patients with severe functional disability (NYHA classes III and

IV). Among patients who came to surgery however, echocardiography was useful in separating patients who would require valve replacement from those in whom valve repair might be successful (26). Plastic reconstruction of the tricuspid valve depended on the presence of a freely mobile and adequate sized anterior leaflet, which could be made to function as a monocusp valve by plication of the atrialised chamber and reduction of the tricuspid annulus by annuloplasty (20). Conversely, the best indicators for valve replacement were tethering and immobility of the anterior leaflet of the tricuspid valve, and a small functional right ventricle (26).

For purposes of surgical repair, Carpentier *et al.* have also proposed four grades (A–D) of increasing severity of the disease based on the morphologic characteristics of the tricuspid valve and right ventricle (17). Grade A was characterised by a mobile anterior tricuspid leaflet with a small contractile atrialised chamber; grade B by a mobile anterior leaflet but a large non-contractile atrialised chamber; grade C by tethering of the distal attachments of the anterior leaflet associated with a large non-contractile atrialised chamber; and grade D where the leaflet tissue formed a continuous sac adherent to the right ventricle. These grades can be recognised echocardiographically, and more severe grades correlate roughly with the adverse echocardiographic features described by Shiina *et al.*(3,20). The mobility of the anterior leaflet is obviously of great importance in assessing severity of the disease, as a tethered leaflet will result in greater degree of tricuspid regurgitation, and a smaller functional right ventricle (2). Plastic repair relies on adequate mobilisation of leaflet tissue to form a competent tricuspid valve.

A combination of transesophageal and precordial echocardiography has been shown to be extremely useful in assessing the functional results after plastic repair of the tricuspid valve. The immediate results of plastic repair by mobilisation of the anterior and posterior leaflets, longitudinal plication of the right ventricle and atrialised chamber, and reattachment of the leaflets at the atrioventricular junction to create a bi-leaflet valve (20) can all be assessed (Fig. 3.51). Colour flow grading of tricuspid regurgitation at subsequent follow-up showed a decrease by at least one grade in all patients with >grade 2 regurgitation preoperatively. Systolic reversal of flow within the hepatic veins could not be recorded after surgery in five of six patients in whom it could be detected preoperatively. Measurement of peak velocity of flow across the pulmonary valve by pulsed Doppler showed a significant increase in peak velocity and a decrease in time to peak velocity after surgery, suggesting improved right ventricular systolic function (14,21). The peak velocity of tricuspid inflow also increased, related to a decrease in valve orifice diameter. All these changes were associated with an improvement in the functional class of the patients and improved exercise capacity.

In conclusion, echocardiography enables the diagnosis of Ebstein's anomaly of the tricuspid valve to be made unequivocally. The morphologic severity can be assessed based on the criteria proposed above, although the precise nature of the distal attachments of the anterior leaflet, and the presence of fenestrations or clefts of the leaflet may be incompletely appreciated (2,3). The severity of tricuspid regurgitation can also be semiquantitatively assessed by colour flow mapping. Until better correlation is achieved between indices of morphologic severity and functional status, surgical repair will be reserved for those with severe symptoms and functional disability.

EBSTEIN'S ANOMALY OF THE MITRAL VALVE

Ebstein's anomaly of the left atrioventricular valve (morphologic tricuspid valve) occurs with discordant atrioventricular connections, and resembles the descriptions of the disease described previously (22). However, Ebstein's malformation of the morphologic mitral valve has been described (23,24), and even more rarely, Ebstein's malformation of both the tricuspid and mitral valves in the same patient (25). Classically, Ebstein's malformation of the morphologic mitral valve does not produce reversed offsetting of the atrioventricular valves. This is because the anterior (aortic) leaflet of the mitral valve, which is in fibrous continuity with the aortic valve, cannot be displaced along the septum or parietal wall of the left ventricle as it is not related to either of these structures (24). Instead, it is the posterior (mural) leaflet that is displaced towards the apex of the left ventricle. There is usually associated dysplasia of the leaflet, with shortened or thickened chordae and physiologically significant mitral regurgitation. These features can all be well recognised by transesophageal imaging (Fig. 3.52) in a manner similar to the corresponding abnormalities of the tricuspid valve described above.

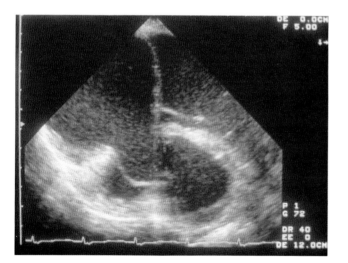

Figure 3.51 *An immediate post-bypass intraoperative transesophageal study from a patient who has undergone tricuspid valve repair for Ebstein's anomaly. Note the lateral plication of the atrioventricular valve ring and the reimplantation of the septal leaflet into its correct position within the atrioventricular junction.*

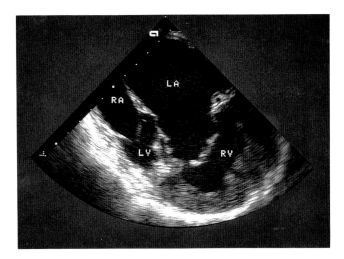

Figure 3.52 *A transverse plane transesophageal study demonstrating an Ebstein malformation of the left atrioventricular valve in a patient with atrioventricular discordance. Note the doming redundant stenotic valve leaflets with their short chordae implanted onto a septal papillary muscle. Colour flow mapping studies in this patient showed the valve to be significantly regurgitant.*

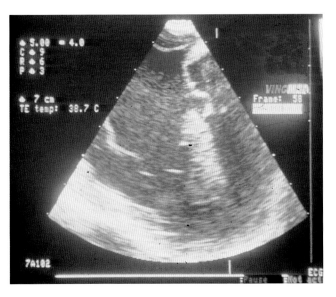

Figure 3.53 *A transverse plane transesophageal study from a patient with overriding and straddling of a right atrioventricular valve. The large ventricular septal defect is well imaged as is the overriding and straddling of the septal leaflet and its chorda.*

STRADDLING AND OVERRIDING ATRIOVENTRICULAR VALVES

Straddling and overriding atrioventricular valves often co-exist with abnormal chamber relations and complex associated congenital malformations. This section will focus on the relative merits of transthoracic and transesophageal echocardiographic identification of the presence and degree of straddling and overriding of atrioventricular valves. It should be remembered that either approach must be complemented by a detailed description of the segmental connections, chamber morphology and relations, and all associated intracardiac defects.

A straddling atrioventricular valve is one whose tensor apparatus arises from both sides of the ventricular septum (26). Overriding of an atrioventricular valve refers to a valve whose annulus is committed to both chambers of the ventricular mass. Straddling therefore refers to a mode of connection, and the degree of override determines the type of connection (27). Although straddling and override often co-exist (Fig. 3.53), it is best to consider them as independent anatomic variables as each can occur without the other. Clinical recognition of straddling has hitherto been difficult as

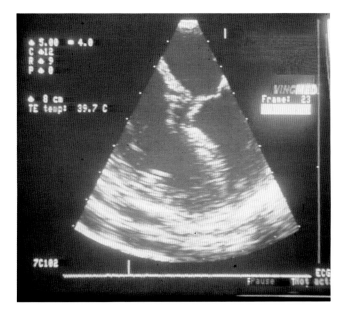

Figure 3.54 *A transverse plane transesophageal study from a patient with a partial atrioventricular septal defect with close packed chordae straddling across the ventricular septum from the left atrioventricular valve component to the right ventricular side of the interventricular septum.*

angiography often fails to identify the chordal insertions or papillary muscle arrangement; it may not also be possible to identify the relation of the atrioventricular valve annulus to the ventricular septum from angiography. With the advent of new surgical techniques for the repair of complex cardiac malformations, the importance of recognising straddling valves preoperatively has increased enormously as the precise surgical option (for example closure of a ventricular septal defect and biventricular repair versus a ventricular exclusion operation) may depend on the presence and degree of straddling.

In hearts with two atrioventricular valves, straddling of either the left, right or both atrioventricular valves may occur, in the setting of biventricular (concordant, discordant or ambiguous atrioventricular connection) or univentricular (double inlet) connections. Straddling is also a feature of a common atrioventricular valve (a valve that drains both atrial chambers to the ventricular mass) such as occurs with an atrioventricular septal defect (Fig. 3.54). Less frequently, straddling can also occur in the setting of an absent left or right connection, or with a univentricular connection through a common atrioventricular valve (28).

Cross-sectional echocardiography permits detailed real time morphologic assessment of the atrioventricular valves, the chordal apparatus and papillary muscle arrangement, and is therefore the technique of choice for investigating suspected chordal straddling. Using the transthoracic approach, multiple cross-sectional views of the atrioventricular junction and sub-valve region are required to diagnose straddle and override reliably. In addition to standard apical four-chamber views and parasternal short axis scans, different transducer positions and planes of section may have to be evolved during the echocardiographic study, to accommodate for abnormal position of the heart within the chest, and abnormal relations of the atrioventricular valves or ventricular chambers which may not be in the same plane relative to one another. The four-chamber view is best suited to recognising abnormal chordal insertions of the valve. Additionally, when the chordae of a leaflet are inserted into the contralateral ventricle (or rudimentary chamber) the free edge of the leaflet involved is often seen to move through the ventricular septal defect into the contralateral chamber in diastole (29). This finding may be useful in diagnosing straddling when the chordae and papillary muscle disposition cannot be identified accurately.

Based on the echocardiographic identification of the precise sites of insertion of the straddling chordae into the contralateral ventricle (or rudimentary chamber), three different types of straddling, of increasing anatomic severity, have been proposed (30) – *Type A*: where the chordae insert into the contralateral ventricle near the crest of the ventricular septum, in close proximity to the midline of the septum (Fig. 3.55); *Type B*: where the chordae insert into the contralateral chamber along the ventricular septum at some distance from the midline; *Type C*: where the chordae insert into the free wall or to a papillary muscle of the contralateral chamber.

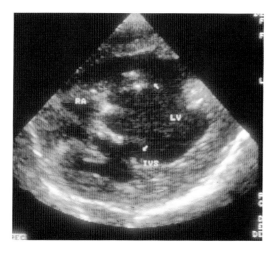

Figure 3.55 *A transverse plane transesophageal study from a patient with a straddling right atrioventricular valve.*

With both straddling and overriding valve, some degree of malalignment between the atrial and ventricular septa is present in the four-chamber views. Transducer positioning is extremely important in diagnosing overriding, as some degree of overriding can be artefactually produced by varying the transducer angulation (29). Additionally, malalignment of the atrial and ventricular septa is a common feature of discordant atrioventricular connection, even in the absence of straddling or override (31). The presence of overriding is therefore best assessed by considering the relation of the crux of the heart (the junction between the atrial septum or interatrial groove and the atrioventricular sulcus) to the interventricular septum. When overriding of an atrioventricular valve exceeds 50% of its annular diameter, it is usually obvious in the four-chamber view. With lesser degrees of override, other views may be necessary to diagnose overriding. This is particularly true when the valve orifices are not in the same plane, as with criss-cross connections or supero-inferior ventricular arrangement. As mentioned previously, the degree of overriding also has a bearing on nomenclature of the type of atrioventricular connection. The atrioventricular valve is assigned to the chamber which receives a greater share of its annulus (33). Hence if the degree of override exceeds 50% and the other valve annulus is entirely committed to the same chamber, the connection is double-inlet, whereas if the degree of overriding is <50%, the connection may be concordant, discordant or ambiguous. With increasing degree of override, there is associated hypoplasia of the chamber to which only a minor portion of the valve annulus is committed.

While straddling may occur with any segmental connection (32), it is best in the interests of simplicity to describe it in terms of straddling of the morphologic tricuspid or mitral valve in the setting of right or left handed ventricular topology (39). Recognition of the morphology of the atrioventricular valve that straddles or overrides has several important implications. It enables prediction of ventricular morphology in patients with biventricular connections. It also helps to predict the disposition of the conducting tissues. In most echocardiographic and pathologic series, the morphologic tricuspid valve appears to straddle more frequently than a morphologic mitral valve (26,27,33,34). This may be partly because of the close anatomic relation of the septal leaflet of the valve and the ventricular septum, with chordae from this leaflet normally attached to the septum (36). The morphology of the straddling valve may be defined as tricuspid from the short axis scan which may demonstrate all three valve leaflets. Alternately, the bileaflet mitral valve when seen in the short axis cut has a characteristic 'fish mouth' appearance. With both concordant and discordant connections, the ventricular septal defect also bears a constant relationship to the straddling valve depending on the morphology of the valve, irrespective of whether the valve is left-sided or right-sided (26). Thus, with a straddling tricuspid valve, the septal defect is usually posterior, and the ventricular septum does not extend to the crux of the heart. As a result, the atrioventricular septum is also deficient, and in the four-chamber view the normal offsetting of the two atrioventricular valves is lost (29). Occasionally, exceptions to this arrangement may exist. In contrast, with a straddling morphologic mitral valve, the ventricular septum invariably extends to the crux of the heart and the defect, and therefore the straddle, are in the anterior portion of the septum. Offsetting

of the two atrioventricular valves will therefore be preserved in the apical four-chamber view.

When the two atrioventricular valves are at the same level with straddling of the tricuspid valve, mild degrees of tricuspid valve override are poorly appreciated in the four-chamber view which may not show displacement of the posterior extent of the ventricular septum. The right ventricular inlet view, with the transducer rotated anticlockwise through approximately 90° from the four-chamber view and angled posteriorly, is useful in these cases (29).

Transesophageal echocardiography would appear to be the definitive technique for the identification of either atrioventricular valve override or chordal straddling in the older patient. These entities are virtually always identified by high-resolution transthoracic imaging in the younger paediatric patient. However, even in this age group, transthoracic imaging may fail to define the precise chordal morphology and a transesophageal study may be indicated. The criteria and methodology used to define either entity are the same as these described above for the transthoracic approach. Transverse plane imaging is the approach of choice when imaging from the oesophagus. Longitudinal plane imaging has little to offer in this respect. The transverse plane approach can define all the relevant malformations thus consistently providing diagnostic information. Multiplane imaging may be of additional benefit as it will allow individual chordae to be followed from their point of origin to their point of insertion in a manner which is often impossible using transverse plane imaging alone.

In summary, straddling of either atrioventricular valve may be conclusively diagnosed when chordae from one of the valves are demonstrated to insert into a papillary muscle in the contralateral ventricle. This is best appreciated in the four-chamber views using either the transthoracic or transesophageal approaches, although additional planes of section may often be required, to adjust for malpositions of the valves and chambers. Straddling of a major degree is associated with movement of the affected leaflet through the ventricular septum and towards the contralateral ventricle in diastole. While direct recognition of the morphology of the straddling valve is feasible, the location of the ventricular septal defect in relation to the straddling valve often enables prediction of the morphology of the valve, irrespective of whether it is left-sided or right-sided. Thus straddling of the tricuspid valve is associated with a common level of attachment of the two atrioventricular valves, and a posterior ventricular septal defect, so that the septum does not reach the crux of the heart. With double-inlet ventricles, it may often be difficult either by echocardiography or even on direct inspection to distinguish tricuspid and mitral valve morphology. The ventricular morphology may therefore have to be predicted either from recognition of the trabecular pattern of the main and rudimentary chambers, or from the relationship of the ventricular septum to the atrioventricular connections on echocardiography.

Straddling valve with absent connection, and straddling of a common atrioventricular valve in univentricular connection

The diagnosis of absent connection can confidently be made on echocardiography, and the clinical picture is determined both by the absent connection and the associated malformations. The diagnostic criteria for straddling are as described for hearts with two atrioventricular valves. Rarely straddling may be a feature of a common atrioventricular valve in the setting of a univentricular connection. The echocardiographic features of the common valve are similar to those of the common atrioventricular valve with biventricular connections (atrioventricular septal defect) (35). In the four-chamber view, the free-floating anterior leaflet appears to move in a supero-inferior plane, disappearing from the plane of section in diastole and reappearing in systole, and is flanked by two lateral leaflets (28).

SURGICAL IMPLICATIONS

Straddling, by definition, is associated with a ventricular septal defect, although a straddling tricuspid valve without associated ventricular septal defect has been recently reported (36). With milder degrees of straddling (type A) repair is relatively easily accomplished by deviation of the ventricular septal defect patch around the straddling chordae. With greater degrees of straddling a ventricular septation procedure may be required to repair the defect without sacrificing the straddling valve. Where either of these is not feasible, and depending on the size and function of the two ventricles, the straddling valve may have to be excised and replaced with a prosthetic valve, particularly if it is regurgitant. Alternately, for univentricular connections associated with major straddling and varying degrees of underdevelopment of one of the chambers in the ventricular mass, a ventricular exclusion procedure

(atriopulmonary or cavopulmonary connection) may be feasible without closing the ventricular septal defect.

The presence of straddling also affects the disposition of the conducting tissue. With a main chamber of left ventricular morphology (usually associated with straddling morphologic tricuspid valve) the ventricular septum does not extend to the crux of the heart, irrespective of the connections (biventricular, or univentricular) or position of the right ventricular chamber (right- or left-sided). The conduction bundle will therefore not arise from the regularly situated atrioventricular node. In contrast, when the main chamber is of right ventricular morphology the course of the conducting tissue will depend on the position of the left ventricular chamber. Prior knowledge of these variations is of obvious benefit when planning surgery.

CONGENITAL MITRAL VALVE LESIONS

Double-orifice mitral valve

Double-orifice mitral valve is rare as an isolated anomaly, and in the majority of patients is an incidental finding at surgery or autopsy (37,38). It may occasionally cause symptoms, arising from either severe regurgitation of the valve, or less commonly stenosis (39–41). It should therefore be suspected in every child who presents with signs of isolated mitral regurgitation or stenosis. It is more commonly associated with atrioventricular septal defects(42), and has been reported to occur in up to 10% of postmortem specimens of atrioventricular septal defects (41); other associated anomalies are obstructive lesions of the left ventricular outflow tract. Double-orifice mitral valve can be correctly diagnosed on cross-sectional echocardiography (43). The short axis views (parasternal or subcostal) are best suited to visualising both valve orifices and the tension apparatus. Three morphologic variants have been described based on echocardiographic appearances and morphologic studies.

The first two categories are where a bridge of tissue separates the two valve orifices. The bridging tissue may be at annulus level, completely partitioning the valve annulus (complete bridge), or may be at leaflet level (incomplete bridge), in which case the valve annulus appears normal. These therefore represent opposite ends of a spectrum where a bridge of tissue connects the two leaflets of the mitral valve. The axes of the two orifices are nearly parallel. The apical four-chamber view will therefore demonstrate the two separate valve orifices particularly if they are partitioned at annulus level. Parasternal short axis scans starting at mitral annulus level and progressively angling downwards towards the apex will demonstrate both orifices (which in the complete type look like a pair of spectacles) and their chordae. The chordae from each of the valve orifices invariably attach to a single papillary muscle, resulting in separate parachute arrangement for each orifice. The papillary muscles themselves are usually located in the normal position. In the incomplete bridge type, the two orifices will not be seen at annulus level on the short axis scan, but will appear as the scan plane is tilted towards the apex. Again, the chordal attachments for each orifice are to a single papillary muscle.

The third type of double-orifice valve that has been distinguished by cross-sectional imaging is where the minor orifice appears as a hole in one or other leaflets of the mitral valve. It does however have distinct chordal attachments to a separate papillary muscle, as for the preceding varieties, which can be identified on serial short axis scans towards the apex of the ventricle. The presence of a distinctive subvalvar apparatus distinguishes this type of double orifice valve from a fenestration or cleft of one of the leaflets (75). The second orifice may only be seen at mid-leaflet level in the short axis view, and may not be in the same plane as the major orifice. On scanning at valve ring level, the appearance is that of a single valve orifice, but with a cleft in one of the valve leaflets.

Colour flow imaging enables best appreciation of the double orifice valve, by identifying two separate streams of inflow into the left ventricle in the four-chamber view. Regurgitation through one or both orifices can also be readily detected, and pulsed Doppler guided by colour flow imaging enables measurement of the peak velocity of inflow.

Thus a successful precordial echocardiographic study of double-orifice left atrioventricular valve can only be accomplished by using an appropriate series of scan planes derived from various transducer positions. These imaging planes are normally readily available in paediatric patients in whom high-quality image resolution can be obtained. Such image resolution can rarely be obtained in adult patients. This was exemplified by our own experience in studying three adult patients with such an anomaly. In the first patient, marked obesity precluded diagnostic transthoracic imaging. In this case, a prior incorrect diagnosis of a partial atrioven-

tricular septal defect had been made. In the second case (with atrioventricular discordance) precordial scanning had suggested there was only a single orifice of the left-sided morphologic tricuspid valve. Precordial imaging identified only chordal attachments of this valve to the crest of the ventricular septum. Transverse plane transesophageal imaging identified a second set of chordae tethered to a single lateral papillary muscle, and this in turn led to the recognition of the second mitral orifice (Fig. 3.56). In the third patient, we presume the relatively small size of the second additional orifice prevented its recognition during precordial scanning.

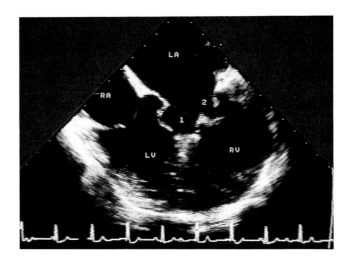

Figure 3.56 *A transverse plane transesophageal study from a patient with atrioventricular discordance who had a double-orifice left atrioventricular valve and a large inlet ventricular septal defect. Both orifices (1, 2) are well visualised.*

In two cases (patient 1 and patient 2), scanning through the four-chamber planes from a low esophageal transducer position clearly demonstrated two components to the left atrioventricular valve which were divided by bridging tissue. The amount of this tissue was more pronounced in the first patient than in the second. In patient 3, in whom biplane transesophageal imaging was available, the longitudinal plane was the only imaging plane in which the second orifice was detected. The second orifice could not be visualised in the transverse plane. Transesophageal studies proved to be superior to the precordial approach in defining the anatomy of the subvalvar apparatus. This was particularly the case with regard to the definition of the disposition and insertion of the chordae tendineae. In every case, the chordae from each orifice were attached separately to their own single papillary muscle, resembling in this respect the chordal insertion of a parachute valve. Colour flow mapping in every case was of value in defining either the competence or the degree of regurgitation of either mitral orifice (Fig. 3.57). In the first patient studied, the mitral regurgitation of the medial orifice was caused by a cleft in its anterior leaflet. The cleft was not defined by transesophageal scanning but could be visualised on subsequent repeat precordial scanning. The substrate for incompetence in the remaining orifices was not defined in any case. Stenosis of any of the valve orifices was not encountered in this series.

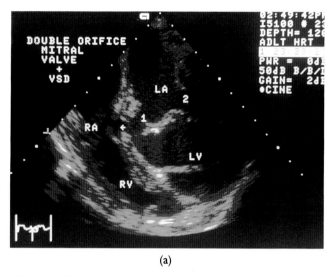

(a)

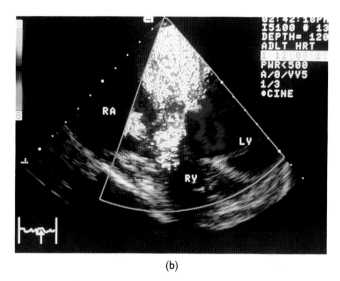

(b)

Figure 3.57 (a) *A transverse plane transesophageal study from a patient with a double-orifice mitral valve, a small perimembranous ventricular septal defect which is partially closed by tricuspid valve pseudoaneurysm (arrowed).* **(b)** *The corresponding transverse plane transesophageal colour flow map from (a). Note here the two jets of regurgitation into the left atrium via either orifice of the double-orifice mitral valve. In addition, there is turbulent flow across the ventricular septum into the right ventricle from the restrictive ventricular septal defect. A small jet of tricuspid regurgitation is also seen entering the right atrium.*

While tranverse plane transesophageal imaging in this series proved a superior diagnostic technique to precordial imaging, it may not give the answer in every case. Transverse plane transesophageal studies do not offer as many imaging planes as the precordial approach and could miss a small second mitral orifice. An adjunct to a transverse plane transesophageal study is to image the heart from the transgastric approach. This approach in theory should always identify the second mitral orifice. However, in our experience, high-resolution transgastric imaging of the mitral valve in its short axis is only possible in a relatively small number of adult patients. It is our opinion that the addition of longitudinal plane imaging or multiplane transesophageal imaging should increase the diagnostic accuracy of transesophageal echocardiography in defining this complex lesion.

In conclusion, in cases with non-diagnostic transthoracic images, transesophageal echocardiography combined with colour flow mapping can offer a better approach to the assessment of a double-orifice left atrioventricular valve. Bi- or multiplane transesophageal imaging may be a more reliable diagnostic technique than the single transverse plane approach. By this means, clear definition of the anatomy and function of each valve component can be obtained.

Congenital mitral stenosis

The normal mitral valve has an anterior (or aortic) leaflet, and a posterior (or mural) leaflet. The two commissures of this bileaflet valve correspond to the subjacent anterolateral and posteromedial papillary muscles, and chordae tendineae run from each leaflet to the two papillary muscles. On the basis of this anatomic arrangement, a primary and secondary orifice of the valve may be defined. The primary orifice is bounded anteriorly and posteriorly by the two valve leaflets, and laterally and medially by the two papillary muscles. The secondary orifices are then the series of openings lying between the chordae tendineae. On functional grounds, the requirements for a non-stenotic and competent valve therefore are: (1) the presence of pliable valve tissue to allow free mobility; (2) the presence of an adequate sized annulus; (3) lack of undue restraint at the commissural junctions; (4) appropriate position and function of the chordae and papillary muscles. Congenital 'mitral stenosis' may therefore be defined as a developmental abnormality of the mitral valve leaflets, the valve commissures, annulus, interchordal spaces, papillary muscles or the immediate supravalvar area that produces obstruction to left ventricular filling.

Isolated congenital mitral stenosis is a rare lesion (44). It is usually associated with other cardiac defects, which are also often left-sided. The physical signs are often subtle, and can go unrecognised in the presence of an associated major cardiac anomaly. Early recognition and treatment are however important, as the natural history is often one of progressive pulmonary hypertension and death.

The exact anatomy of the obstruction may remain unclear even after cardiac catheterisation and angiography. Although the role of M-mode echocardiography in the diagnosis of acquired mitral stenosis is well established, it has been found to be less useful in defining the precise site or severity of obstruction in congenital mitral stenosis. Driscoll et al.(45) analysed the M-mode echocardiograms of children known to have congenital mitral stenosis using both qualitative and quantitative criteria. Mitral stenosis was associated with anterior movement of the posterior leaflet of the mitral valve in diastole (suggesting chordal fusion), absence of the A wave of mitral valve reopening with atrial systole, and diastolic vibration of both mitral leaflets (probably reflecting turbulent diastolic flow across pliable leaflet tissue). Quantitatively, the rate of early diastolic closure (E-F slope) of the anterior leaflet and the amplitude of excursion of the anterior leaflet (vertical D-E distance) were reduced in some patients, suggesting limited valve motion and prolonged filling through an obstructive valve. Others have also reported on the presence of abnormal echoes behind the mitral valve (within the left atrium) associated with supramitral membranes (46,47). Overall however, while the diagnosis of mitral stenosis could be correctly made even in the presence of other associated lesions, none of these variables was useful in delineating the precise anatomy of the left ventricular inflow obstruction, or in predicting its severity. Calculation of the rate of left ventricular filling using digitised left ventricular echocardiography (by measuring the rate of dimension change of the ventricle in diastole) (48,49), was also of limited value in the assessment of severity of congenital mitral stenosis (50). Cross-sectional echocardiography has enabled better definition of some of the more commonly recognised malformations of the mitral valve apparatus that result in mitral stenosis. These will be discussed in turn, following the basic scheme of lesions primarily affecting different levels of the left ventricular inflow tract. Although the echocardiographic features of some of these entities is individually presented, it is important to remember that several of these malformations may co-exist.

'Typical' mitral stenosis

This is the commonest form of isolated congenital mitral stenosis (51), and the abnormality consists of hypoplasia and thickening of the valve leaflets (associated with increased echodensity of the leaflets on echocardiography) with a reduced valve orifice, reduced leaflet motion in diastole, and a small mitral valve annulus. The orifice of the mitral valve is best evaluated in the short axis views (parasternal or subcostal). Starting from the apex of the ventricle and angulating upwards, the two papillary muscles are initially seen, typically in the 3 o'clock and 8 o'clock positions. With further upward angulation the two leaflets of the mitral valve are visualised with a typical 'fish-mouth' appearance. In congenital mitral stenosis, the effective valve orifice is often lower than expected, and often eccentric (and therefore not in the plane of the short axis of the left ventricular cavity). Careful adjustment of the transducer position will be required to image the orifice in its true short axis plane. Calculation of the valve orifice area by planimetry have been found to correlate with the severity of stenosis assessed at cardiac catheterisation in a small group of patients (52).

Commissural fusion

Isolated commissural fusion is a rare cause of congenital mitral stenosis, and is frequently associated with dysplasia of the valve leaflets and the sub-valve apparatus. The appearances of the valve are similar to those of rheumatic mitral valve disease, with restricted mobility of both leaflets, and a funnel-shaped mitral orifice in the parasternal long axis view. The leaflets themselves are frequently thickened, but may appear thin and pliable. In both the parasternal long axis and four-chamber views, the subvalvar apparatus may also appear abnormally dense, representing shortened and thickened chordae with obliteration of the interchordal spaces. The valve annulus diameter is usually normal. In sequential short axis views towards the apex of the ventricle from the level of the annulus, the mitral orifice may be visualised at a much lower level than expected, giving the appearance of a funnel (50).

Annulus hypoplasia

With most varieties of congenital mitral stenosis the annulus dimensions are usually preserved within the normal range (50). Annular hypoplasia is usually associated with variants of the hypoplastic left-heart syndrome (51). The mitral annulus is best measured in the parasternal long axis projection, as this view is easily reproducible and standard landmarks are available. The annulus is measured during maximum diastolic excursion of the leaflets. The anterior landmark is the point of continuity of the anterior mitral leaflet and the posterior wall of the aortic root, and the posterior landmark the point where the posterior leaflet is inserted at the atrioventricular junction (50).

Accessory mitral valve tissue

This appears as an accessory mass attached to the atrial surface of one of the leaflets (usually the mural leaflet), and may produce inflow obstruction. Occasionally, accessory valve tissue on the ventricular aspect of the leaflet may herniate into the left ventricular outflow tract and produce outlet obstruction (53).

Parachute mitral valve

In a parachute mitral valve, a single papillary muscle (usually the posteromedial papillary muscle) is pre-

sent in the left ventricle, into which the chordae from both mitral valve leaflets insert. Often the two papillary muscles are fused together and function as a single muscle. Mitral stenosis may be the result of several anatomic features. The chordae tendineae are frequently thickened and shortened, and hold the anterior and posterior leaflets together in diastole. With a single posteromedial papillary muscle, the anterior diastolic movement of the aortic leaflet is often severely restricted (54). The primary orifice of the valve is therefore diminished by both the restricted leaflet mobility, and convergence of all the chordae to the single papillary muscle. Ventricular filling must therefore occur through the secondary orifices (interchordal spaces) which are frequently obstructed by thickened and fused chordae.

The parasternal short axis view is ideal for demonstrating the number of papillary muscles. The subcostal four-chamber view will also demonstrate the papillary muscle arrangement and their chordal attachments (50). Even when two papillary muscle groups are identified, one of them may be hypoplastic and the chordae attach to only the other one (50). Functionally, these lesions and situations where the two papillary muscles are fused are similar to the classic parachute mitral valve with a true single papillary muscle.

SURGICAL CONSIDERATIONS

In view of the difficulties associated with prosthetic valve replacement in children, precise knowledge of the morphology of the obstructive lesion is of obvious benefit in planning surgical repair, and the optimal method of valve reconstruction (55,56).

CONGENITAL MITRAL REGURGITATION

The following lesions are associated predominantly with mitral regurgitation, and will be classified according to whether they primarily affect the valve leaflets, annulus or sub-valve apparatus.

Isolated cleft of the mitral valve

Isolated clefts of the mitral valve are an uncommon cause of congenital mitral regurgitation. It is however important to recognise the lesion, as it is potentially correctible by surgery, without requirement for prosthetic mitral valve replacement (57). The cleft usually involves the anterior leaflet of the mitral valve, although clefts of the posterior leaflet have also been described (58). Cross-sectional echocardiography is superior to other investigative techniques such as angiography in the diagnosis of the lesion (57,59).

The cleft is best seen in the parasternal short axis view. Starting from the aortic root, as the transducer is angled down towards the mitral valve orifice, the anterior leaflet will appear as an unbroken echo, spanning the area of fibrous continuity between the aortic root and mitral valve. With a cleft of the anterior leaflet a break in the continuity of the leaflet will be seen, and during diastole the leaflet separates into medial and lateral portions. The cleft is directed anteriorly towards the left ventricular outflow tract, and usually extends from the leaflet edge to the annulus of the mitral valve. This is the most important aspect of a true cleft of the mitral valve, and distinguishes it from the cleft (the space between the anterior and posterior bridging leaflets) of an atrioventricular septal defect which is always directed medially towards the right ventricle. Additionally, with an isolated cleft the atrioventricular septum is intact, with normal offsetting of the tricuspid and mitral valves in the apical or subcostal four-chamber views, to further distinguish the two lesions (57). The break in continuity of the anterior leaflet can also often be seen in the four-chamber view, as the edges of the cleft move apart in diastole.

The tissue at the edge of the cleft often appears denser than the surrounding valve leaflet tissue, and may be thickened and rolled towards the left ventricle (60). Careful attention needs to be paid to the chordal and papillary muscle arrangement in the parasternal short axis scan, as it is often possible to have anomalous chordae attached to the edges of the cleft and connecting to an abnormally situated papillary muscle on the septum or anterior wall of the left ventricle, resembling an additional commissure (60). Rarely, a fold of a redundant anterior leaflet, or an abnormally septated anterior leaflet, may mimic the appearance of a cleft (61).

Additional features to be documented on echocardiography include the dimensions of the left atrium and ventricle, which provide an indication of the degree of regurgitation. Both pulsed Doppler (with the sample volume located within the left atrium) and colour flow imaging will confirm the presence of mitral regurgitation. Colour flow imaging in the short axis will also demonstrate that the regurgitation occurs through the cleft. With colour

flow imaging in the parasternal long axis view, the regurgitant jet is often seen to be directed posteriorly, giving the appearance of mitral regurgitation due to prolapse of the anterior leaflet.

The majority of patients with isolated clefts of the mitral valve remain clinically well, as mitral regurgitation is often well tolerated. The results of surgical correction by suture closure of the cleft have however been good, and most patients with isolated clefts can be referred to surgery on the basis of non-invasive investigations alone, before the onset of cardiac decompensation.

Anomalous mitral arcade

This is a rare lesion wherein the papillary muscles appear to extend up to the leaflets of the mitral valve, and in the more severe forms are continuous with the mitral leaflets (62,63). The chordae are considerably shortened and thickened, and the leaflets are held open in systole, with resultant mitral regurgitation. Cross-sectional echocardiography has proved helpful in defining this lesion (64,65). In the parasternal long axis view, a mass of tissue may be seen in the sub-valve region from which multiple short chordae extend to the anterior and posterior leaflets of the mitral valve. In short axis scans multiple short papillary muscle heads may be identified, giving rise to the chordae (65).

Other rare anomalies producing congenital mitral regurgitation

These include abnormalities of the chordae such as being too short (when the leaflet is held open in systole) or too long (when the leaflet prolapses into the left atrium), and papillary muscle dysfunction. Papillary muscle dysfunction may be the result of an abnormal position of the muscle (for example when it is attached to the upper third of the left ventricular wall) or infarction of one or both muscles either due to anomalous origin of the left coronary artery from the pulmonary trunk, or due to endocardial fibroelastosis. An abnormal position of the papillary muscle is often identified when the papillary muscle and one of the leaflets of the mitral valve are visualised in the same short axis plane. The mitral valve may be eccentrically positioned (closer to the ventricular septum or the left ventricular free wall) in the short axis, although the orifice itself may appear circular (66). Anomalous origin of the left coronary artery from the pulmonary trunk may present with clinical features of myocardial infarction in infancy. The diagnosis can often be established by cross-sectional and Doppler ultrasound examination (67–70). With longstanding infarction and fibrosis the affected papillary muscle appears more echodense than normal, and occasionally calcification of the papillary muscle may be evident. There may be associated left ventricular dilatation and dysfunction, which may often be segmental depending on the infarcted area.

REFERENCES

1. SCHIEBLER GL, GRAVENSTEIN JC, VAN MIEROP LHS. Epstein's anomaly of the tricuspid valve: translation of original description with comments. Am J Cardiol 1968; **22:** 867–73.

2. LEUNG MP, BAKER EJ, ANDERSON RH, ZUBERBUHLER JR. Cineangiographic spectrum of Ebstein's malformation: its relevance to clinical presentation and outcome. J Am Coll Cardiol 1988; **11:** 154–61.

3. SHIINA A, SEWARD JB, EDWARDS WD, HAGLER DJ, TAJIK AJ. Two-dimensional echocardiographic spectrum of Ebstein's anomaly: detailed anatomic assessment. J Am Coll Cardiol 1984; **3:** 356–70.

4. MATSUMOTO M, MATSUO H, NAGATA S, et al. Visualization of Ebstein's anomaly of the tricuspid valve by two-dimensional and standard echocardiography. Circulation 1976; **53:** 69–79.

5. PORTS TA, SILVERMAN NH, SCHILLER NB. Two-dimensional echocardiographic assessment of Ebstein's anomaly. Circulation 1978; **58:** 336–43.

6. GUSSENHOVEN WJ, SPITAELS SEC, BOM N, BECKER AE. Echocardiographic criteria for Ebstein's anomaly of tricuspid valve. Br Heart J 1980; **43:** 31–7.

7. KAMBE T, ICHIMIYA S, TOGUCHI M, et al. Apex and subxiphoid approaches to Ebstein's anomaly using cross-sectional echocardiography. Am Heart J 1980; **100:** 53–8.

8. NIHOYANNOPOULOS P, MCKENNA W, SMITH G, FOALE R. Echocardiographic assessment of the right ventricle in Ebstein's anomaly: relation to clinical outcome. J Am Coll Cardiol 1986; **8:** 627–35.

9. BROWN AK, ANDERSON V. Two dimensional echocardiography and the tricuspid valve. Leaflet definition and prolapse. Br Heart J 1983; **49:** 495–500.

10. LÜNDSTROM NR. Echocardiography in the diagnosis of Ebstein's anomaly of the tricuspid valve. Circulation 1973; **47:** 597–605.

11. DANIEL W, RATHSACK P. WALPURGER G, et al. Value of M-mode echocardiography for non-invasive diagnosis of Ebstein's anomaly. Br Heart J 1980; **43:** 38–44.

12. MONIBI AA, NECHES WH, LENOX CC, PARK SC, MATHEWS RA, ZUBERBUHLER JR. Left ventricular anomalies associated with Ebstein's malformation of the tricuspid valve. Circulation 1978; **57:** 303–6.

13. ROBERTS WC, GLANCY DL, SENINGEN RP, MARON BJ, EPSTEIN SE. Prolapse of the mitral valve (floppy valve) associated with Ebstein's anomaly of the tricuspid valve. Am J Cardiol 1976; **38:** 377–82.

14. QUAEGEBEUR JM, SREERAM N, FRASER AG, et al. Surgery for Ebstein's anomaly: the clinical and echocardiographic evaluation of a new surgical technique. J Am Coll Cardiol 1991; **17**(3): 722–9.

15. HARDY KL, MAY IA, WEBSTER CA, KIMBALL KG. Ebstein's anomaly: a functional concept and successful surgical repair. J Thorac Cardiovasc Surg 1964; **48:** 927–40.

16. DANIELSON GK, FUSTER V. Surgical repair of Ebstein's anomaly. Ann Surg 1982; **196:** 499–504.

17. CARPENTIER A, CHAUVAUD S, MACE L, et al. A new reconstructive operation for Ebstein's anomaly of the tricuspid valve. J Thorac Cardiovasc Surg 1988; **96:** 92–101.

18. BARNARD CN, SCHRIRE V. Surgical correction of Ebstein's malformation with prosthetic tricuspid valve. Surgery 1963; **54:** 302–8.

19. MCFAUL RC, DAVIS Z, GIULIANI ER, RITTER DG, DANIELSON GK. Ebstein's malformation: surgical experience at the Mayo Clinic. J Thorac Cardiovasc Surg 1976; **72:** 910–15.

20. SHIINA A, SEWARD JB, TAJIK AJ, HAGLER DJ, DANIELSON GK. Two-dimensional echocardiographic-surgical correlation in Ebstein's anomaly: preoperative determination of patients requiring tricuspid valve plication vs replacement. Circulation 1983; **68:** 534–44.

21. SCHMIDT KG, CLOEZ J-L, SILVERMAN NH. Assessment of right ventricular performance by pulsed Doppler echocardiography in patients after intraatrial repair of aortopulmonary transposition in infancy or childhood. J Am Coll Cardiol 1989; **13:** 1578–85.

22. ANDERSON KR, DANIELSON GK, MCGOON DC, LIE JT. Ebstein's anomaly of the left-sided tricuspid valve. Pathological anatomy of the valvular malformation. Cardiovasc Surg 1978; **58:** 1-87–91.

23. RUSCHHAUPT DG, BHARATI S, SEV M. Mitral valve malformation of Ebstein type in absence of corrected transposition. Am J Cardiol 1976; **38:** 109–12.

24. LEUNG M, RIGBY ML, ANDERSON RH, WYSE RKH, MACARTNEY FJ. Reversed offsetting of the septal attachment of the atrioventricular valves and Ebstein's malformation of the morphologically mitral valve. Br Heart J 1987; **57:** 184–7.

25. DUSMET M, OBERHANSLI I, COX JN. Ebstein's anomaly of the tricuspid and mitral valves in an otherwise normal heart. Br Heart J 1987; **58:** 400–4.

26. MILO S, HO SY, MACARTNEY FJ, et al. Straddling and overriding atrioventricular valves: morphology and classification. Am J Cardiol 1979; **44:** 1122–34.

27. TYNAN MJ, BECKER AE, MACARTNEY FJ, QUERY-JIMENEZ M, SHINEBOURNE EA, ANDERSON RH. The nomenclature and classification of congenital heart disease. Br Heart J 1979; **41:** 544–53.

28. SMALLHORN JF, TOMMASINI G, MACARTNEY FJ. Two-dimensional echocardiographic assessment of common

atrioventricular valves in univentricular hearts. *Br Heart J* 1981; **46:** 30–4.

29. SMALLHORN JF, TOMMASINI G, MACARTNEY FJ. Detection and assessment of straddling and overriding atrioventricular valves of two dimensional echocardiography. *Br Heart J* 1981; **46:** 254–62.

30. RICE MJ, SEWARD JB, EDWARDS WD, *et al.* Straddling atrioventricular valve: two-dimensional echocardiographic diagnosis, classification and surgical implications. *Am J Cardiol* 1985; **55:** 505–13.

31. SUTHERLAND GR, SMALLHORN JF, ANDERSON RH, RIGBY ML, HUNTER S. Atrioventricular discordance; cross-sectional echocardiographic-morphological correlative study. *Br Heart J* 1983; **50:** 8–20.

32. ANDERSON RH, HO SY. Straddling and overriding valves – segmental morphology. In: Wenink ACG (ed.), *The ventricular septum of the heart.* Boerhaave series vol 21. The Hague: Martinus Nijhoff, 1981: 157–73.

33. OSTERMEYER J, KORFER R, FRENZEL H, BIRCKS W. Straddling atrioventricular valves in biventricular hearts: observations made in five cases. *Thorac Cardiovasc Surg* 1980; **28:** 233–8.

34. WENINK ACG, GITTENBERGER de GROOT AC. Straddling mitral and tricuspid valves: morphologic differences and developmental backgrounds. *Am J Cardiol* 1982; **49:** 1959–71.

35. SMALLHORN JF, TOMMASINI G, ANDERSON RH, MACARTNEY FJ. Assessment of atrioventricular septal defects by two dimensional echocardiography. *Br Heart J* 1982; **47:** 109–21.

36. ISOMATSU Y, KUROSAWA S, IMAI Y. Straddling tricuspid valve without a ventricular septal defect. *Br Heart J* 1989; **62:** 222–4.

37. WIGLE ED. Duplication of the mitral valve. *Br Heart J* 1957; **19:** 296–300.

38. KENAAN G, NEUFELD HN, DEUTSCH V, SHEM-TOR A. Isolated congenital double-orifice mitral valve. *Isr J Med Sci* 1974; **10:** 743–7.

39. MERCER JL, TUBBS OS. Successful surgical management of double orifice mitral valve with subaortic stenosis. *J Thorac Cardiovasc Surg* 1974; **67:** 440–2.

40. YURDAKUL Y, BILGIC A, SAYLAM A, SANOGLU T, KOSKER S, AYTAC A. Congenital double-orifice mitral valve. *Jpn Heart J* 1980; **21:** 545–60.

41. WAKAI CS, EDWARDS JE. Pathologic study of persistent common atrioventricular canal. *Am Heart J* 1958; **56:** 779–94.

42. WARNES C, SOMERVILLE J. Double mitral valve orifice in atrioventricular defects. *Br Heart J* 1983; **49:** 59–64.

43. ROWE DW, DESAI B, BEZMALINOVIC Z, DESAI JM, WESSEL RJ, GRAYSON LH. Two-dimensional echocardiography in double orifice mitral valve. *J Am Coll Cardiol* 1984; **4:** 429–33.

44. COLLINS-NAKAI RL, ROSENTHAL A, CASTANEDA AR, BERNHARD WF, NADAS AS. Congenital mitral stenosis. A review of 20 years' experience. *Circulation* 1977; **56:** 1039–47.

45. DRISCOLL DJ, GUTGESELL HP, McNAMARA DG. Echocardiogarphic features of congenital mitral stenosis. *Am J Cardiol* 1978; **42:** 259–66.

46. CHUNG KS, MANNING JA, LIPCHIK EO, *et al.* Isolated supravalvar stenosing ring of left atrium: diagnosis before operation and sucecssful surgical treatment. *Chest* 1974; **65:** 25–8.

47. LACORTE M, HARADA K, WILLIAMS R. Echocardiographic features of congenital left ventricular inflow obstruction. *Circulation* 1976; **54:** 562–6.

48. GIBSON DG, BROWN D. Measurement of instantaneous left ventricular dimension and filling rate in man, using echocardiography. *Br Heart J* 1973; **35:** 1141–9.

49. UPTON MT, GIBSON DG. The study of left ventricular function from digitised echocardiograms. *Prog Cardiovasc Dis* 1978; **20:** 359–84.

50. SMALLHORN J, TOMMASINI G, DEANFIELD J, DOUGLAS J, GIBSON D, MACARTNEY F. Congenital mitral stenosis. Anatomical and functional assessment by echocardiography. *Br Heart J* 1981; **45:** 527–34.

51. RUCKMAN RN, VAN PRAAGH R. Anatomic types of congenital mitral stenosis: Report of 49 autopsy cases with consideration of diagnosis and surgical implications. *Am J Cardiol* 1978; **42:** 592–601.

52. RIGGS TW, LAPIN GD, PAUL MH, *et al.* Measurement of mitral valve orifice area in infants and children by two-dimensional echocardiography. *J Am Coll Cardiol* 1983; **1:** 873–8.

53. MELDRUM-HANNA WG, CARTMILL TB, HAWKER RE, CELERMAJER JM, WRIGHT CM. Accessory mitral valve tissue causing left ventricular outflow tract obstruction. *Br Heart J* 1986; **55:** 376–80.

54. MACARTNEY FJ, SCOTT O, IONESCU MI, DEVERALL PB. Diagnosis and management of parachute mitral value and supravalvar mitral ring. *Br Heart J* 1974; **36:** 641–52.

55. CARPENTIER A, BRANCHINI B, COUR JC, *et al.* Congenital malformations of the mitral valve in children. Pathology and surgical treatment. *J Thorac Cardiovasc Surg* 1976; **72:** 854–66.

56. BERRY BE, RITTER DG, WALLACE RB, McGOON DC, DANIELSON GK. Cardiav valve replacement in children. *J Thorac Cardiovasc Surg* 1974; **68:** 705–10.

57. SMALLHORN JF, DELEVAL M, STARK J, *et al.* Isolated anterior mitral cleft. Two dimensional echocardiographic assessment and differentiation from 'clefts' associated with atrioventricular septal defect. *Br Heart J* 1982; **48:** 109–16.

58. GOODMAN DJ, HANCOCK EW. Secundum atrial septal defect associated with a cleft mitral valve. *Br Heart J* 1973; **35:** 1315–20.

59. MACARTNEY FJ, BAIN HH, IONESCU MI, DEVERALL PB, SCOTT O. Angiographic/pathologic correlations in congenital mitral valve abnormalities. *Eur J Cardiol* 1976; **4:** 191–211.

60. DI SEGNI E, BASS JL, LUCAS RV, EINZIG S. Isolated cleft mitral valve: A variety of congenital mitral regurgitation identified by 2-dimensional echocardiography. *Am J Cardiol* 1983; **51:** 927–31.

61. ORTIZ E, SOMERVILLE J. Assessment by cross sectional echocardiography of surgical 'mitral valve' disease in children and adolescents. *Br Heart J* 1986; **56:** 267–71.

62. LAYMAN TE, EDWARDS JE. Anomalous mitral arcade. A

type of congenital mitral insufficiency. *Circulation* 1967; **35:** 389–95.

63. DAVACHI F, MOLLER JH, EDWARDS JE. Diseases of the mitral valve in infancy. An anatomic analysis of 55 cases. *Circulation* 1971; **43:** 565–79.

64. PARR GVS, FRIPP RR, WHITMAN V, BHARATI S, LEV M. Anomalous mitral arcade: echocardiographic and angiographic recognition. *Ped Cardiol* 1983; **4:** 163–5.

65. GRENADIER E, SAHN DJ, VALDES-CRUZ LM, ALLEN HD, LIMA CO, GOLDBERG SJ. Two-dimensional echo Doppler study of congenital disorders of the mitral valve. *Am Heart J* 1984; **107:** 319–25.

66. CELANO V, PIERONI DR, MORERA JA, ROLAND J-M, GINGELL RL. Two-dimensional echocardiographic examination of mitral valve abnormalities associated with coarctation of the aorta. *Circulation* 1984; **69:** 924–32.

67. FISHER EA, SEPEHRI B, LENDRUM B, LUKEN J, LEVITZKY S. Two-dimensional echocardiographic visualization of the left coronary artery in anomalous origin of the left coronary artery from the pulmonary artery. *Circulation* 1981; **63:** 698–704.

68. KING DH, DANFORD DA, HUHTA JC, GUTGESELL HP. Noninvasive detection of anomalous origin of the left main coronary artery from the pulmonary trunk by pulsed Doppler echocardiography. *Am J Cadiol* 1985; **55:** 608–9.

69. SCHMIDT KG, COOPER MJ, SILVERMAN NH, STANGER P. Pulmonary artery origin of the left coronary artery: diagnosis by two-dimensional echocardiography, pulsed Doppler ultrasound and color flow mapping. *J Am Coll Cardiol* 1988; **11:** 396–402.

70. SREERAM N, HUNTER S, WREN C. Acute myocardial infarction in infancy: unmasking of anomalous origin of the left coronary artery from the pulmonary artery by ligation of an arterial duct. *Br Heart J* 1989; **61:** 307–8.

Ventricular septal defects

G. R. Sutherland

INTRODUCTION

THE ROLE OF TRANSTHORACIC ULTRASOUND IN VENTRICULAR SEPTAL DEFECT EVALUATION

Cardiac ultrasound has an important role to play in the evaluation of defects within the ventricular septum, both in the initial diagnosis and the definition of the haemodynamics associated with the defect, as well as in the intra- and perioperative (early and late) assessment of successful defect closure. In infants and young children, the combination of precordial and subcostal cross-sectional imaging will identify and correctly classify the majority of moderate or large ventricular septal defects (1). Cross-sectional imaging has a low sensitivity for the identification of small trabecular septal defects (especially those located at the apex or in the anterior trabecular septum) and for small muscular outlet defects. Imaging combined with colour flow mapping will normally identify the presence of such small trabecular septal defects as well as multiple defects within the septum in cases where the defects are restrictive (2,3). The additional use of pulsed and continuous wave Doppler studies will normally define the trans-septal pressure gradient (if any is present) and can thus allow an accurate indirect estimation of pulmonary artery peak systolic pressure. Pulsed Doppler evaluation of the respective volume flows in the left ventricular outflow tract and pulmonary artery will give a clinically useful evaluation of the degree of left-to-right shunting. The only haemodynamic parameter which is not adequately defined by routine precordial ultrasound studies in the unoperated infant or young child with a ventricular septal defect is pulmonary vascular resistance.

In the operating theatre, epicardial cross-sectional imaging allied to the use of all available Doppler modalities plus the use of intraoperative contrast echocardiography will allow the surgeon a precise evaluation of defect morphology prior to surgical closure and an immediate accurate method of appraising results after bypass has been discontinued (4).

What, then, might be the role of the transesophageal approach, if any, in the clinical evaluation of ventricular septal defects?

THE POTENTIAL ROLE OF TRANSOESOPHAGEAL IMAGING

Precordial ultrasound will fail to characterise a small proportion of moderate or large ventricular septal defects in the unoperated older child, adolescent and adult (figs. 3.58 and 3.59). In these patients, the precordial or subcostal ultrasound windows are frequently restricted by either chest deformity, lung disease, cardiac malposition or a combination of the above. An alternative ultrasound approach that could accurately identify a ventricular septal defect and define its associated haemodynamics would be of value in this patient group. In addition, in the early or late postoperative patient in whom a residual defect is suspected, the thoracotomy may preclude any ultrasound evaluation from the precordium. In addition, many cardiac surgeons are reluctant to allow intraoperative epicardial

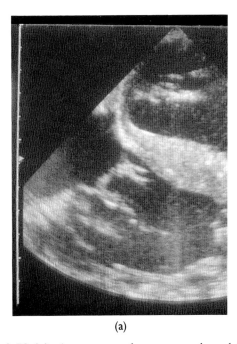

(a)

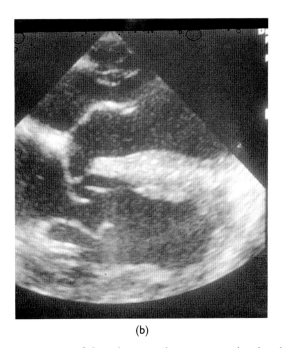

(b)

Figure 3.58 (a) *A transverse plane transesophageal image of the posterior portion of the inlet muscular septum and trabecular septum. Both are intact.* **(b)** *In this transverse plane image from the same patient, a large perimembranous inlet septal defect is seen. The defect is bounded superiorly by the central fibrous body into which both atrioventricular valve septal leaflets insert at a common level. The lower margin of the defect is the crest of the trabecular septum. Note that the chordae of the tricuspid valve insert below the defect into the trabecular septum.*

ultrasound probes into the sterile operative field and are more attracted to the concept of monitoring ventricular septal defect repair from within the oesophagus. Finally, one area where transeso-phageal imaging would seem to be an essential alternative to precordial imaging is in the immediate postoperative period in the intensive care unit when the chest has been closed and precordial imaging is very limited in the information that it can yield (5,6). In comparison, a thoracotomy has little if any effect on the image quality obtained from the oeso-phagus.

Having thus defined the areas in which transeso-phageal imaging might provide a better or an alternative imaging approach, the question must now be answered; just how much information on ventricular septal defects can be obtained by the use of either single or biplane (multiplane) transeso-phageal imaging?

THE MEMBRANOUS SEPTUM AND PERIMEMBRANOUS VENTRICULAR SEPTAL DEFECTS

With the probe introduced and positioned at the level at which the aortic root and valve leaflets are visualised in the transverse plane, then, with slight further introduction of the probe, the left ven-tricular outflow tract will be brought into view. In this view, the thin interventricular portion of the membranous septum will be visualised immediately below the aortic valve ring on its medial aspect. In hearts in which the aortic valve is normal, this structure is relatively well visualised; but where

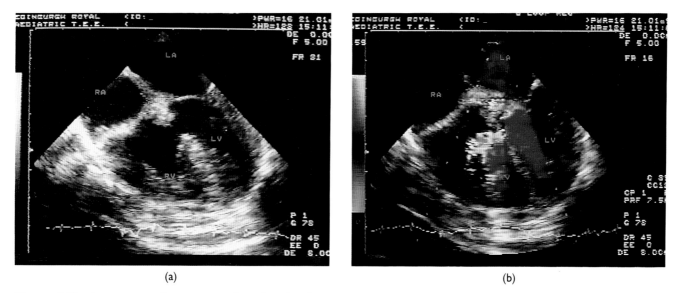

Figure 3.59 *A transverse plane transesophageal study of a muscular inlet ventricular septal defect.* **(a)** *The muscular inlet defect is well seen. The upper border of the defect is a projection of muscle extending down from the central fibrous body. There is normal offsetting of the septal leaflets of the atrioventricular valves as they insert into the central fibrous body. The lower margin of the defect is the crest of the trabecular septum.* **(b)** *The corresponding colour flow image from the above case. The turbulent jet exiting from the inlet muscular defect into the right ventricle is well seen.*

there is either a well developed fibrous element to the aortic ring, where there is calcium in the aortic valve leaflets or in the aortic root, or where there is a prosthetic aortic valve, then ultrasound shadowing due to the highly echo-reflective nature of the aortic root may either create a region of false positive echo 'drop out' within the area of the membranous septum or may obscure this area altogether. Furthermore, in a percentage of patients, the area of the membranous septum will constantly move in and out of the transesophageal imaging plane and this motion can cause further problems in the imaging evaluation of the integrity of the membranous septum by creating the appearance of echo 'drop out'. Colour flow mapping studies may be of help in such cases where there is doubt about the integrity of the membranous septum, as small restrictive membranous septal defects will be associated with widespread turbulent flow on the right ventricular aspect of the defect. In the younger patient, where the right ventricular cavity is not at great depth in the transesophageal imaging field, then colour flow mapping will reliably identify or exclude defects in the membranous septum by either identifying the characteristic systolic flow disturbance within the right ventricle or excluding it. In addition, a detailed colour flow examination of the left ventricular

aspect of the region of the membranous septum will often confirm the presence of flow across the defect by identifying the presence of flow convergence (the PISA effect) into the defect within the left ventricular outflow tract; this being more prominent in systole when the majority of transseptal flow occurs, but convergent flow may also be present during diastole in some cases where there is a high-volume left-to-right shunt (Fig. 3.60). However, problems do exist when using transesophageal colour flow mapping to evaluate the right ventricle. In adult cases, the right ventricle may lie outside the depth range at which effective colour flow mapping studies may be carried out and thus they may be of little additional benefit. Similar problems with the depth of interrogation will be encountered when using pulsed Doppler studies to define the exit point of the systolic turbulent jet into the right ventricular cavity. Many of the current generation transesophageal probes have the ability to perform continuous wave Doppler studies, and in theory this modality could be used to identify the high-velocity trans-septal jet associated with a restrictive defect. However, both perimembranous defects and trabecular defects have jets which are exiting into the right ventricle either at 90 degrees to the interrogating transesophageal continuous wave beam or

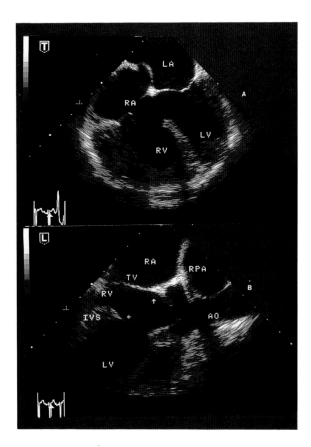

Figure 3.60 *A biplane transesophageal study of a perimembranous confluent defect.* **(a)** *A transverse plane transesophageal study of the large perimembranous confluent defect. The defect is seen to be roofed by the central fibrous body and atrioventricular valve septal leaflets which are inserted into the central fibrous body at a common level. The large defect is bounded inferiorly by the crest of the trabecular septum.* **(b)** *A longitudinal plane study of the same defect. This is a slightly unusual transesophageal cut with the probe tip angulated towards the right ventricle. In this case, the tricuspid valve septal leaflet is seen to be in fibrous continuity with the aortic root. In the longitudinal plane, the defect is seen to be bounded superiorly by the central fibrous body and inferiorly by the crest of the ventricular septum. It is unusual to see the outlet extension of a perimembranous defect in this view. This indicates that the defect is very large.*

are, at best, very poorly aligned to it. It has been our experience that such transesophageal continuous wave studies are of little practical value in unoperated patients with restrictive ventricular septal defects.

Where transesophageal imaging may be of more benefit in the study of perimembranous defects is in the evaluation of their mechanisms of closure. The degree and nature of accessory tricuspid tissue ingrowth around the defect margins (Fig. 3.61) is frequently better defined in the older child and adult using the transesophageal as opposed to the precordial approach, as is any interraction of the defect with a prolapsing right coronary leaflet. This latter entity, including the characteristic 'tear-drop' malformation of the right coronary sinus, is well defined from the oesophagus (Fig. 3.62). Indeed, in the older patient where image definition from the oesophagus is excellent, the esophageal approach may be the technique of choice (compared with angiography) in distinguishing between a ruptured Sinus of Valsalva and the combination of a perimembranous ventricular septal defect with associated aortic incompetence.

All the information to be obtained on perimembranous defects from the oesophagus will normally be obtained from a transverse plane study. The longitudinal transesophageal plane is aligned for the most part parallel to the ventricular septum and thus is of little value. The thin membranous septum can be visualised in a small number of cases using longitudinal scanning by rotating the probe from the long axis of the left ventricular outflow tract plane clockwise towards the tricuspid valve view. In perimembranous inlet defects, the exit of the turbulent jet into the inlet of the right ventricle just inferior to the tricuspid valve septal leaflet, may also be well defined in a number of cases. Only large perimembranous outlet defects will be visualised in the longitudinal plane.

TRABECULAR VENTRICULAR SEPTAL DEFECTS

The transesophageal transverse plane can rarely scan the whole of the trabecular septum. With the probe tip positioned to image the membranous septum (see above) and with subsequent slight probe advancement and tip ante-flexion, then an imaging plane which appears to correspond to a precordial apical four-chamber plus aortic root view will be

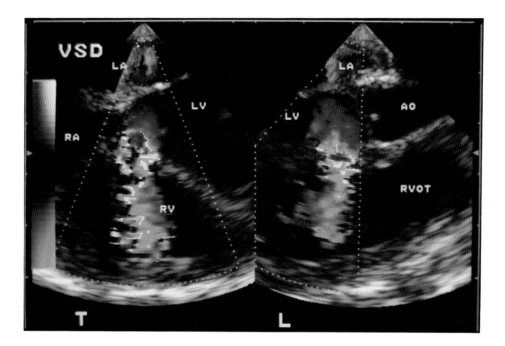

Figure 3.61 *A biplane transesophageal study of a perimembranous outlet defect. In the left panel, a transverse plane colour flow mapping image is seen in which accelerative flow (the Pisa effect) into the defect is well visualised on the left ventricular surface of the defect and the extensive right ventricular turbulent jet seen on the right hand aspect of the defect. In the right hand panel, a longitudinal plane view of the same defect is seen. Again, note the accelerative flow into the defect which is well seen on its left ventricular aspect as well as flow through the defect and the turbulent exiting flow from the defect into the right ventricle. In this case, the jet exits into the outlet portion of the right ventricle below the right ventricular outflow tract.*

obtained. What appears to be the cardiac apex in this imaging plane (Fig. 3.59) is in fact a portion of the anterior surface of the left ventricle cut at mid-cavity level. Thus, the true antero-apical area of the trabecular septum will rarely be scanned from within the oesophagus. This is especially true when carrying out studies in the older patient. However, because of the larger esophageal window in the child, it may be possible to view the true cardiac apex in a proportion of cases. Thus apical trabecular septal defects may be visualised in the younger patient but will be missed in a high proportion of older children or adult patients. This problem is well illustrated by the relatively low sensitivity with which moderate or large apical post-infarction septal defects are visualised from an intraesophageal probe tip position.

To better profile the antero-apical trabecular septum, the probe tip should be advanced to the fundus of the stomach and then manipulated to image a transverse plane view which is a direct equivalent of a precordial four-chamber plus aortic root view. In this view, the portion of the interventricular septum nearest to the transducer will normally be the true anteroapical septum. This view is the optimal one to identify or exclude small single apical trabecular ventricular septal defects, multiple ('Swiss-cheese') defects and post-infarction apical acquired ventricular septal defects. Even using this view, small apical ventricular septal defects can be missed. The longitudinal plane equivalent of this view is of little value in the definition of apical defects as it images in a plane parallel to the septum.

Defects in the mid or posterior portions of the

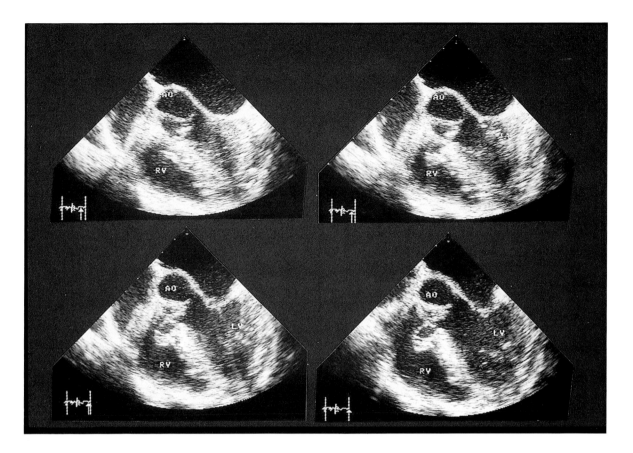

Figure 3.62 *Four images taken from a transverse plane transesophageal study from a patient with a perimembranous inlet defect partially closed by a tricuspid valve pseudoaneurysm. In the upper left panel taken in diastole, the defect is not visualised. In the upper right panel taken slightly later in the cardiac cycle, there appears to be a protruding aneurysm from the interventricular septum. In the lower left panel, the ventricular septal defect is seen and the tissue partially closing the defect on its right ventricular aspect is seen to arise from the septal leaflet of the tricuspid valve with chordae packed onto the crest of the trabecular septum. In the lower right image asystolic frame, the defect is well seen with again the chordae clearly seen to partially close the defect off on its right ventricular aspect.*

trabecular septum are normally well characterised from within the oesophagus using a combination of imaging and colour flow mapping, and so the use of transgastric imaging is rarely required.

MUSCULAR INLET DEFECTS

These defects lie within the smooth muscular inlet septum which is located between the inlet valves of the two ventricles. Such defects are separated superiorly from the central fibrous body by a muscle ridge and do not extend to involve the membranous septum (Fig. 3.63). Thus the mode of implantation of the septal leaflet of each atrioventricular valve into the central fibrous body is normal as the atrioventricular septa are normal (cf. perimembranous inlet defects). Such defects are best visualised during a transesophageal imaging study using the transverse plane. They are rarely visualised using longitudinal plane scanning. They may also be visualised by a transgastric transverse plane study.

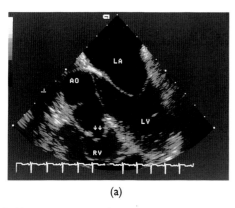

(a)

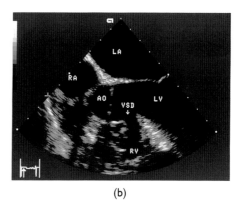

(b)

Figure 3.63 *A transverse plane transesophageal study from a patient with an abnormal right aortic root sinus and a ventricular septal defect. In this patient, the aortic valve right coronary cusp prolapsed into the defect in systole rather than diastole presumably due to the Venturi effect of systolic flow through the ventricular septal defect. In* **(a)** *the abnormal aortic sinus is clearly visualised but not the ventricular septal defect. With slight probe advancement* **(b)**, *the ventricular septal defect is well seen with the right coronary cusp prolapsing into the defect in systole.*

MUSCULAR OUTLET DEFECTS

The muscular outlet septum (a remarkably small but important septal structure) is relatively poorly characterised by precordial ultrasound studies. Single (or multiple) defects within this septum may easily be missed. The muscular outlet septum can be visualised using transverse plane transesophageal imaging but this approach is still not optimal. It appears to be the longitudinal transesophageal plane which best visualises this septal structure and which best defines its defects. Our experience with this defect group has been limited as isolated muscular outlet defects are relatively rare, and so this initial impression awaits confirmation. In addition, the longitudinal plane can best delineate any associated anterior or posterior deviation of the outlet septum while any medial or lateral deviation of the outlet septum is best characterised by a transgastric transverse plane study.

DOUBLY COMMITTED SUB-ARTERIAL DEFECTS

These are invariably large ventricular septal defects and are rarely missed even in the poorest precordial imaging subject. The defects are characterised by the abnormal fibrous continuity of the aortic and pulmonary valve rings which roof the defect in the septum. Such defects may or may not extend to involve the membranous septum. Transesophageal imaging in the transverse plane can characterise all the morphologic features of these defects, but esophageal longitudinal plane imaging will give a better visualisation of the fibrous continuity of the aortic and pulmonary valve rings. The ventricular septal defect will be equally well seen using either esophageal imaging plane. Transgastric imaging in the transverse plane should be equally effective in defining the defect but is of additional advantage (as with all outlet defects) in that it can best identify any degree of aortic override above the septal defect. (Aortic override is poorly characterised by the transesophageal transverse plane but any anterior aortic displacement above the defect is well defined using the transesophageal longitudinal plane.) The use of the biplane approach and the combination of imaging from both the oesophagus and the fundus of the stomach should overcome the problems which Muhiudeen *et al.*(7) found when using only the transesophageal transverse plane approach to define these defects (7).

INTRAOPERATIVE EVALUATION OF VENTRICULAR SEPTAL DEFECT CLOSURE FROM THE ESOPHAGUS

The above descriptions of how to define each type of ventricular septal defect using a transesophageal probe should have indicated that this is frequently an examination which requires both skill and experience and in general is a technique which is a poor substitute for high-resolution precordial imaging (even when using a bi- or multiplane probe).

However, in the operating theatre, the esophageal approach has many advantages which appeal to the surgeon, not the least of which being that it does not invade the sterile operative field.

Prior to attempted surgical closure, it has been our experience that epicardial imaging remains superior in a number of ways to esophageal imaging: in image quality, in the wide range of imaging planes in which the defect and its relationships can be assessed, and in the ability to align all the Doppler modalities to the intracardiac flows to allow a more accurate intraoperative evaluation of haemodynamics. The multiplane epicardial approach allows the surgeon a greater three-dimensional concept of the defect than single or biplane esophageal imaging and this may be of clinical value. However, it is in the evaluation of the postoperative patient that problems arise when using the esophageal approach. Any prosthetic material sewn into the heart will produce a greater or lesser degree of 'ultrasound masking' owing to its relative reduced permeability to sound waves. This is the case with both biologic (pericardium) or non-biologic (Dacron) patches used to close ventricular septal defects. To identify a residual ventricular septal defect from the oesophagus, the investigator must demonstrate one of two things: (1) the actual defect itself, and (2) the trans-septal jet and the resultant diagnostic area of turbulent systolic flow within the right ventricular cavity. An additional useful diagnostic feature may be the identification

Table 3.4 *The relative value of the differing transesophageal or transgastric imaging positions in the visualisation of ventricular septal defects*

	Perimembranous	Trabecular			Muscular		Doubly committed sub-arterial
		Apical	Mid	Posterior	Inlet	Outlet	
Intraesophageal							
(a) Transverse plane	++	+	++	+++	+++	+	++
(b) Longitudinal plane	+	++	++	+	+	+++	+++
Transgastric							
(a) Transverse plane	++	+++	++	++	++	−	+
(b) Longitudinal plane	−	−	−	+	−	−	++

+++ = Excellent
++ = Good
+   = Limited value
−   = Not of value

Note that optimum evaluation of the integrity of the ventricular septum requires a combination of scanning positions and the use of both imaging planes.

of a zone of flow convergence on the left ventricular aspect of the patch indicating the site of flow into the defect. (Neither turbulent trans-septal or right ventricular flow nor a flow convergence zone will be present where there is a large residual non-restrictive ventricular septal defect.)

Direct imaging of the defect around the patch margins from the oesophagus may only be possible in approximately half the cases. This is due in part to the relatively small size of many residual defects and their obliquity to the imaging planes available. Thus much reliance has to be placed on the sensitivity of esophageal or transgastric colour flow mapping. In the child of less than 20 kg and with an imaging probe with a frequency of some 5 MHz, then colour flow information on flows can normally be obtained from the whole of the right ventricular cavity. However, in the older paediatric patient, and especially in the adult, the depth at which the right ventricular cavity lies in the transesophageal imaging field often means that no useful colour flow information may be obtained from this cavity. In addition, the ventricular septal defect patch, especially if large, and made of non-biologic material, may cast a complete ultrasound shadow over the whole of the right ventricular cavity and thus no useful colour flow information will be obtained. A coexisting prosthesis in either the aortic or mitral valve positions may also cast a similar shadow and preclude visualisation of both the patch and the right ventricular flow characteristics.

Given the above caveats, it is surprising that there is much current enthusiasm for the use of transesophageal imaging in the determination of ventricular septal defect closure as opposed to the much more versatile (and accurate) technique of epicardial imaging. Certainly our limited experience in the infant and young child would suggest that the transesophageal approach may be almost as effective in the definition of residual important trans-septal shunting as the epicardial approach but that as patient weight increases it becomes an increasingly less effective technique. Currently we would strongly advocate that any immediate post-bypass study of ventricular septal defect patch integrity should be carried out from the epicardium and should involve the use of imaging, colour Doppler, colour M-mode, continuous wave Doppler and left atrial contrast studies as described previously in our

work (3,8). Such an approach should provide the surgeon with the maximum information on the success of surgery prior to chest closure. Transesophageal imaging then becomes the technique of choice to define any patch dehiscence in the ventilated patient in the intensive care unit. This perhaps is the most valuable role of the technique in the evaluation of ventricular septal defects.

REFERENCES

1. SUTHERLAND GR, GODMAN MJ, SMALLHORN JF, GUITTERAS P, ANDERSON RH, HUNTER S. Ventricular septal defects – two dimensional echocardiographic and morphological correlations. *Br Heart J* 1982; **47:** 316–28.

2. SUTHERLAND GR, SMYLLIE JH, OGILVIE BC, KEETON BR. Colour flow imaging in the diagnosis of multiple ventricular septal defects. *Br Heart J* 1989; **62:** 43–9.

3. LUDOMIRSKY A, HUHTA JC, VICK GW, MURPHY DJ, DANFORD DA, MORROW WR. Colour Doppler detection of multiple ventricular septal defects. *Circulation* 1986; **74:** 1317–22.

4. STÜMPER O, FRASER AG, ELZENGA NJ, VAN DAELE M, FROHN-MULDER I, HERWERDEN L, QUAGEBEUR J, SUTHERLAND GR. The assessment of ventricular septal defect closure by intraoperative epicardial ultrasound. *J Am Coll Cardiol* 1990; **16:** 1672–9.

5. SREERAM N, SUTHERLAND GR, KAULITZ R, STÜMPER OFW, HESS J, QUAEGEBEUR JM. The comparative roles of intraoperative epicardial and early postoperative precordial echocardiography in the assessment of surgical repair of congenital heart defects. *J Am Coll Card* 1990; **16:** 913–20.

6. STÜMPER O, KAULITZ R, ELZENGA NJ, BOM N, ROELANDT JRTC, HESS J, SUTHERLAND GR. The value of transesophageal echocardiography in children with congenital heart disease. *J Am Soc Echo* 1991; **4:** 164–76.

7. MUHIUDEEN IA, ROBERTSON DA, SILVERMAN NH, et al. Intraoperative echocardiography in infants and children with congenital cardiac shunt lesions – transesophageal versus epicardial echocardiography. *J Am Coll Cardiol* 1990; **16:** 1687.

8. STÜMPER OFW, KAULITZ R, SREERAM N, FRASER AG, HESS J, ROELANDT JRTC, SUTHERLAND GR. Intraoperative transoesophageal versus epicardial ultrasound in surgery for congenital heart disease. *J Am Soc Echo* 1990; **3:** 392–401.

The left ventricular outflow tract and the aortic valve

G. R. Sutherland

INTRODUCTION

Congenital lesions of the left ventricular outflow tract can be sub-divided into three main groups: those at sub-valve level, lesions of the valve itself and the much rarer supra-valve lesions. This chapter will deal with both of the former sub-groups and will attempt to assess the current role and relative merits of the transesophageal approach in defining lesions at both of these levels. Precordial imaging using 5 or 7 mHz transducers will normally give excellent image resolution of left ventricular outflow tract structures in unoperated infants or children, and this will seldom be bettered by the use of the current range of paediatric transesophageal probes with their single plane approach and limited powers of resolution (related to their reduced element numbers). It is only where there has been prior cardiac surgery (with a resultant impairment of precordial imaging) a chest deformity or lung disease that esophageal imaging may provide a better approach in this age group. However, as the patient's weight increases to above 15–20 kg, precordial imaging becomes more difficult and the left ventricular outflow may be better imaged from the oesophagus. In addition, above the weight of 20–40 kg, adult size transesophageal probes can be introduced with care in the intubated, anaesthetised child. These probes (able to image at 5.0 and 7.0 mHz) with these increased element numbers (64) and imaging in a biplane or multiplane modality offer many imaging advantages over the precordial approach. However, they remain limited in their

spectral Doppler capabilities to determine accurate gradients within the left ventricular outflow because of frequent poor alignment to the jet direction from an intraesophageal position. (Transgastric imaging offers much better alignment to left ventricular outflow tract flow.) In the adult patient, it is now clear that in the majority of cases, the left ventricular outflow will be better imaged from the oesophagus – that is if any doubt persists about the morphologic diagnosis after a precordial imaging examination.

IMAGING OF LEFT VENTRICULAR OUTFLOW

Standard tranverse plane transesophageal imaging normally provides excellent imaging of all the structures which form the boundaries of the subvalvar portion of the left ventricular outflow. The optimal imaging plane obtained by tip manipulation in the antero-posterior direction will often parallel the sub-valve outflow tract and thus alignment to flow may be good in a proportion of cases. The left ventricular outflow tract is that area of the left ventricle which is bounded laterally by the area of aortomitral fibrous continuity and the anterior mitral valve leaflet (in diastole), medially by the upper portion of the trabecular septum and membranous septum and the inferior aspect of the fibrous aortic ring, anteriorly by a combination of the trabecular and muscular outlet septa, and posteriorly by the aortic

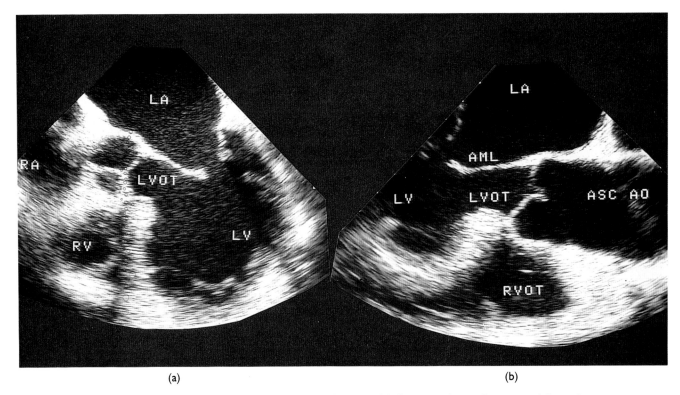

(a)   (b)

Figure 3.64 *The transverse and longitudinal plane images of a normal left ventricular outflow tract.* **(a)** *In this transverse plane image, the left ventricular outflow tract is seen to be foreshortened when compared to the image of the left ventricular outflow tract in the longitudinal plane. The outflow tract is bounded laterally by the anterior mitral leaflet, medially by the crest of the trabecular septum and the membranous ventricular septum and ends at the coapted aortic valve leaflets. There is no evidence of any obstruction within this outflow tract.* **(b)** *The longitudinal plane image of a normal left ventricular outflow tract. In this image, the left ventricular outflow tract is seen in its true long axis. Posteriorly, it is bounded by the anterior mitral leaflet and anteriorly by the trabecular and membranous septa. Note that in both the transverse and longitudinal planes, the membranous septum is foreshortened and poorly seen.*

fibrous curtains as they extend down from the aortic annulus. These structures and their relationships to one another are easily visualised in every case by standard single plane transesophageal scanning (Fig. 3.64 (a)). The precise antero-posterior relationships of the various components are not always well appreciated when using this transverse plane; to determine these, the additional use of the longitudinal or multiplane approach is required.

To visualise the left ventricular outflow tract, the transesophageal probe should be advanced in the oesophagus until a standard view is obtained in which the inflow tract of the left ventricle (i.e. both leaflets of the mitral valve and their sub-valve apparatus) is visualised. Slight clockwise rotation of the probe and slight withdrawal of the probe will bring

the whole left ventricular outflow tract into view. In some cases, the outflow tract will initially appear in a rather foreshortened cut. In such cases, antero-posterior flexion of the probe tip will frequently open up the long axis of the outflow tract. All the structures forming its medial and lateral margins will be well visualised. In some cases (especially in the adult population) highly echo-reflective fibrous tissue present in the medial portion of the aortic root and central fibrous body may give rise to ultrasound shadowing in the region of the membranous portion of the ventricular septum thus creating false positive areas of echo 'drop out' which may simulate the appearance of perimembranous ventricular septal defect.

The addition of the longitudinal transesophageal

plane offers advantages when studying lesions of the left ventricular outflow tract. This plane will better visualise the antero-posterior relationships of structures which border onto or obstruct the out-flow tract (Fig. 3.64 (b)). Indeed, obstructive lesions which are poorly characterised by transverse plane scanning may often be well characterised in the longitudinal plane (Figs 3.65 and 3.66).

The longitudinal scan of the left ventricular out-flow tract is best commenced with the probe tip inserted at a depth and in a position where the stan-dard long axis images of the interatrial septum, for-amen ovale and superior vena cava are visualised in the one plane. The probe should then be rotated in a counterclockwise manner to bring the aortic root and proximal ascending aorta into view. With this tip angulation (i.e. with the lateral steering mech-anism in the neutral position) the left ventricular outflow tract is cut in an oblique plane and is not normally well imaged. It is with the use of appro-priate lateral tip flexion (using the lateral steering mechanism) that the whole left ventricular outflow tract will be opened out. In this imaging plane, the chamber visualised nearest to the transducer is the left atrium. The anterior mitral leaflet is visualised as the posterior structure bordering on the cresentic left ventricular outflow tract, and the ventricular septum (both trabecular and muscular outlet components) is seen to form the anterior border. Lying anterior to the ventricular septum, the right ventricular outflow tract, pulmonary valve and main pulmonary artery are visualised. With further counterclockwise probe rotation a scan can be made from the left ventricular outflow to the mitral valve which will demonstrate the antero-posterior re-lationships of the outflow tract of the left ventricle to both mitral valve leaflets and the long axis of the left ventricle.

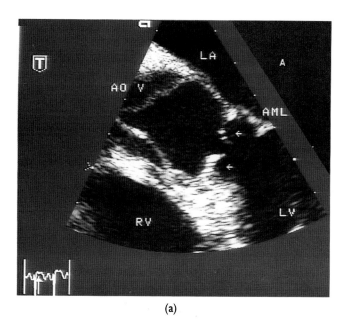

(a)

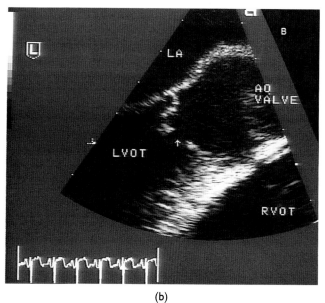

(b)

Figure 3.65 (a) *A transverse plane transesophageal image of the left ventricular outflow tract in a patient with a discrete subaortic fibromuscular obstruction (arrowed). The medial aspect of the obstruction is seen to take rise from the crest of the trabecular septum, the lateral insertion is on to the anterior mitral valve leaflet.* **(b)** *The longitudinal long axis plane from the same patient. Again, the discrete fibromuscular obstruction is well seen with its central orifice. Again, the anterior and posterior sites of insertion are well visualised.*

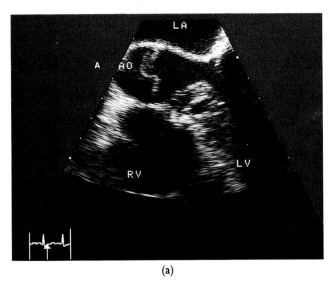

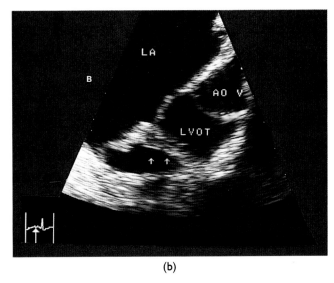

(a)

(b)

Figure 3.66 *Subaortic obstruction caused by accessory chordal tissue implanting into the left ventricular outflow tract in a patient with a partial atrioventricular septal defect. In (a) (the transverse plane study) a mass of proliferative tissue is imaged within the outflow tract below the aortic valve. This has the appearance not unlike that of discrete fibromuscular obstruction. It was, however, the longitudinal plane study in (b) which demonstrated that the obstruction was due to accessory chordae (arrowed) inserting across the left ventricular outflow tract into the septum in a subaortic position.*

TRANSGASTRIC IMAGING OF THE LEFT VENTRICULAR OUTFLOW TRACT

The left ventricular outflow tract may also be studied by positioning the transesophageal probe tip in the fundus of the stomach to produce what are essentially the equivalent of the transthoracic four-chamber plus aortic root (transgastric transverse axis) (Fig. 3.67) and long axis left ventricular (transgastric longitudinal) views of the left ventricular outflow tract (1). These transgastric views are much less easy to obtain than the transesophageal views described above. To obtain the transverse plane transgastric view, the probe tip should be advanced to a position near the fundus of the stomach and the probe then retro-flexed in the antero-posterior plane to obtain the equivalent of the transthoracic four-chamber aortic root view which will allow visualisation of the left ventricular outflow tract.

This series of probe manoeuvres will normally require insertion of the probe to a depth greater than that normally necessary when attempting to obtain the transgastric short-axis cut of the ventricles. This manoeuvre may be poorly tolerated by awake or sedated patients. In the anaesthetised patient, this view can be obtained in the majority.

When the transgastric four-chamber aortic root view has been obtained using the transverse plane of a biplane probe, then by switching to the longitudinal plane a transthoracic left ventricular outflow tract long axis equivalent cut can sometimes be obtained. However, because of the differing positions of the imaging elements on the shaft of a biplane transesophageal probe, direct switching to obtain the longitudinal transgastric view of the left ventricular outflow tract is seldom possible and further transducer manipulation is usually required to obtain this view. In the older patient, this is frequently a very difficult view to obtain.

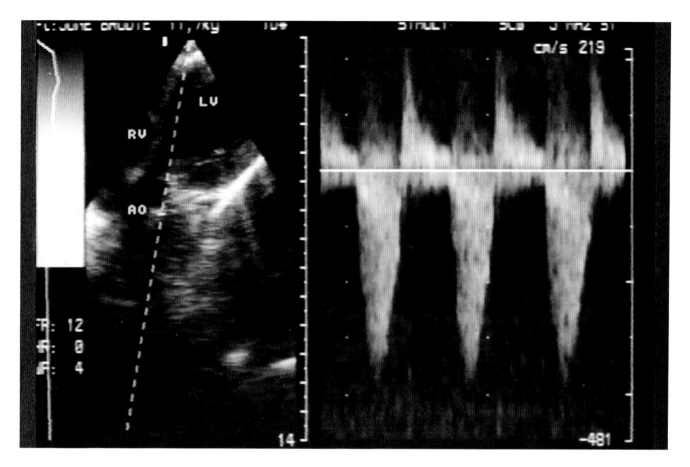

Figure 3.67 *A transgastric 4-chamber plus aortic root image of the left ventricular outflow tract and aortic valve in a patient with valvar aortic stenosis. Note that in this projection, the imaging plane is well aligned to the outflow tract and thus can allow accurate continuous wave Doppler interrogation of the left ventricular outflow tract flow obstruction.*

In general, the use of the transgastric views of the left ventricular outflow tract do not contribute additional information on outflow tract obstruction where the aortic and mitral valves are normal. Because of the increased distance when imaging from the stomach, the image quality obtained from this position is usually markedly reduced when compared to imaging from the oesophagus. However, where there is calcium in either valve or either valve has been replaced by a prosthesis, then any ultrasound masking of the left ventricular outflow tract which occurs using an intraesophageal imaging position can be circumvented using the combined transgastric views.

Colour flow mapping studies of the normal left ventricular outflow tract are remarkably uniform in their appearance. With appropriate velocity and variance settings (at above 0.5 metre/sec) for the velocity range to be encoded, the flow in the left ventricular outflow tract will be seen to be laminar in systole with little or no appearance of turbulent flow. In diastole aortic regurgitation is a very rare finding in the apparently 'normal' patient and in our opinion such regurgitation is always a pathologic finding and is not physiologic (*vis-à-vis* 'physiologic' tricuspid regurgitation). Pulsed Doppler studies commencing in the body of the left ventricle with subsequent positioning of the sample volume in a series of positions within the left ventricular outflow tract until the transaortic flow is reached will demonstrate a normal mild acceleration of flow within the normal left ventricular outflow tract from some 0.5–0.6 metre/sec to 0.8–1 metre/sec. The peak velocity of flow within the normal left ventricular outflow tract rarely exceeds 1.2 metre/sec even in cases where cardiac output is significantly increased.

OBSTRUCTIVE LESIONS OF THE LEFT VENTRICULAR OUTFLOW TRACT

The spectrum of lesions which may cause obstruction within the left ventricular outflow tract in patients with congenital heart disease is very wide (2) (Table 3.5). Various classifications of this group of lesions have been proposed. Fibromuscular obstruction within the outflow tract may be present either as a discrete lesion (often referred to as a subaortic membrane) or as diffuse involvement of the whole outflow tract (3). Discrete fibromuscular obstruction is the most common form of left ventricular outflow tract obstruction encountered in patients with congenital heart disease. Other less common causes of obstruction are (1) hypertrophic obstructive cardiomyopathy, (2) obstruction caused by (a) reduplication of the anterior mitral leaflet or (b) anomalous insertion of sub-valve chordae into the ventricular septum (the latter occurring most commonly in the setting of an atrioventricular septal defect), (3) obstruction caused by tumors or connective tissue disorders and obstruction caused by the protrusion of an aneurysm of the ventricular septum into the left ventricular outflow (this latter entity only occurs when the right ventricle is at higher pressure than the left and thus will normally only be encountered in patients with classical transposition of the great vessels).

Table 3.5 *Obstructive lesions of the left ventricular outflow tract encountered in patients with congenital heart disease*

Discrete fibromuscular obstruction. 'Subaortic membrane')
Diffuse fibromuscular obstruction
Hypertrophic obstructive cardiomyopathy
Accessory mitral valve tissue
Anomalous insertion of the mitral sub-valve apparatus into the ventricular septum
Tumours or connective tissue masses
Aneurysm (or pseudo-aneurysm) of the ventricular septum (TGA)
Leftwards and downward deviation of the outlet septum (i.e. TGA / VSD)

DISCRETE FIBROMUSCULAR OBSTRUCTION

In the infant and child, this lesion is normally a crescentic thin fibromuscular ridge sited one to five millimetres below the aortic valve leaflets. Its medial insertion is normally into the junction of the trabecular and fibrous membranous septa and is more prominent than its lateral insertion which is at the junction of the base of the anterior mitral leaflet and the aortic valve fibrous ring. In this age group, multiple sites of insertion of the fibromuscular tissue are uncommon. The degree of obstruction caused by the fibromuscular ridge is variable as is its propensity to develop progressively severe obstruction (4). Associated lesions are aortic incompetence (of varying severity and progression), mild mitral incompetence and concentric left ventricular hypertrophy (often of a severity out of all proportion to the measured resting outflow tract gradient).

In the adolescent or adult patient, the lesion may be much more complex than a simple single fibromuscular ridge. The fibromuscular outgrowths may be multiple with complex insertions both medially and laterally into the structures which bound the outflow tract such as the aortic valve leaflets and the chordae and papillary muscles of the mitral valve. Such complex lesions are much more difficult to remove surgically. The complexity of the lesion in this sub-group of adult patients would appear to be another manifestation of the progressive nature of discrete fibromuscular obstruction which occurs in a subset of the patient population.

THE TRANSOESOPHAGEAL APPEARANCE

A single discrete shelf will normally be imaged by transverse plane scanning lying some 1–5 mm below the aortic valve leaflets (5,6). The structure normally appears highly echogenic (probably reflecting its fibrous nature). The single septal insertion will normally be at the junction of the trabecular and membranous components of the ventricular septum. The ridge will appear thicker at its septal insertion and will become thinner as it protrudes into the outflow tract. The lateral insertion is normally much less prominent and is sited either at the fibrous junction of the aortic and mitral valve rings or is into the anterior leaflet of the mitral valve. The level of insertion of the lateral component may vary considerably. Neither the anterior nor posterior involvement of the outflow tract is well characterised by single transverse plane scanning. These are best defined using either the longitudinal plane of a biplane probe or a single multiplane probe (Figs 3.65).

It is rare for a single fibromuscular obstruction to have a lateral insertion into other than the area of aorto-mitral fibrous continuity or the anterior mitral valve leaflet, but where a lateral insertion is not visualised in this area then the whole sub-valve apparatus of either leaflet should be scanned very carefully.

In the adolescent or adult patient, the lesion may be much more complex. In our own prospective study involving 28 patients in whom precordial ultrasound imaging had suggested the presence of a possible isolated or co-existing discrete fibromuscular subaortic obstruction, a wide range of new information on the morphology of the obstruction was provided by a single plane transesophageal study (7). The prior clinical diagnosis, the diagnosis following the precordial study and the diagnosis established by the transesophageal study in each of the 28 patients is given in Table 3.6. From these findings, we established that precordial imaging is a good but not perfect technique for the identification of discrete subaortic obstruction. Transesophageal imaging is clearly better. However, the real benefit of transesophageal imaging is illustrated in Table 3.7 which compares the accuracy with which precordial and transesophageal imaging defined the complexity of the medial and lateral insertions, and in Table 3.8 which compares the accuracy with which both modalities identified the co-existing range of abnormalities. Over the whole range of patient ages, transesophageal imaging was consistently better at defining the site and multiplicity of the medial and lateral insertions of the fibromuscular tissue, the presence of multilevel fibromuscular obstruction, the involvement of the aortic valve leaflets, the presence of co-existing dynamic obstruction within the outflow tract and the presence of mitral regurgitation. Aortic regurgitation was equally well characterised by the precordial and the transesophageal techniques. As a result of this study, it has now become our practice to refer all older patients (i.e. adolescents and adults) in whom precordial echocardiography either confirms or suggests the presence of discrete fibromuscular obstruction for a transesophageal examination in an attempt to define the detailed morphology of the lesion. In infants and young children (in whom precordial im-

Table 3.6 *Fibromuscular subaortic obstruction: diagnostic comparisons*

Morphology	Clinical diagnosis on referral	Diagnosis following precordial study	Diagnosis following transesophageal echocardiography
Isolated aortic valvar disease	9	0	0
Aortic valvar stenosis + discrete fibromuscular obstruction	0	4*	4*
Isolated discrete fibromuscular obstruction	12	20	23
Isolated hypertrophic cardiomyopathy	4	0	0
Hypertrophic cardiomyopathy + discrete fibromuscular obstruction	0	4	1
Ventricular septal defect + aortic regurgitation	3	0	0
Total	28	28	28

*= 1 false-positive diagnosis.

aging is normally of higher definition than current generation paediatric probe transesophageal imaging) a transesophageal study will seldom be required. It is only in the older child where precordial imaging may be poor, or diagnostic doubts exist, that the decision to proceed to a transesophageal study under general anaesthesia rather than to cardiac catheterisation may be contentious. It has been our experience that transoesphageal imaging in this age group almost invariably will provide more information on the morphology of the lesion than multiplane angiography. Transesophageal imaging can also be used to monitor the surgical enucleation of the fibromuscular obstruction. Our own experience in using the transverse plane technique and

Table 3.7 *Fibromuscular subaortic obstruction: comparison of precordial imaging and TEE (patients as in Table 3.6)*

	Continuous wave Doppler waveform			Colour flow mapping		
	Fixed obstruction	Dynamic obstruction	Fixed + dynamic obstruction	Left ventricular outflow tract turbulence	Aortic regurgitation	Mitral regurgitation
Precordial echocardiography	23	3	1	26	20	6
Transesophageal echocardiography	Not applicable	Not applicable	Not applicable	27	27	22

Table 3.8 *Fibromuscular subaortic obstruction: co-existing abnormalities (patients as in Table 3.6)*

	Septal insertion		Lateral insertion	
Precordial echocardiography	Single	17	Single	8
	Multiple	2	Multiple	2
		19		10
Transesophageal echocardiography	Single	21	Single	15
	Multiple	6	Multiple	12
		27		27

direct epicardial imaging of the outflow tract resulted in the conclusion that high-frequency multiplane epicardial imaging was of great help to the surgeon both in assessing the morphology of the lesion and in assessing the immediate results of surgical resection (8). We have, as yet, had no opportunity to compare bi- or multiplane transesophageal imaging with the epicardial approach in such lesions, but we would expect the transesophageal multiplane approach to be a significant improvement on transverse plane imaging alone but to remain inferior to epicardial imaging in the range of imaging and Doppler information that it would provide.

HYPERTROPHIC OBSTRUCTIVE CARDIOMYOPATHY

Hypertrophic obstructive cardiomyopathy is a rare lesion in infants and young children but its incidence increases in the adolescent population. The spectrum of morphologic and haemodynamic abnormalities associated with this condition are normally well documented by a precordial ultrasound study. Transesophageal studies are rarely indicated in this patient group except in those in whom precordial imaging is non-diagnostic. Single transverse plane studies can give additional information on (1) the nature of the obstruction by defining the precise interraction of the mitral valve anterior leaflet and sub-valve apparatus with the interventricular septum, and (2) the presence, morphology and severity of co-existing mitral regurgitation (Fig. 3.68) (9). The degree of septal hypertrophy will be overestimated in a significant number of cases because the transesophageal imaging plane will normally cut the septum obliquely and thus give the appearance of an increased septal thickness. In addition, the transverse plane approach normally cannot image the antero-apical or outlet septal components and thus co-existing intracavitary, apical or right ventricular obstruction due to hypertrophy of these septal areas will be poorly defined. The use of the longitudinal plane will add significant new information when studying patients with hypertrophic cardiomyopathies. Using this plane, the dynamic relationships in the antero-posterior plane of the mitral valve and the septum will be defined (compared with the transverse plane which defines the medial-lateral relationships). The degree of hypertrophy of the subaortic portion of the trabecular and outlet septae is better defined as is any obstruction of the right ventricular outflow tract by hypertrophy of the outlet septum.

The transesophageal longitudinal view will also allow visualisation of the cavity and apex of the left ventricle and thus can be used to identify mid-cavity and apical areas of obstruction. Thus, if a diagnostic transesophageal study is to be contemplated in such patients, a biplane study would be the approach of choice.

Currently, the main role of transesophageal echo in patients with hypertrophic obstructive cardiomyopathy is in the monitoring of surgical interventions (10). Imaging from the oesophagus has been used in the operating theatre to guide the surgeon in both surgical myectomy of the septal hypertrophy and in repair or replacement of the mitral valve. Biplane transesophageal imaging should be an important advantage in monitoring such surgical procedures. Quite what the relative advantages and disadvantages of transesophageal versus epicardial imaging are in the surgery of this lesion is yet to be established.

OTHER FORMS OF SUBAORTIC OBSTRUCTION

DIFFUSE (TUNNEL) FIBROMUSCULAR OBSTRUCTION

This rare lesion is normally well characterised by precordial imaging. Where imaging from the precordium is non-diagnostic, a transesophageal study will define the morphology of the lesion. Occasionally areas of discrete obstruction will co-exist within the tunnel-like narrowing of the outflow tract. These may be better defined (or excluded) by an appropriate transesophageal study. Tunnel fibromuscular obstruction will be best characterised by a biplane transesophageal study.

OTHER RARE FORMS OF SUBAORTIC OBSTRUCTION

Any other obstructive lesions within the left ventricular outflow tract will be well characterised by a transesophageal study. Examples of lesions causing

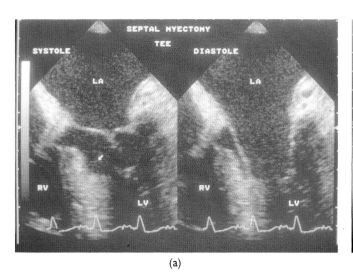

(a)

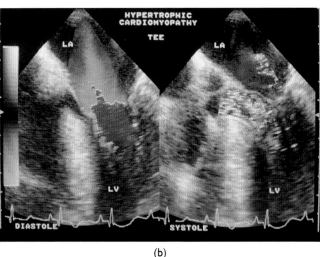

(b)

Figure 3.68 (a) *A transverse plane transesophageal study of a patient with hypertrophic obstructive cardiomyopathy who has had a previous septal myectomy (arrowed). In the left-hand panel, the systolic frame is shown and in the right-hand panel the diastolic frame. There has been adequate relief of the left ventricular outflow tract obstruction by the resection. **(b)** A transverse plane transesophageal colour flow mapping study from a patient with hypertrophic obstructive cardiomyopathy. Note the thickened upper end of the ventricular septum and the turbulent flow within the left ventricular outflow tract indicating obstruction. In addition, this patient has trivial associated mitral regurgitation.*

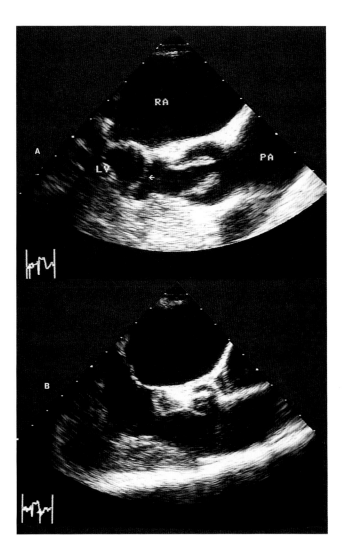

such obstruction include (1) benign tumors or tissue outgrowths, (2) reduplication of the anterior mitral leaflet, (3) abnormal implantation of part of the mitral sub-valve into the septum (Fig. 3.66), (4) protrusion of a true aneurysm of the ventricular septum or tricuspid valve pseudoaneurysm through a ventricular septal defect (both in the context of classical transposition) to cause left ventricular outflow (i.e. sub-pulmonary) obstruction (Figs 3.69 and 3.70).

Figure 3.69 *A longitudinal plane transesophageal study from a patient with atrioventricular discordance and a sub-pulmonary discrete fibromuscular obstruction (arrowed).*

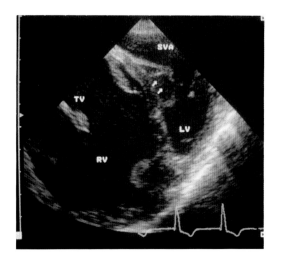

Figure 3.70 *A transverse plane transesophageal study from a patient with transposition of the great vessels and a small perimembranous ventricular septal defect who has undergone a Mustard procedure. In the late postoperative period, the patient developed the signs of increasing left ventricular outflow tract obstruction. Precordial imaging was unhelpful in this patient. Transesophageal imaging demonstrated a true aneurysm of the membranous septum around the edges of the ventricular septal defect which was bulging forward in right ventricular systole to occlude the left ventricular outflow tract.*

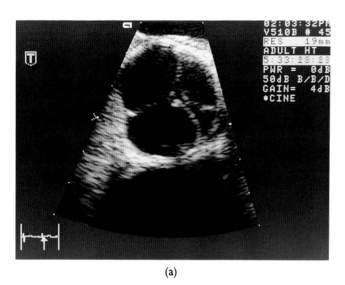

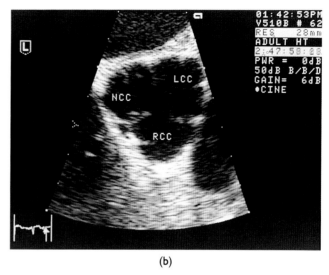

(a) (b)

Figure 3.71 (a) *A transverse plane transesophageal diastolic image of a normal tricuspid aortic valve. The individual aortic valve leaflets are indicated.* **(b)** *The corresponding longitudinal plane short axis image of a normal tricuspid aortic valve. The leaflets are marked as above. L = left coronary cusp, R = right coronary cusp, NC = non-coronary cusp.*

EVALUATION OF THE AORTIC VALVE

Transverse plane transesophageal imaging is a less than optimal technique with which to image the morphology and function of the aortic valve. Transverse plane imaging sections the aortic root and valve in an oblique plane. In the majority of patients, the three leaflets of the valve can be imaged but not in their same scan plane (7). However, by using a scanning technique, the three leaflets can be correctly identified and related to the corresponding aortic sinus (Fig. 3.71). Longitudinal plane imaging has been a major advance in the transesophageal evaluation of aortic valve morphology. Using a combination of both steering mechanisms, the left ventricular outflow tract, the aortic root and the ascending aorta can be sectioned in both their long and short axes. The long axis image of the aortic valve is of additional value in defining the motion of the valve leaflets, their thickness, the presence of any lesion on the valve leaflet (such as an infective vegetation), the presence of leaflet prolapse and (using colour flow mapping) the width of any aortic regurgitant jet within the left ventricular outflow tract.

The short axis image of the aortic valve is obtained using the longitudinal scanning plane and directing the transducer tip to the patient's left by using full rotation of the lateral tip steering mechanism. Using fine adjustments of the degree of lateral tip flexion and with modifications in the level of probe insertion, the aortic valve can be imaged in its true cross section in virtually every case. (This is only rarely possible using transverse plane scanning.) In this imaging plane (Fig. 3.72), the leaflet morphology, the commissures and the orifice area in systole are all well appreciated when there is no heavy calcification of the valve leaflets (11,12). In a haemodynamic multiplane transesophageal imaging correlative study, Hoffman *et al.* demonstrated excellent results for the use of the transesophageal imaging in planimetry of the stenotic orifice area (11). This technique should be of maximal value in the paediatric, adolescent or young adult patient in whom valve calcification is rarely a problem. In these patients, the optimal information on valve leaflet morphology, the cause of the stenosis, the valve orifice area and the suitability or nonsuitability of the valve for balloon dilatation may all be obtained from longitudinal plane transesophageal scanning. This technique may, in the future, become invaluable in assessing the feasibility of balloon valvuloplasty in the adolescent and young adult age group.

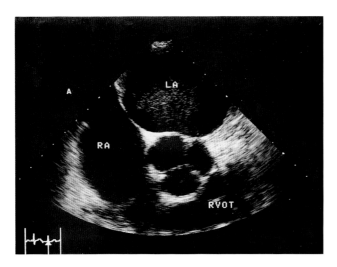 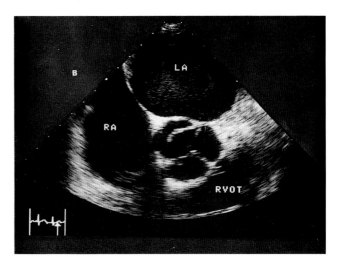

Figure 3.72 *A longitudinal plane transesophageal study from a patient with a structurally tricuspid aortic valve which is functionally bicuspid. In the left-hand panel taken in diastole, there are obviously three leaflets to the aortic valve. In early systole, only two of the leaflets are seen to open with complete fusion of the anterior commissure. Longitudinal plane imaging of the aortic valve is an excellent technique for defining both the morphology and effective orifice area of non-calcified aortic valves.*

Accurate estimation of the aortic valve gradient by continuous wave Doppler from within the oesophagus is rarely possible. However, in a few patients, the use of the esophageal longitudinal imaging plane may appear to allow excellent alignment of the interrogating Doppler beam to the transvalve jet visualised on colour flow imaging and, in these patients, the correct peak jet velocity may be obtained. This is the exception. In contrast, we have found the transgastric approach to be of value in determining the peak and mean transaortic gradient. From this transducer position, and by using transverse plane imaging with an integrated continuous wave Doppler capability, excellent alignment to transaortic flow can be obtained in the majority of paediatric patients (1). This is only to be expected as the transgastric transducer position used to interrogate the aortic valve is essentially the same as in the subcostal approach which is known to be excellent for use in gradient evaluation in children.

ASSESSMENT OF AORTIC REGURGITATION

Transesophageal echocardiography is limited in the evaluation of native valve aortic regurgitation. When there is calcification within the aortic valve,

flow masking may occur in the left ventricular outflow tract and severe aortic regurgitation may be missed. However, when the valve is non-calcified, excellent images of the regurgitant jet may be obtained (13). The regurgitant jet morphology may be imaged in both the transverse and longitudinal planes. The longitudinal plane short axis view of the aortic valve leaflets is of value in determining the precise site or sites of origin of the regurgitation. It is relatively easy to determine whether this is from the central orifice or is located in one or more of the commissures. This information may be of value in identifying patients to be considered for aortic valve repair. In addition, the longitudinal plane long axis view of the left ventricular outflow tract is the best transesophageal plane in which to image the aortic regurgitant jet. Colour M-mode studies in either transesophageal plane are of value in determining the relative jet area with regard to the total area of the left ventricular outflow tract. The jet dimensions should be measured as close as possible to the point of origin of the jet on the left ventricular aspect of the aortic valve.

Where the aortic valve is heavily calcified and there is flow masking within the left ventricular outflow tract, the transgastric imaging approach may provide additional information on the origin and severity of aortic regurgitation.

In summary, transesophageal echocardiography is only an adjunct to precordial echocardiography in the assessment of aortic regurgitation. Its main role is in defining the underlying cause of the regurgitation (i.e. discrete leaflet perforation etc.) rather than defining its severity. Precordial echocardiography, especially in patients with calcific aortic stenosis or aortic valve prostheses, remains a superior technique to transesophageal echocardiography in this respect.

REFERENCES

1. HOFFMAN P, STÜMPER OFW, RYDLEWSKA-SADOWSKA W, SUTHERLAND GR. Transgastric Imaging – a valuable addition to the assessment of congenital heart disease by transverse plane transoesophageal echocardiography. *J Am Soc Echo* 1993; **6**(1): 35–44.
2. EDWARDS JE. Pathology of left ventricular outflow obstruction. *Circulation* 1965; **31:** 586–99.
3. SUNG CS, PRICE EC, COOLEY DA. Discrete subaortic stenosis in adults. *Am J Cardiol* 1978; **42:** 283–90.
4. FREEDOM RM, PELECH A, BRAND A, et al. The progressive nature of subaortic stenosis in congenital heart disease. *Int J Cardiol* 1985; **8:** 137–43.
5. STÜMPER O, KAULITZ R, ELZENDA NJ, SREERAM N, HESS J, SUTHERLAND GR. Left ventricular outflow tract obstruction in infancy – improved diagnosis by paediatric transoesophageal echocardiography. *Int J Cardiol* 1990; **28:** 107–9.
6. MÜGGE A, DANIEL WG, WOLPERS HG, et al. Improved visualisation of discrete subvalvular aortic stenosis by transesophageal color-coded Doppler echocardiography. *Am J Cardiol* 1989; **117:** 474–5.
7. SUTHERLAND GR, ROELANDT JRTC, FRASER AG, ANDERSON RH. *Transesophageal echocardiography in clinical practice.* London: Gower Medical Publishing, 1991: 7.1–7.9.
8. SREERAM N, SUTHERLAND GR, BOGERS AJJC, STÜMPER O, HESS J, BOS E, QUAEGEBEUR JM. Subaortic obstruction: intraoperative echocardiography as an adjunct to operation. *Ann Thor Surg* 1990; **50:** 579–85.
9. WIDIMSKY P, FOLKERT J, CATE T, VLETTER W, VAN HERWERDEN L. Potential applications for transesophageal echocardiography in hypertrophic cardiomyopathies. *J Am Soc Echo* 1992; **5:** 163–7.
10. STENLEY TE, RANKIN JS. Idiopathic hypertrophic subaortic stenosis and ischemic mitral regurgitation: the value of intraoperative transesophageal echocardiography and Doppler color flow imaging in guiding operative therapy. *Anesthesiology* 1990; **72:** 1083–5.
11. HOFMANN T, KASPAR W, MEINERTZ T, et al. Determination of aortic valve orifice area in aortic valve stenosis by two-dimensional transesophageal echocardiography. *Am J Cardiol* 1987; **59:** 330–5.
12. CHANDRASEKERAN K, FOLEY R, WEINTRAUB A, et al. Evidence that transesophageal echocardiography can reliably and directly measure the aortic valve area in patients with aortic stenosis – a new application that is independent of LV function and does not require Doppler data (abstract). *J Am Coll Cardiol* 1991; **17:** 20.
13. SMITH MD, HARRISON M, PINTON R, et al. Regurgitant jet size by transesophageal compared with transthoracic Doppler color flow imaging. *Circulation* 1991; **83:** 79–86.

The right ventricular outflow tract and pulmonary arteries

O. Stümper and P. Hoffman

INTRODUCTION

Precordial cross-sectional echocardiography allows a detailed non-invasive assessment of right ventricular outflow tract obstruction in the vast majority of patients. In infants and young children a complete evaluation of this range of lesions can be performed from subcostal scan positions (1,2). However, this approach may be limited in the older child or adolescent and adult patients (3). Parasternal and suprasternal scan positions, used in the paediatric patient, can provide a detailed evaluation of the anatomy and function of the central pulmonary artery system. But again, this approach is frequently of limited value in the older patient with poor transthoracic ultrasound windows. The additional use of colour flow mapping techniques, finally, has contributed to a better understanding of pulmonary artery perfusion in children with complex pulmonary atresia (4). Nevertheless, in cases in whom diagnostic difficulties are encountered using ultrasound, angiocardiography remains the gold standard in the preoperative evaluation.

More recently, magnetic resonance imaging has been shown to provide very accurate morphologic insights into complex lesions involving the right ventricular outflow tract and the central pulmonary artery system (5,6). In addition, the technique has been reported to yield excellent results in the follow-up evaluation of palliative shunt procedures (7). Thus, magnetic resonance imaging can now be recommended as a first choice investigative technique for this spectrum of lesions in centres where facilities are readily available.

The transverse axis transesophageal ultrasound approach to lesions of the right ventricular outflow tract and the pulmonary arteries is prone to a multitude of difficulties and limitations. Firstly, transverse axis imaging of the right ventricular outflow tract produces short axis cuts. Thus, because of the failure to demonstrate the right ventricular outflow tract in its long axis, a detailed assessment of obstructive lesions is not feasible (Fig. 3.73). Secondly, the right ventricular outflow tract lies in the far field when assessed from within the oesophagus. Conclusively cross-sectional imaging is limited in terms of both penetration and resolution. Moreover, colour flow mapping and Doppler studies suffer from marked ultrasound attenuation. Thirdly, the trachea and the bronchial tree are interposed between the oesophagus and the central pulmonary artery system. Although the main pulmonary artery can be visualised in virtually every patient studied, as can be the proximal right pulmonary artery, the left pulmonary artery is most often not adequately visualised. In particular the mid section of this vessel is routinely hidden behind the left main bronchus, and only a distal segment will be visualised anterior to the descending aorta. These limitations are even more marked in the adolescent and adult patient. This is mainly related to the more cranial position of the pulmonary arteries relative to the bronchial tree in the older age group. In contrast, in patients with left atrial enlargement excellent images of the central pulmonary artery system can be obtained.

The recent addition of longitudinal plane transesophageal imaging has much improved the visualisation of the right ventricular outflow tract. It is now possible to assess the entire right ventricular

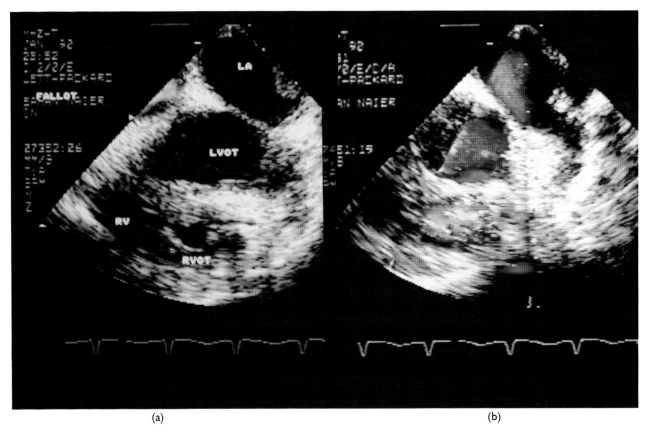

(a) (b)

Figure 3.73 *Transesophageal transverse axis study in a child with tetralogy of Fallot. From a scan plane through the right ventricular outflow tract (just above the superior margin of the ventricular septal defect) the outflow tract obstruction can be diagnosed both on (a) cross-sectional imaging and (b) colour flow mapping studies. Whereas the sagittal dimension of the outflow tract can be assessed, no information on the deviation of the outlet septum and the degree of aortic override is obtained. Doppler alignment to flow is poor.*

outflow tract, the pulmonary valve and the proximal portion of the main pulmonary artery on the same scan plane (8,9). Both branch pulmonary arteries are seen in cross-section, which in turn allows the accurate assessment of vessel diameters. In addition, the left pulmonary artery is generally better visualised by this technique.

In this chapter the transesophageal assessment of congenital lesions involving the right ventricular outflow tract, the pulmonary valve and the central pulmonary artery system will be outlined. In addition, the transesophageal ultrasound evaluation following palliative surgical procedures will be discussed.

RIGHT VENTRICULAR OUTFLOW TRACT OBSTRUCTION

The underlying morphologic substrates which cause this wide range of lesions include, firstly, hypertrophy of the septomarginal trabeculations of the right ventricle, secondly, a malorientation of the outlet or infundibular septum (as occurs classically in tetralogy of Fallot), and, thirdly, hypoplasia of the outlet portion of the right ventricle with its extreme represented by infundibular pulmonary atresia. Frequently valvar pulmonary stenosis or its extreme valvar atresia is associated with these lesions and will therefore be discussed here.

Mid-cavity right ventricular obstruction

When scanning transesophageal four-chamber views, the body of the right ventricle is readily demonstrated. From a low esophageal scan position the right ventricular apex is demonstrated. Obstructions within the cavity of the right ventricle are thus readily diagnosed on these views (Fig. 3.74). When compared with transthoracic ultrasound techniques

it is in particular an improved definition of the relationship of the tricuspid valve apparatus to these obstructive lesions which may warrant transesophageal studies prior to surgical correction. Involvement of the medial papilary muscle of the septal leaflet of the tricuspid valve will be readily identified and thus may alter the surgical approach.

Infundibular pulmonary stenosis

On transesophageal transverse axis imaging the right ventricular outflow tract is seen on scan planes which demonstrate the left ventricular outflow tract and the aortic root. It is visualised as an oval chamber since image orientation is in an almost oblique fashion. On slight withdrawal of the probe the pulmonary valve will be visualised lying to the left of the aortic valve. In children it is always possible to visualise the anterior free wall of the right ventricle. However, this may be difficult in the adult patient. The internal sagittal dimension of the outflow tract can be measured on routine imaging studies and an M-mode recording rapidly identifies changes in dimension during the cardiac cycle (see Fig. 3.73). Hypertrophic muscle bundles can be identified by this technique, as can hypertrophy of the anterior free wall. In addition, cross-sectional imaging can detect the presence of fibrous tissue layers, which are identified by their marked increase

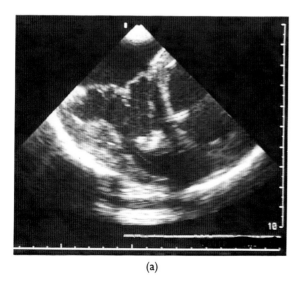

(a)

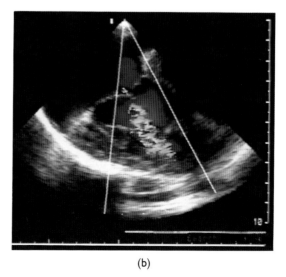

(b)

Figure 3.74 (a) and **(b)** *Mid-cavity right ventricular outflow obstruction taking the form of a double-chambered right ventricle. The attachment of the tricuspid valve and any involvement of the chordal apparatus in the obstruction is readily documented on low esophageal views. Alignment to flow patterns across the obstruction is excellent.*

in echogenicity. Although this information to be derived is of some value to the surgeon, and can sometimes be more detailed than that obtained by parasternal imaging, the transverse axis planes do not allow for a reliable assessment of the length of the obstruction (10). Moreover, colour flow mapping studies and Doppler interrogation are largely limited owing to poor alignment, the direction of flow being always perpendicular to the interrogating Doppler beam. It is only the advent of longitudinal axis imaging that has allowed the visualisation of the entire right ventricular outflow tract from within the oesophagus. This has provided a more detailed evaluation of this area than hitherto possible. However, alignment to the direction of blood flow remains unsatisfactory using the longitudinal plane.

In patients with tetralogy of Fallot the principal underlying lesion is an antero-superior deviation of the outlet septum. Whereas this was difficult to ascertain with the use of transverse axis imaging planes, it is now much better evaluated by the use of longitudinal imaging planes (Fig. 3.75). The deviated outlet septum is demonstrated together with the distal portion of the right ventricular outflow tract, and the actual chamber dimensions can be assessed. The relationship to the tricuspid valve and its chordal apparatus can be delineated as well as the relationship of the right ventricular outflow tract to the aortic root. This information contributes to the accurate planning of the surgical repair. Thus, with the provision of biplane imaging the transesophageal evaluation of this wide range of lesions is now much more rewarding and can be conducted with good results in patients in whom precordial and subcostal imaging is inadequate.

Recently, in patients with right ventricular outflow tract obstruction, we have developed a practice of expanded transgastric imaging, in an attempt to improve the demonstration of this spectrum of lesions. This technique involves a deep introduction of the transesophageal probe into the stomach. Following maximal anteflexion of the tip, the probe is then rotated in a clockwise fashion and is slightly withdrawn, so as to maintain contact between the transducer and the stomach wall. The images produced with such a technique closely resemble those obtained from the subxiphoid position used in standard transthoracic imaging (Fig. 3.76). The initial current experience with this technique suggests that a detailed insight into the morphology and the function of the right ventricular outflow tract can be obtained using transverse axis imaging on its own. Furthermore, transgastric imaging appears to be the only transesophageal technique which allows for a

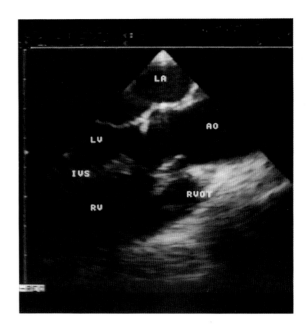

Figure 3.75 *Longitudinal plane imaging in a patient with tetralogy of Fallot. The morphology of the infundibular obstruction is clearly visualised, as is the relationship to the pulmonary valve. Using a sweep of longitudinal plane images, both the deviation of the outlet septum and the resulting aortic override can be documented.*

good alignment to flow within the right ventricular outflow tract, thus enabling the accurate calculation of pressure gradients. Clearly, this adjunct to standard transesophageal imaging is of major importance in patients with poor subcostal ultrasound windows, as in the majority of adolescent and adult patients.

Lesions frequently associated with tetralogy of Fallot are branch pulmonary artery stenosis, a persistent left superior caval vein, and coronary artery anomalies. Stenoses of the right pulmonary artery will be readily identified on both transverse and longitudinal axis imaging, as is the presence of a left persistent superior caval vein. However, proximal stenosis of the left pulmonary artery is frequently difficult to ascertain and in most cases cannot be definitely ruled out. Finally, our experience would suggest that it is currently not possible to exclude surgically important coronary artery anomalies (such as a conal branch artery arising from the right coronary artery) with any transesophageal imaging technique.

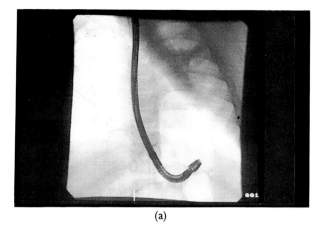

(a)

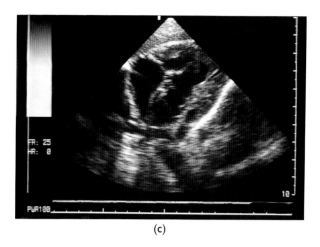

(c)

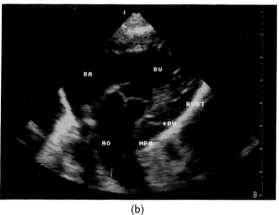

(b)

Figure 3.76 *Transgastric imaging in a patient with tetralogy of Fallot.* **(a)** *Gastric probe position and orientation.* **(b)** *The corresponding image documents the aortic override and the considerable narrowing of the right ventricular outflow tract.* **(c)** *Further counterclockwise rotation and tip angulation demonstrate the pulmonary artery bifurcation and a long segment of the right pulmonary artery.*

Valvar pulmonary stenosis

The pulmonary valve is commonly only poorly visualised by transverse axis imaging. In fact, the normal pulmonary valve leaflets are often not appreciated on routine scanning because of their thin structure and the considerable amount of ultrasound attenuation when examining more anterior cardiac structures from within the oesophagus. In cases with a thickened, fibrotic pulmonary valve, dense echos can be demonstrated in this area, but it remains virtually impossible to assess the precise morphology of either the valve cusps or their commissures (12). In contrast, pronounced doming of the pulmonary valve will seldom be missed by transverse axis imaging of adequate quality. Colour flow mapping studies will allow the determination of the level of obstruction; i.e. truly valvar or subvalvar. Only continuous wave or high pulse repetition Doppler studies can allow an estimation of the pressure gradient. However, alignment of the Doppler beam to blood flow remains poor in cases where marked tip angulation has to be used for adequate imaging.

Longitudinal plane transesophageal imaging provides an improved evaluation of this range of lesions. Only by using this technique will the anterior leaflet of the pulmonary valve be demonstrated. Doming of the pulmonary valve is readily visualised and valve motion can be observed. Nonetheless, far-field limitations persist, and, as pointed out above, the Doppler ultrasound evaluation of any valvar obstruction is limited because of continued poor alignment to the direction of blood flow.

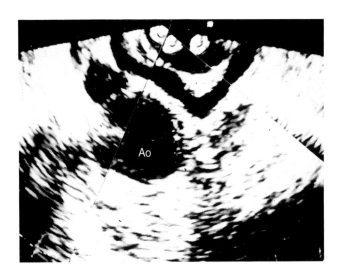

Figure 3.77 *Composite picture of the central pulmonary artery system in a child with pulmonary atresia, as assessed by a sequence of transverse axis transesophageal images. Note the absence of a patent right ventricular infundibulum.*

Pulmonary atresia

Although strictly speaking these lesions are anomalies of the ventriculo-arterial junction (Chapter 3.9), their close relation with the above mentioned entities permits their brief discussion in this chapter. The morphologic correlate of pulmonary atresia, whether with or without a ventricular septal defect, can be either complete atresia of the right ventricular outflow tract or, more rarely, an imperforate pulmonary valve. Transthoracic ultrasound is the diagnostic technique of first choice in infancy. Transesophageal imaging in these patients allows a good visualisation of the main central pulmonary arteries (Fig. 3.77) and can reliably document isolated valvar pulmonary atresia. This latter contribution of transesophageal ultrasound may be of benefit in the selection of patients for newer interventional catheter procedures, such as laser assisted balloon dilatation which can replace surgical valvotomy (13).

In the older child or adolescents and adult patient the main contribution of transesophageal imaging techniques would appear to lie in evaluation of the central pulmonary artery system. Nonetheless the exact role of transesophageal echocardiography in the assessment of these complex lesions is still ill-defined, and studies should only be undertaken in cases where the technique is likely to answer specific questions. Both angiocardiography and magnetic resonance imaging (5) are certainly superior to transesophageal ultrasound studies in the complete evaluation of patients with pulmonary atresia.

LESIONS OF THE PULMONARY ARTERIES

Transesophageal evaluation of the morphology of the central pulmonary artery system is limited by the interposition of the bronchial tree between the oesophagus and these structures. Whereas the right

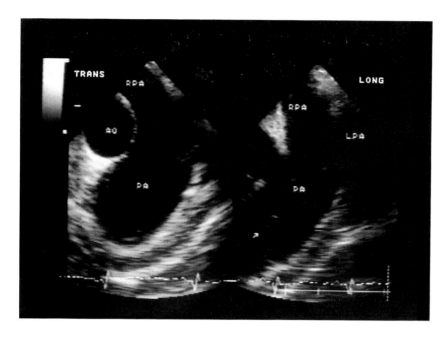

Figure 3.78 *Longitudinal axis imaging of the pulmonary artery bifurcation. In particular the proximal left pulmonary artery is better visualised than by transverse axis imaging, thus allowing for exclusion of proximal stenosis.*

pulmonary artery routinely can be scanned as far distally as its first bifurcation, this is not possible for the left pulmonary artery. The left aspect of the bifurcation of the main pulmonary artery is frequently difficult to visualise on transverse axis transesophageal imaging. Although the advent of longitudinal plane imaging has slightly decreased these limitations (Fig. 3.78), routine transesophageal studies, to date, cannot be recommended in the evaluation of suspected pulmonary artery pathology.

Stenotic lesions of the central pulmonary artery system can be identified by appropriate transesophageal studies. Stenoses of the right pulmonary artery and of the main pulmonary artery can be visualised on transverse axis imaging, and the underlying morphology can be defined. Transverse axis imaging of these lesions allows for optimal Doppler alignment to flow patterns distal to the obstruction and thus estimation of the obstructing gradient. The addition of longitudinal plane imaging allows an accurate determination of right pulmonary artery diameter at the site of obstruction and immediately proximal and distal to the obstruction. This could prove to be of value in the selection of patients who may benefit from subsequent stent placement for relief of the obstruction. Assessment of obstructive lesions of the left pulmonary artery is much more difficult using transesophageal imaging studies. On transverse axis imaging the proximal portion of this vessel is frequently inadequately

demonstrated. However, in our experience, visualisation of the distal portion of the left pulmonary artery as it passes just anterior to the descending aorta should be feasible in the vast majority of cases. Subsequent combined colour flow mapping and Doppler ultrasound studies then allow the reliable exclusion or the detection of left pulmonary artery stenosis. When longitudinal imaging equipment is available for study, a better visualisation of the anatomy of the proximal left pulmonary artery is frequently obtained.

Evaluation of pulmonary venous flow patterns of right and left sided pulmonary veins is often helpful in the assessment of branch pulmonary artery obstruction. The time velocity integral of pulmonary venous return from the obstructed artery is generally much reduced when compared with the contralateral lung. In our experience, the finding of almost equal pulmonary venous return from either lung (Fig. 3.79) excludes the presence of haemodynamically significant obstruction. The complete occlusion of one pulmonary artery can be diagnosed on the finding of only to and fro flow within the corresponding pulmonary vein.

In patients who had previously undergone banding of the pulmonary artery for the palliation of complex congenital heart disease with increased pulmonary blood flow, precordial evaluation of the distal main and the branch pulmonary arteries will often be hampered by the presence of dense fibrous tissue adhesions, precluding adequate imaging. In

In this respect, transesophageal ultrasound is frequently superior to precordial imaging. Nonetheless, it remains a technique with major limitations when compared to angiography or magnetic resonance imaging.

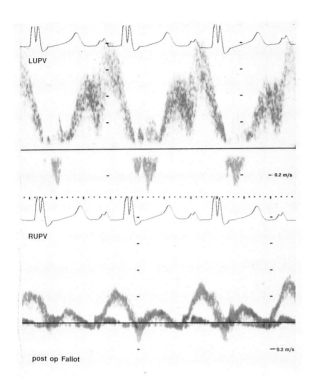

Figure 3.79 *Pulsed wave Doppler assessment of pulmonary venous flow profiles in a child following total correction of tetralogy of Fallot. The marked differences in pulmonary venous return from the left and the right lung reveal haemodynamically significant obstruction within the right pulmonary artery system.*

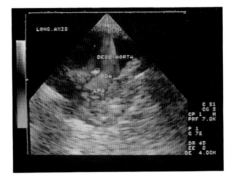

Figure 3.80 *Longitudinal plane colour flow mapping study in a patient with a large patent ductus arteriosus. Both the aortic and the pulmonary end of the duct are visualised.*

these instances transesophageal imaging is frequently extremely helpful in excluding any obstruction at the branching of the pulmonary arteries. Especially in patients with transposed great vessels, excellent image quality of this area is obtained by transverse axis imaging. This allows definition of the precise position of the band, and the exclusion or identification of any obstruction at the site of the bifurcation. High pulse repetition or continuous wave Doppler studies can reliably predict the resulting gradient across the band or at the orifice of one of the branch pulmonary arteries. In patients with pulmonary atresia the presence and the size of a confluent central pulmonary artery system can rapidly be identified, and the existence or absence of multiple stenoses can be confirmed (Fig. 3.78).

PATENT DUCTUS ARTERIOSUS

Determination of the precise morphology of a patent ductus arteriosus is of value in planning a transcatheter device closure. Precordial imaging is frequently limited in its ability to define the morphology and the length of the patent duct (14). In our experience, these limitations cannot be solved by the use of transesophageal imaging. The close relation of the patent duct to the trachea and to the left main bronchus precludes adequate transverse axis imaging in the vast majority of cases. On such scans only the aortic ampulla will be recognised. The duct itself, coursing above the left main bronchus and in front of the trachea, is not visualised. In addition its site of drainage into the pulmonary artery which is in most cases to the superior aspect and left to the pulmonary artery bifurcation, is hidden by the trachea. Moreover small ducts may be missed entirely both on transesophageal colour flow mapping and pulsed wave Doppler studies. Longitudinal plane imaging allows an improved visualisation of the duct together with its aortic and pulmonary end (Fig. 3.80). However, it is unlikely that even longitudinal plane imaging will visualise the duct in every case.

SYSTEMIC–PULMONARY SHUNTS

Transesophageal evaluation of systemic-pulmonary shunts is again limited because of the constraints imposed by the interposition of the bronchial tree. Especially in patients with longstanding Blalock-Taussig shunts there is frequently a cranial shift of the corresponding pulmonary artery, which in turn precludes an adequate visualisation of the anastomotic site on transverse axis imaging studies. Nonetheless, pulsed wave Doppler sampling within both the proximal and distal segments of the pulmonary artery allows an assessment of shunt function in the majority of patients studied. Such studies will reveal continuous flow patterns in the distal pulmonary arteries. The adjunct of pulsed Doppler interrogation of the pulmonary venous return allows the detection of obstructions or complete occlusion of the pulmonary artery distal to the shunt anastomosis. The problems encountered in direct shunt and anastomosis visualisation are markedly less in infants and young children, and transesophageal ultrasound studies have been reported to be useful in the evaluation of immediate shunt dysfunction in this particular age group (15).

The transesophageal ultrasound evaluation of Waterston shunts (ascending aorta to right pulmonary artery) is more rewarding and frequently allows an improved visualisation of shunt morphology and size when compared to transthoracic ultrasound studies. The dimensions of the anastomosis can be measured accurately by combined transverse and longitudinal plane imaging. The integrity of the proximal right pulmonary artery and the adequate peripheral run-off can be documented on combined imaging and colour flow mapping studies (Fig. 3.81). Our experience in the transeso-

phageal evaluation of other types of systemic-pulmonary shunt procedures is limited. However, it may be expected that the technique yields detailed information on the morphology and function of a Potts shunt (descending aorta to left pulmonary artery) which might occasionally still be encountered in the adolescent patient population.

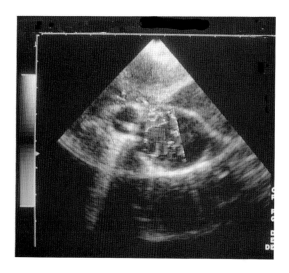

Figure 3.81 *Transverse axis colour flow mapping study in a child following a Waterston shunt. There is good shunt patency towards the right pulmonary artery, but complete occlusion towards the main pulmonary artery.*

SUMMARY

Transverse axis transesophageal imaging is limited in the assessment of congenital cardiac lesions involving the right ventricular outflow tract. It is only the addition of transgastric and longitudinal imaging planes that can allow the acquisition of detailed morphologic and haemodynamic information. The transesophageal evaluation of lesions involving the central pulmonary artery system is limited by the interposition of the bronchial tree between the oesophagus and the pulmonary arteries. Whereas the main and the right pulmonary arteries can be assessed in detail in all patients studied, this is not the case for the left pulmonary artery.

Currently transesophageal ultrasound studies are not indicated in patients with isolated congenital lesions of either the right ventricular outflow tract or the pulmonary arteries.

REFERENCES

1. SANDERS SP, BIERMAN FZ, WILLIAMS RG. Conotruncal malformations: diagnosis in infancy using sub-xiphoid 2-dimensional echocardiography. *Am J Cardiol* 1982; **50:** 1361–7.

2. SILOVE ED, DE GIOVANNI JV, SHIU MF, MYINT YI. Diagnosis and right ventricular outflow obstruction in infants by cross-sectional echocardiography. *Br Heart J* 1983; **50:** 416–20.

3. BANSAL RC, TAJIK AJ, SEWARD JB, OFFORD KP. Feasibility of detailed two-dimensional echocardiographic examination in adults. *Mayo Clin Proc* 1980; **55:** 291–308.

4. SMYLLIE J, SUTHERLAND GR, KEETON BR. The value of color flow mapping in determining pulmonary blood supply in infants with pulmonary atresia with ventricular septal defect. *J Am Coll Cardiol* 1989; **14:** 1759–65.

5. REES RSO, SOMERVILLE J, UNDERWOOD SR, WRIGHT J, FIRMIN DN, KLIPPSTEIN RH, LONGMORE DB. Magnetic resonance imaging of the pulmonary arteries and their systemic connections in pulmonary atresia: comparison with angiographic and surgical findings. *Br Heart J* 1987; **58:** 621–6.

6. WESLEY VICK G, ROKEY R, HUHTA JC, MULVAGH SL, JOHNSTON DL. Nuclear magnetic resonance imaging of the pulmonary arteries, subpulmonary region, and aorticopulmonary shunts: a comparative study with two-dimensional echocardiography and angiography. *Am Heart J* 1990; **119:** 1103–10.

7. JACOBSTEIN MD, FLETCHER BD, NELSON AD, GLAMPITT M, ALFIDI RJ, RIEMENSCHNEIDER TA. Magnetic resonance imaging: evaluation of palliative systemic-pulmonary artery shunts. *Circulation* 1977; **56:** 473–9.

8. STÜMPER O, FRASER AG, HO SY, *et al.* Transoesophageal echocardiography in the longitudinal axis: correlation between anatomy and images and its clinical implications. *Br Heart J* 1990; **64:** 282–8.

9. SEWARD JB, KHANDHERIA BK, EDWARDS WD, OH JK, FREEMAN WK, TAJIK AJ. Biplanar transesophageal echocardiography: anatomic correlations, image orientation, and clinical applications. *May Clin Proc* 1990; **65:** 1193–213.

10. STÜMPER O, ELZENGA NJ, HESS J, SUTHERLAND GR. Transesophageal echocardiography in children with congenital heart disease – an initial experience. *J Am Coll Cardiol* 1990; **16:** 433–41.

11. HOFFMAN P. Echocardiographic morphology of the heart from the gastric fundus: description of two new projections. *Kard Pol* 1991; **35:** 346–52.

12. STÜMPER O, WITSENBURG M, SUTHERLAND GR, CROMME-DIJKHUIS A, GODMAN MJ, HESS J. Transesophageal echocardiographic monitoring of interventional cardiac catheterization in children. *J Am Coll Cardiol* 1991; **15:** 1506–14.

13. QURESHI SA, ROSENTHAL E, TYNAN M, ANJOS R, BAKER EJ. Percutaneous laser assisted balloon pulmonary valve dilatation in pulmonary valve atresia. *J Am Coll Cardiol* 1991; **17:** 18A (abstract).

14. KRICHENKO A, BENSON LN, BURROWS P, MOES CAF, MCLAUGHLIN P, FREEDOM RM. Angiographic classification of the isolated, persistently patent ductus arteriosus and implications for percutaneous catheter occlusion. *Am J Cardiol* 1989; **62:** 1089–92.

15. KYO S, KOIKE K, TAKANAWA E, *et al.* Impact of transesophageal Doppler echocardiography on pediatric cardiac surgery. *Int J Card Imag* 1989; **4:** 41–2.

Ventriculo-arterial junction anomalies

O. Stümper

INTRODUCTION

Complex congenital cardiac defects are frequently associated with anomalies of the ventriculo-arterial junction. The ventriculo-arterial connection can be concordant, discordant, double-outlet or single-outlet (1). A schematic representation of the various types of ventriculo-arterial connections is given in Fig. 3.8.2. Although these lesions may be isolated, such as typically in complete transposition of the great arteries, they are frequently associated with other abnormalities, in particular in hearts with abnormal atrioventricular connections.

Because of the complexities of congenital lesions involving the ventriculo-arterial junction, the vast majority of patients will present in early infancy. The diagnosis of an abnormal ventriculo-arterial junction is normally made by precordial ultrasound studies (2,3). In fact, the clarity with which such lesions are documented by transthoracic imaging usually obviates the need for further preoperative diagnostic tests. It is only in the older child, the adolescent and the adult patient that transesophageal ultrasound studies may be indicated. In such patients the major contribution of the transesophageal approach lies in the exclusion or the definition of frequently associated lesions which may interfere with subsequent surgical correction, rather than in a detailed assessment of the ventriculo-arterial junction itself.

Using a sequence of high esophageal transverse axis scans, obtained by varying the level of probe insertion, the type of ventriculo-arterial connection can be determined by documenting the relation of the arterial trunks relative to the ventricular chambers. However, as transverse axis imaging rarely allows the simultaneous visualisation of both arterial valves and the crest of the ventricular septum in patients with a ventricular septal defect, definition of arterial override by this technique is unsatisfactory (4). The introduction of biplane imaging has to some extent overcome this problem. In fact, the use of the additional longitudinal plane appears to be a prerequisite in the detailed transesophageal evaluation of the ventriculo-arterial junction. Nonetheless, transthoracic ultrasound studies and angiography remain the diagnostic techniques of choice.

Discussion of the contribution of transesophageal imaging in the assessment of congenital anomalies of the ventriculo-arterial junction will be limited to (1) complete transposition and (2) double outlet of the right ventricle. The evaluation of congenitally corrected transposition has been described in detail in Chapter 3.4 and pulmonary atresia in Chapter 3.8. The remaining two lesions to be considered are truncus arteriosus, which is rarely seen beyond infancy, and double outlet of the left ventricle, an exceedingly rare lesion.

VA CONNECTIONS

concordant

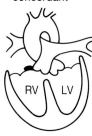

discordant

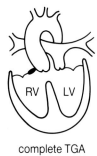

complete TGA

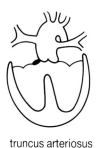

congenitally corrected TGA

double outlet

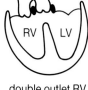

double outlet RV

single outlet

truncus arteriosus

Figure 3.82 *Diagram summarising the different types of ventriculo-arterial connections.*

COMPLETE TRANSPOSITION

Transesophageal studies will normally only be considered in the older child, in whom the intracardiac morphology has precluded surgical correction at an early age. The majority of such patients will have significant subpulmonary obstruction and a ventricular septal defect. In patients with subpulmonary obstruction and an intact ventricular septum, the obstruction is most often related to a combination of both a dynamic obstruction (due to bulging of the interventricular septum) and an organic or fixed obstruction caused by either a fibromuscular membrane or an abnormality of the mitral valve apparatus (Fig. 3.83). As discussed in Chapter 3.7, the transesophageal evaluation of this wide range of lesions which cause left ventricular outflow obstruction is frequently superior to transthoracic imaging. This is particularly true in older patients in whom the left ventricle has a rather banana shaped appearance, and thus may be difficult to visualise adequately from the chest wall. In patients with transposition of the great arteries in whom there is an associated ventricular septal defect, subpulmonary obstruction occurs in about one-third of the cases. The degree of obstruction in these cases tends to be more-severe and more complex than in cases with an intact ventricular septum. A commonly encountered form of obstruction includes a rather tunnel-like fibromuscular narrowing or muscular obstruction, which is caused by posterior deviation of the outlet septum. Using transesophageal ultrasound studies, such lesions can be differentiated with ease from other types of obstructions which are produced by abnormalities of the atrioventricular valves. In this latter category in particular two lesions are noteworthy: firstly, attachment of the anterior mitral valve leaflet to the muscular outlet septum, and, secondly, redundant tricuspid valve tissue which prolapses through the ventricular septal defect in systole (Fig. 3.84). Further atrioventricular valve abnormalities which may be encountered include dysplastic valves and chordal straddling (see Chapter 3.5). Although these latter lesions may not produce outflow obstruction, they may preclude surgical correction (5). The overall incidence of atrioventricular valve anomalies in patients with complete transposition is about 20%. Transthoracic ultrasound studies frequently may not identify these lesions in children beyond infancy (6). Thus, it is our current policy to perform transesophageal ultrasound studies to exclude such lesions in every child with complete transposition in whom surgical correction has been delayed.

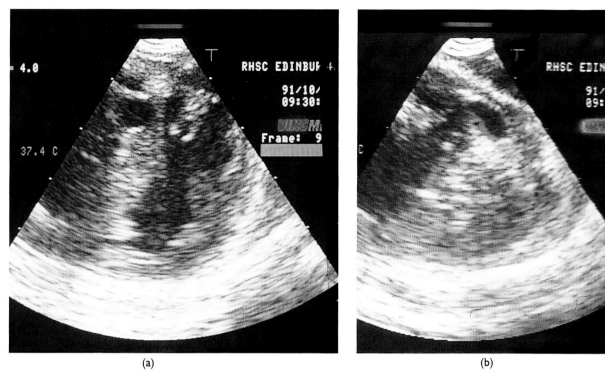

(a)   (b)

Figure 3.83 *Transesophageal ultrasound study in a child with complete transposition and left ventricular outflow obstruction.* **(a)** *on low four-chamber views, abnormal chordal implantation of the mitral valve is readily recognised.* **(b)** *More cranial scan positions allow definition of the subvalve area with evidence of a fibromuscular tunnel-like obstruction.*

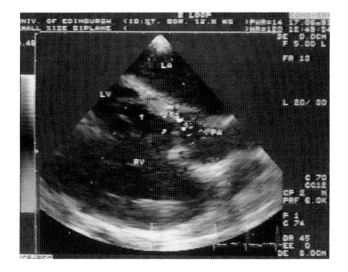

Figure 3.84 *Longitudinal plane image in a patient with complete transposition and left ventricular outflow obstruction caused by a redundant septal leaflet of the tricuspid valve, which prolapses through the ventricular septal defect.*

DOUBLE-OUTLET RIGHT VENTRICLE

In hearts in which both great arteries originate primarily from the right ventricle the haemodynamic disturbances, and thus the clinical picture, entirely depends on (1) the relation of the great arteries to one another and to the ventricular septal defect, and (2) the presence of subpulmonary or subaortic obstruction. At one end of the spectrum the haemodynamic situation may be similar to a tetralogy of Fallot, and at the other end it may be similar to complete transposition. Precordial ultrasound studies are the diagnostic technique of choice and normally allow a comprehensive assessment of the underlying morphology (7). Recently, magnetic resonance imaging has also been shown to be a most accurate imaging technique in the preoperative evaluation (8). Transverse axis transesophageal imaging in these patients allows a clear demonstration of the relation of the arterial trunks to one another. However, as indicated above, the technique does not allow definition of the degree of arterial override, as it is rarely able to delineate the relation of the great arteries to the crest of the ventricular septal defect (Fig. 3.85). Although the addition of expanded transgastric views as described in Chapter 3.8 did hold some promise for an improved definition of the ventriculo-arterial junction, this is not always the case. In fact, because of a lack of anatomic landmarks, transgastric imaging is often unable to clearly define the relation of the arterial trunks to the ventricular chambers. The major contribution of transgastric scan planes therefore lies in an improved alignment to flow patterns when using continuous wave Doppler interrogation in the quantification of outflow obstruction. The current experience with biplane imaging technology in the assessment of these complex lesions is still limited. However, it appears that again the additional longitudinal plane is a prerequisite in a detailed assessment of such lesions from within the esophagus.

As with the experience with transesophageal imaging in patients with complete transposition, the indications for studies in patients with double outlet of the right ventricle would appear to be only in the preoperative exclusion or detailed definition of either coexisting atrioventricular valve anomalies or left ventricular outflow obstruction. It is particularly important to exclude chordal straddling commonly associated with this group of lesions, as it normally precludes definitive surgical correction (9). The morphology of any coexisting posterior (left) ventricular outflow tract obstruction is usually well demonstrated on transverse axis imaging planes, whereas the definition of anterior (right) ventricular outflow obstruction is generally ill-defined by transesophageal imaging.

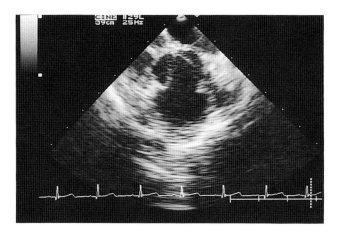

Figure 3.85 *Transverse axis image of the level of the ventriculo-arterial junction in a patient with double outlet from the right ventricle. The transverse plane does not allow definition of the degree of override and a detailed assessment of the relationship between the arterial trunks and the ventricular septal defect.*

REFERENCES

1. TYNAN MJ, BECKER AE, MACARTNEY FJ, QUERO-JIMENEZ M, SHINEBOURNE EA, ANDERSON RH. Nomenclature and classification of congenital heart disease. *Br Heart J* 1979; **41:** 544–53.

2. HENRY WL, MARON BJ, GRIFFITH JM. Cross-section echocardiography in the diagnosis of congenital heart disease: identification of the relation of the ventricles and the great arteries. *Circulation* 1977; **56:** 267–73.

3. HAGLER DJ, TAJIK AJ, SEWARD JB, MAIR DD, RITTER DG. Wide-angle two-dimensional echocardiographic profiles of conotruncal abnormalities. *Mayo Clin Proc* 1980; **55:** 73–82.

4. STÜMPER O, ELZENGA NJ, HESS J, SUTHERLAND GR. Transesophageal echocardiography in children with congenital heart disease – an initial experience. *J Am Coll Cardiol* 1990; **16:** 433–41.

5. HUHTA JC, EDWARDS WD, DANIELSON GK, FELDT RH. Abnormalities of the tricuspid valve in complete transposition of the great arteries with ventricular septal defect. *J Thorac Cardiovasc Surg* 1982; **83:** 569–76.

6. DASKALOPOULOS DA, EDWARDS WD, DISCROLL DJ, SEWARD JB, TAJIKAJ, HAGLER DJ. Correlation of two-dimensional echocardiographic and autopsy findings in complete transposition of the great arteries. *J Am Coll Cardiol* 1983; **2:** 1151–7.

7. MACARTNEY FJ, RIGBY ML, ANDERSON RH, STARK J, SILVERMAN NH. Double outlet right ventricle: cross-sectional echocardiographic findings, their anatomical explanation and surgical relevance. *Br Heart J* 1984; **52:** 164–77.

8. PARSONS JM, BAKER EJ, ANDERSON RH, et al. Double-outlet right ventricle: morphologic demonstration using magnetic resonance imaging. *J Am Coll Cardiol* 1991; **18:** 168–78.

9. RICE MJ, SEWARD JB, EDWARDS WE, et al. Straddling atrioventricular valve: two-dimensional echocardiographic diagnosis, classification and surgical implications. *Am J Cardiol* 1985; **55:** 505–13.

The coronary arteries and the thoracic aorta

G. R. Sutherland

TRANSTHORACIC IMAGING OF CORONARY ARTERIES

High-frequency transthoracic imaging will identify the aortic origin of both the left and right main coronary vessels in the majority of infants and children. In some cases, the bifurcation of the left main system into its anterior descending and circumflex branches can also be visualised. The remainder of the distal coronary tree is more difficult to visualise. Congenital abnormalities of the main coronary tree which can be visualised include (1) an intermural course of either main coronary artery, (2) a coronary artery which arises from an inappropriate sinus, (3) single origin of the whole coronary arterial system and (4) absence of the left main vessel with separate orifices from the left coronary sinus of the anterior descending and circumflex vessels. In addition, numerous reports have appeared on the role of transthoracic ultrasound in the identification of (1) an anomalous origin of the left coronary artery from the pulmonary trunk or (2) coronary artery fistulae. The role of transthoracic ultrasound in the investigation of acquired lesions of the coronary arteries in Kawasaki's disease have also been much studied. The role of either transthoracic or transesophageal imaging in the evaluation of coronary atherosclerosis and its sequelae is outwith the remit of this chapter.

As with other lesions, the ability of transthoracic imaging to confirm a morphologic diagnosis is to a large extent related to patient age, weight and the presence of an adequate ultrasound window.

Accurate visualisation of the coronary arteries and their anomalies is dependent on 5.0 or 7.0 mHz imaging. Lower imaging frequencies are often inadequate to define these relatively small structures. Thus an alternative high-frequency imaging window such as transesophageal echocardiography could be of benefit in certain clinical situations.

TRANSESOPHAGEAL IMAGING OF THE NORMAL CORONARY VESSELS AND THEIR MORPHOLOGIC VARIANTS

In adult patients, the origin of the two main coronary arteries can be imaged from the oesophagus in a significant number of patients (1–8). Using *transverse* plane imaging, the left main stem will be imaged in 90–95% of patients, the proximal anterior descending in some 75–80% and the proximal circumflex in some 80–85% (Fig. 3.86). The origin of the right coronary artery is much more difficult to visualise. This will be imaged in some 40–50% of adult patients with normal right-heart pressures and flows but may be imaged in a much higher percentage when either right ventricular pressure or volume flow is increased. The distal coronary vessels will not be imaged at all. In our experience at Edinburgh, the addition of *longitudinal* plane imaging has not added significantly to the visualisation of the proximal coronary arteries.

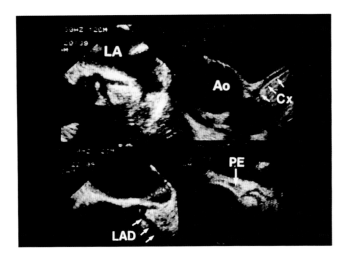

Figure 3.86 *A composite transverse plane transesophageal image of a normal left coronary arterial system. In the upper left panel, the left main vessel is seen to take origin from the aortic root and to divide into the circumflex and anterior descending vessels. In the upper right panel, the transducer has been rotated to image the proximal circumflex coronary artery (arrowed). In the lower left panel, the transducer has been angled to image the proximal anterior descending vessel prior to the first diagonal branch. In the lower right panel, the anterior descending can be seen to divide into two vessels, the first being the proximal diagonal and the second being the first septal perforator. Care must be taken in all these studies not to misinterpretate a small pericardial effusion for a coronary vessel (PE = pericardial effusion).*

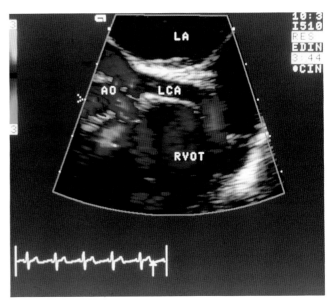

Figure 3.87 *A normal colour flow mapping image of flow within the left main coronary artery (LCA).*

However, on occasion, the origin of the right main vessel may be seen using the longitudinal plane whereas it had been missed using transverse plane scanning.

In infants and children, transesophageal image quality is less good than that acquired in the adult. To date, no large prospective series has been reported which has investigated the frequency with which normal coronary anatomy may be identified, but it is our impression that the figures would be similar for those reported for adults (see above). Similarly, no series has reported on the comparative values of precordial and transesophageal imaging in identifying coronary artery abnormalities in the paediatric age group.

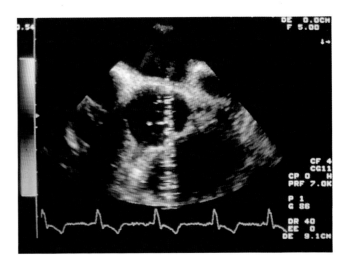

Figure 3.88 *A transverse plane transesophageal image from a patient with a normal right coronary artery demonstrating flow within the proximal vessel.*

THE TECHNIQUE USED TO VISUALISE THE PROXIMAL CORONARY ARTERIES

Transverse plane imaging should be used. The probe should be inserted to the level at which the aortic valve is imaged in an oblique cross-section. The probe should then be slowly withdrawn to image the aortic sinuses. Because of the obliquity of the sectioning plane and the orientation of the

right and left coronary sinus to this plane, the proximal left coronary system will almost always be imaged (Fig. 3.86) whereas the proximal right is less often seen (see above). To image the complete proximal left system, the probe may have to be rotated to the left and minor modifications in both antero-posterior and lateral steering may have to be made to allow a complete scan of the proximal vessels. Using such a scanning technique, the origin of the left main vessel will be seen arising from the left coronary sinus. The left main stem may be of variable length prior to its bifurcation into its anterior descending and circumflex branches. The anterior descending artery can then be imaged over a short course until its first major branch (the diagonal or first septal). The circumflex artery can normally be imaged over a greater distance (sometimes as far as the lateral aspect of the heart) until it passes immediately below the left atrial appendage. The circumflex artery may then be followed further laterally (in cross-section) by switching to the longitudinal plane.

Having imaged the proximal left system, the proximal right coronary artery should now be sought. The transducer should be orientated towards the right and the right coronary sinus scanned to identify the origin of this vessel. As indicated above, this may not be visualised in a high proportion of cases. The addition of colour Doppler imaging is an adjunct to the visualisation of the proximal coronary vessels (Figs 3.87 and 3.88) (6,7). With appropriate velocity settings, flow in the majority of normal vessels will appear laminar throughout the whole proximal coronary tree. However, areas of turbulence may be encoded in normal vessels as well as in vessels with regional stenoses. Pulsed Doppler may also be used to determine the velocity waveform within the vessels (Fig. 3.89). This is of most value in interrogating anterior descending flow as this vessel is virtually parallel to the insonnating beam.

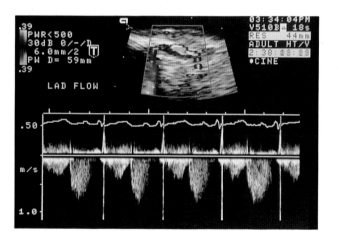

Figure 3.89 *A transverse plane transesophageal colour flow mapping image with a pulsed Doppler study of normal flow in the left anterior descending coronary artery. Note that flow is both in systole and diastole with the majority of flow occurring in diastole.*

Morphologic variants

As yet, there is little published data on the accuracy with which transesophageal imaging can identify morphologic variants of coronary artery anatomy. However it has been our experience that such variants as (1) absence of the left main stem with separate sinus orifices of the anterior descending and circumflex, (2) origin of a main coronary artery from an abnormal sinus, and (3) an intramural course of a coronary artery, can all be reliably identified. More complex distal morphologic variants cannot be visualised from the oesophagus.

CORONARY ARTERY FISTULAE

A coronary artery fistula is a rare disorder (normally congenital but may be acquired) characterised by a communication between a coronary artery and a cardiac chamber. Although rare, they are still the most common of coronary artery anomalies (9). Fistulae may arise from the right coronary system (60%), or left coronary system, or may have multiple origins (10). Drainage will be to right ventricle in 41%, to right atrium in 26%, to pulmonary artery in 12%, to left ventricle in 3%, and to superior vena cava in 1% (9). They tend to enlarge with time, but spontaneous closure has occasionally been reported (11,12). The occurrence of symptoms will depend on the magnitude of the shunt, the chamber into which the fistula drains, and whether myocardial ischaemia occurs due to coronary 'steal' (13). Coronary artery fistulae may be associated with other congenital anomalies of the heart.

Traditionally fistulae have been diagnosed by coronary angiography. However, the difficulty in the identification of the chamber(s) of drainage is an important limitation of the angiographic technique. Transthoracic 2-D-echo combined with pulsed Doppler and colour flow imaging have been found useful in: (i) identifying a coronary artery fistula as the cause of a continuous murmur (14); (ii) in defining the origin, course and site of drainage of the fistulae (15), and (iii) in assessing their surgical closure (15,16). However, limitations both in patient echogenicity and in the spatial resolution of transthoracic imaging (8) create difficulties when trying to detect small shunts (15), or the sites of drainage (16).

There have been a few isolated reports on the use of transesophageal imaging in the detection of coronary fistulae (17–23) which suggest that the esophageal approach might offer a better identification of the origin, course and chamber of drainage of the fistulous vessel. This may be particularly true with the use of biplane probes (20).

During the past five years, we have studied 15 patients with coronary artery fistulae using transesophageal echocardiography (24) and have compared the findings at this study with both the results of precordial ultrasound imaging and selective coronary angiography. Of the 15 patients, 12 were adults and three were children. Eleven had single plane transesophageal studies and four had biplane studies. The morphology of the fistulae studied included: 2 left main → pulmonary artery; 2 left main → left atrium; 2 circumflex → left atrium; 2 circumflex → pulmonary artery; 1 circumflex- 1f coronary sinus; 1 anterior descending → pulmonary artery; 1 right coronary → left atrium; 1 right coronary → right ventricle; 1 right coronary → right atrium; and 2 right coronary → neo-left atrium (both in post-Fontan patients). All had had prior precordial echo studies and 11 had had prior cardiac catheterisation. In 8 cases, the diagnosis of a coronary fistula was known prior to the transesophageal study and, in 7, was made only by TEE. In 5/8 cases in whom prior coronary angiography had demonstrated a fistulous communication, the precise drainage site(s) had not been well defined. In only 3 cases could esophageal imaging define the entire course of the fistulous vessel and define its drainage site. In contrast, colour flow mapping could correctly (correlative angiography – 8 pts, correlative surgery – 4 pts) demonstrate the turbulent flow associated with the exit point(s) of the fistula in all 15 (multiple sites in 3). In 2 cases, (1 left main → left atrium, 1 right main → left atrium) there was a large atrial sized chamber interposed between the two normal atria through which fistula flow occurred. In one case, this cavity was partially thrombosed. Transesophageal pulsed Doppler studies defined three basic patterns of fistula exit flow which were related to fistula size: (1) continuous flow with a dominant diastolic phase (large fistulae); (2) continuous flow with a dominant systolic phase (moderate fistulae); and (3) flow only in systole (filamentous end stage connections). In summary, the combination of coronary angiography and transesophageal colour flow imaging would appear to offer the optimal combination for the complete preoperative evaluation of a coronary fistula. Transesophageal echo alone may be of value in monitoring in real-time intraoperative or coil embolisation closure.

When using the transesophageal approach to study a patient with a suspected coronary artery fistula, the initial step should be to examine the relative dimensions of the proximal coronary arteries. Where either the left or right coronary arterial system is involved in a haemodynamically significant fistulous communication, the respective proximal coronary arterial tree will show marked vessel dilatation (Fig. 3.90). Conversely, the proximal arterial tree may remain entirely normal in size in cases where the fistulous shunt is small and peripheral. Where the origin of the fistulous communication is from the proximal coronary arteries the proximal segment of the fistulous vessel itself can normally be visualised (Fig. 3.90). However, it is rare to be able to follow the course of this vessel. More distal points of origin will not be visualised. Once the origin has been determined, all the cardiac chambers should then be interrogated to determine the exit point(s). A combination of imaging, colour Doppler and pulsed Doppler modalities should be used (Fig. 3.91). The fistulous vessel may exit into one of the four cardiac chambers, into one of the great veins (including coronary sinus (Fig. 3.90)) or into an accessory chamber (Fig. 3.92) interposed between the atria. The flow exiting from the fistula may be turbulent and of relatively high velocity or may be laminar. The precise nature of the exiting flow is dependent on both the size of the shunt and the degree of restriction at the exit point. As indicated above, the pulsed Doppler velocity waveform of the exit flow can be used as a semiquantitative guide to volume flow. In all cases, a detailed study should be carried out to exclude multiple drainage sites. In rare cases, the fistulous vessel will not arise from the normal native coronary circulation but will be an accessory vessel arising from the aortic root (Fig. 3.93).

In summary, our experience has indicated that the combination of transesophageal imaging and selective coronary angiography (to define the course of the fistulous vessel) would appear to offer the optimal combination for the complete evaluation of a coronary artery fistula. Transesophageal imaging would appear to be of value in monitoring successful surgical closure. It may also have a future role in the real-time monitoring of coil embolisation of appropriate fistulae. It is likely that either bi- or multiplane imaging will prove superior to single transverse plane imaging in this regard.

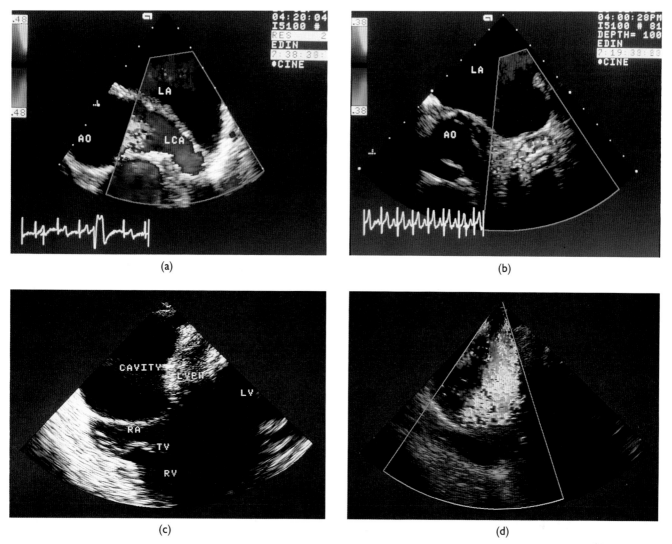

Figure 3.90 *A composite series of images from a transverse plane transesophageal study from a patient with a large circumflex coronary artery to coronary sinus fistula. (a) demonstrates marked dilatation of the left main coronary artery (LCA). (b) demonstrates the fistulous vessel arising from the circumflex coronary artery. The flow in this vessel is turbulent. (c) is a transverse plane posterior four-chamber view demonstrating a large cavity in the place where the coronary sinus would be expected. The right atrium is compressed by this fistulous expansion. (d) demonstrates the turbulent flow from the fistulous vessel entering the grossly enlarged coronary sinus.*

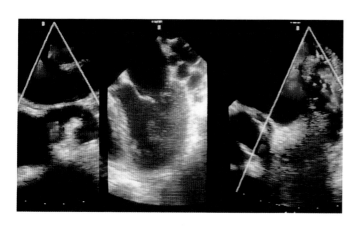

Figure 3.91 *A transverse plane transesophageal study from a patient with a circumflex coronary artery to left atrial fistula. The left-hand image demonstrates the dilated left main and circumflex coronary arteries and the origin of the large fistulous vessel. The middle panel demonstrates the fistula cut in multiple cross sections lying laterally in the left atrioventricular groove. The right-hand image is a colour flow map demonstrating laminar flow from the fistula into the left atrium.*

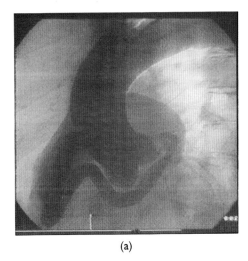

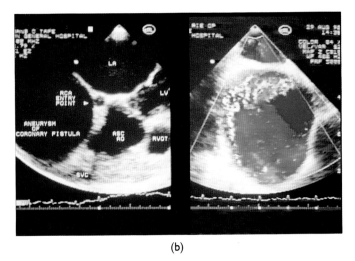

(a)

(b)

Figure 3.92 (a) *is an aortogram shown in the anteroposterior projection from a patient with a right coronary artery to right atrial fistula. The fistulous vessel is seen to enter a large atrial-size cavity lying posterior to the aortic root.* **(b)** *demonstrates the transverse plane transesophageal study from the same patient. In the left-hand image, the entry point of the right coronary artery fistula into the coronary artery aneurysm is seen. The aneurysmal chamber is placed between the left atrium and the superior vena cava. In the right-hand panel, the flow exiting from the right coronary artery into the aneurysmal chamber is well seen. This chamber then demonstrated flow draining to the right atrium.*

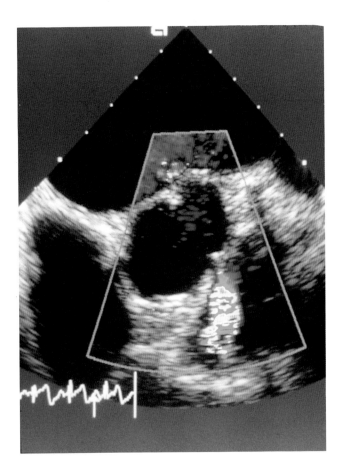

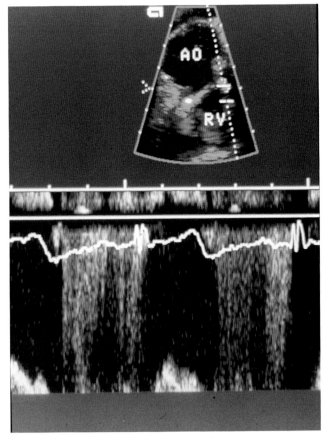

Figure 3.93 *A transverse plane transesophageal study from a patient who has a direct aortic root RVOT coronary fistula. This vessel was anomalous coronary artery not arising from either the right or the left native circulations. In the right-hand panel, the pulsed Doppler study is seen which demonstrates flow into the right ventricular outflow tract in diastole only.*

ANOMALOUS ORIGIN OF A CORONARY ARTERY

Anomalous origin of the left coronary artery from the pulmonary artery is usually identified during the first few weeks or months of life and rarely presents in the older child or adult. Transthoracic ultrasound imaging will normally identify the abnormal origin of the coronary artery from the pulmonary trunk, and colour flow mapping will define the flow exiting from the left main system into the main pulmonary artery. In some cases, doubt may arise about the diagnosis and further investigation may be required. Transesophageal imaging (especially using a bi- or multiplane approach) can identify such abnormal communications, but reports have been limited and the problems inherent in consistently diagnosing this anomaly by transesophageal imaging have not been defined. It is likely that selective coronary angiography will always remain a superior diagnostic technique in this patient group.

THE CORONARY ARTERIES IN TRANSPOSITION OF THE GREAT ARTERIES

The role of transesophageal imaging in the evaluation of anomalies of the coronary arteries prior to an arterial switch procedure and the subsequent evaluation of the surgically reimplanted coronary arteries is discussed in Chapter 4.1.

KAWASAKI'S DISEASE

As with the congenital coronary lesions discussed above, transesophageal imaging has both benefits and limitations when used to investigate the progression of the coronary artery lesions in this disease. The proximal aneurysms within the coronary arterial tree can be imaged and their expansion monitored, as can the development of thrombus within them. However, peripheral lesions cannot be imaged. Coronary angiography remains the investigation of choice in this condition.

CONGENITAL LESIONS OF THE THORACIC AORTA

Transthoracic imaging is limited in its ability to image the whole of the thoracic aorta. In all patients, the immediate supravalvar portion of the ascending aorta is normally well imaged from the precordial approach. In infants and small children, a combination of precordial and subcostal imaging may visualise the majority of the ascending aorta but there usually remains a blind spot in the upper third of the ascending aorta. By using the suprasternal ultrasound window, this blind spot is often overcome but this is not always the case. Suprasternal imaging can visualise the entire aortic arch and the origins of individual head and neck vessels in virtually all young children. This is frequently not the case in the older child and adult. The upper descending aorta to below the level at which the arterial duct takes origin will also be well visualised. The lower half of the descending thoracic aorta is rarely seen from the suprasternal approach but may be visualised in some children from a high lateral precordial position (in both its long and short axes) and from a subcostal position. In the older child and adolescent, this is normally impossible. Using a combination of both colour flow mapping and pulsed Doppler studies, haemodynamic lesions in the aorta can be characterised(25). What then is the role of transesophageal imaging in congenital lesions of the thoracic aorta? This section will deal both with the pathologic changes in the thoracic aorta associated with Marfan's syndrome and with the spectrum of abnormalities associated with coarctation of the aorta. The subject of vascular rings will not be discussed as the investigation of such anomalies in our opinion is outwith the diagnostic capability of transesophageal imaging. Such vascular rings are far better investigated by either CT or MRI imaging or by appropriate angiographic techniques.

The normal thoracic aorta

Transverse plane transesophageal echocardiography can produce excellent images of most of the intrathoracic course of the aorta. The only limitation is that it is impossible to obtain images of the upper half of the ascending aorta and the proximal third of the aortic arch because of the interposition of the trachea between these structures and the esophagus.

A scan of the aorta should be commenced by identifying the ascending aorta just above the aortic valve. It should then be followed superiorly by slowly withdrawing the probe until images are lost once the transducer is above the level of the carina. In patients with annuloaortic ectasia or a tortuous proximal aortic root, the initially more horizontal and rightward course of the aorta than normal allows the proximal portion of the ascending aorta to be seen, together with the aortic valve, in a standard basal view, with some added flexion of the tip of the probe.

The descending thoracic aorta and the oesophagus are closely related. The upper descending aorta is lateral to the oesophagus but the two structures coil around each other so that the aorta lies more posterior to the oesophagus at the level of the diaphragm. It is very easy to scan the whole course of the descending thoracic aorta in the transverse plane if it is first identified by rotating the probe in an anticlockwise direction from a position high in the stomach. The aorta can be imaged for a short distance below the diaphragm, and then kept in view by slowly rotating the probe as it is withdrawn. Once the upper descending thoracic aorta is reached, the lumen of the aorta broadens out into the distal part of the transverse aortic arch. In order to image as much of the arch as possible, the tip of the probe should then be extended and rotated in a clockwise direction. Occasionally, the brachiocephalic vein can be identified in front of the aorta. The demonstration of continuous laminar flow at low velocity confirms that this structure is a vein rather than, for example, a false lumen in a patient with aortic dissection.

Longitudinal plane (or multiplane) scanning has added to the ability of transesophageal echo to visualise virtually all the thoracic aorta. Appropriate use of the longitudinal plane will reduce the size of the 'blind area' in the upper ascending aorta and in some patients may eliminate it altogether. However, in the majority of older children and adults, a small 'blind area' in the upper ascending aorta will persist. Longitudinal plane scanning offers new information on the normal descending aorta but may allow a better evaluation of the arterial duct or on the origin of descending aortic collateral vessels in patients with complex pulmonary atresia. In congenital heart disease, the aorta may be within the left or right chest. In both positions, biplane scanning can be used with equal effectiveness to image the aorta.

An alternative approach to imaging the whole of the ascending aorta is to use the transgastric window. In some cases where the esophageal window is limited, the whole of the ascending aorta

and the arch may be visualised from the sub-costal window using bi- or multiplane probe. This manoeuvre is often possible in smaller children.

The aorta in Marfan's syndrome

The widespread changes in the blood vessels and cardiac valves associated with Marfan's syndrome are most commonly expressed in changes in the ascending thoracic aortic walls. The process of cystic medial necrosis results in aneurysmal dilatation of the aortic root (both the valve ring and sinuses), the ascending aorta and the aortic arch. Dilatation of the ascending aorta most commonly is first expressed in the intrapericardial portion with the initial feature being dilatation of the sinuses of Valsalva (Fig. 3.94). These changes predispose to the formation of dissecting aneurysms. Both the descending thoracic aorta and abdominal aorta may demonstrate similar changes with resultant dissection of the vessel walls but this is much rarer.

Precordial ultrasound imaging is a valuable technique in imaging the morphologic changes in the proximal aorta associated with Marfan's syndrome. Aortic valve abnormalities, dilatation of the aortic root and proximal dissections within the ascending aorta can all be imaged with relative ease within the younger paediatric population. However, the majority of aortic dissections occur in the adolescent and adult age group where precordial imaging of the whole ascending aorta is at best difficult. That is not to say that the accurate identification of complex aortic dissections using the precordial approach is impossible.

Transesophageal imaging has been shown to be a major advance in the diagnosis and definition of aortic pathology in adult patients (26,27). The main area of benefit has been in the study of aortic dissection (28–33). In both de Bakey type I and III dissections, it has been demonstrated to have a diagnostic sensitivity and specificity approaching 100%. It is only in de Bakey type II dissections which are localised to the upper ascending aorta that there are diagnostic difficulties due to the transesophageal 'blind-spot'. These diagnostic difficulties have not been wholly overcome by the introduction of bi- or multiplane scanning. To diagnose an aortic dissection, the intimal flap must be identified within the aortic lumen as must its origin and its extension within the thoracic aorta. Of less relevance is the identification of the entry and exit tears and the definition of the flow profiles in the true and false lumens. Where the aortic root is involved (as will be the case in virtually all patients with Marfan's

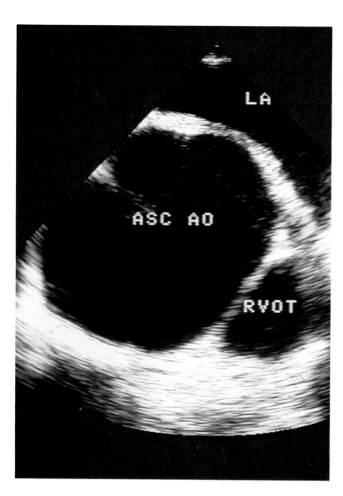 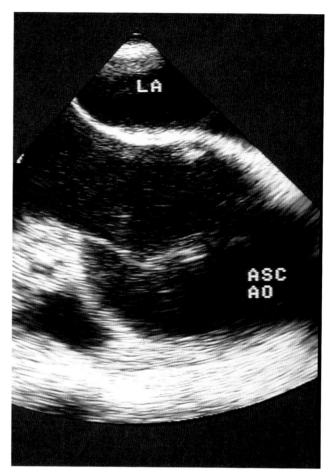

Figure 3.94 *A biplane transesophageal study from a patient with Marfan's Syndrome and a dilated aortic root but no dissection. In the left-hand panel, the transverse plane image is seen demonstrating the cross-sectional dimension of the aorta. In the right-hand panel, the longitudinal plane demonstrates the dilatation to involve the first 5 cm of the ascending aorta with the upper ascending aortic lumen being normal in dimension.*

syndrome), the proximity to or involvement of the intimal flap with the coronary orifices must be determined as must the mechanism for and the degree of aortic valve incompetence. Aortic root rupture with bleeding into the pericardial sac must also be excluded. Single or biplane transesophageal imaging can identify all these complications with ease and accuracy. The longitudinal plane is of special value in identifying any acute anterior dilatation of the aortic sinuses (Fig. 3.95). The transverse plane is the optimal approach to identifying coronary ostial involvement. Both planes are required to provide an optimal assessment of aortic valve pathophysiology. In every case, the aortic arch and descending aorta must be carefully evaluated to identify the distal extent of the dissection and to exclude any second discrete area of dissection (Figs 3.96–3.98). With such a scanning technique, it has been our experience that transesophageal imaging can accurately define the aortic abnormalities in Marfan's syndrome in both the paediatric and adult age groups. Its precise clinical role versus either CT or MRI scanning remains to be assessed, but in the future a logical appraisal may lead to the use of transesophageal imaging as the technique of choice where an acute dissection is suspected (time here is often of the essence) and MRI as the preferred technique when the dissection is known or suspected to be chronic or where follow-up studies are being carried out. Angiography would now appear to have little role to play in the investigation of such patients.

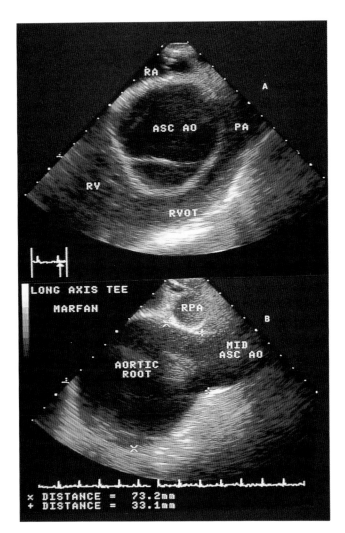

Figure 3.95 *A biplane transesophageal study from a patient with Marfan's Syndrome and an acute dissection of the ascending aorta. The dissection flap is best visualised in the transverse plane (upper panel) while the anterior aortic root and proximal ascending aortic dilatation was best imaged in the longitudinal plane (lower panel).*

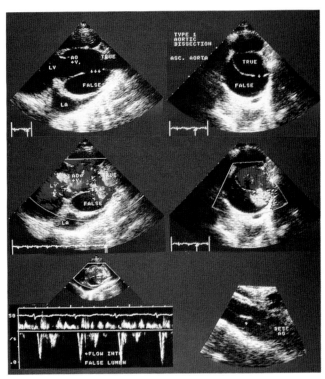

Figure 3.96 *A transverse plane transesophageal study from a patient with a type III aortic dissection. The three images in the right-hand panel demonstrate a scan of the descending aorta with the dissection flap clearly extending throughout the width of the thoracic aorta. The entry point (arrowed) is well seen in the upper right-hand image.*

Pitfalls in the transesophageal diagnosis of aortic dissection must be avoided. The most common of these is the presence of linear or curvilinear reduplication echoes within the aortic lumen which mimic dissection flaps. These echoes are most commonly reduplications of strong echoes within the aortic wall due to the deposition of calcium within athersclerotic plaques. It has been our experience that these reduplication echoes do not pose a problem to the experienced operator. A very useful rule-of-thumb is that if the investigator is not 100% certain that an intraluminal echo is a dissection flap then it is an artefact.

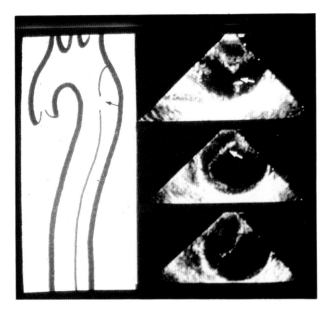

Figure 3.97 *A composite series of images from a patient with Marfan's Syndrome who had an old type III dissection and an acute type 1. The dissection flap can be seen to extend from the aortic root to the descending aorta.*

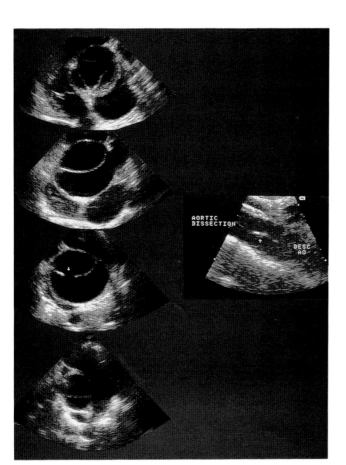

Figure 3.98 *A transverse plane transesophageal study of the ascending aorta in a patient with Marfan's Syndrome and a type 1 dissection.*

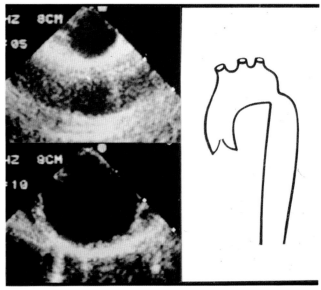

Figure 3.99 *A transverse plane transesophageal study from a patient with a localised aortic coarctation. In the upper panel, the descending aortic lumen at the site of the coarctation is seen to be 1.2 cm in diameter compared to the descending aortic dimension in the lower image (2.4 cm) measured just above the level of the diaphragm.*

AORTIC COARCTATION

Transesophageal imaging using either single transverse plane or multiplane imaging can reliably identify the majority of simple coarctations of the descending aorta. To scan the descending aorta, the transverse plane probe should be positioned so that the descending aorta is imaged in cross-section just above the diaphragm. The probe should then be gradually withdrawn to image the aortic dimen-sions at a series of levels (in adults at 1 cm intervals) until the aortic arch is reached. A discrete aortic coarctation will normally be positioned just below the aortic arch opposite to the origin of the left subclavian artery. This will be recognised as an area of discrete narrowing on cross-sectional imaging with a variable area of pre-coarctation hypoplasia and a variable area of post-coarctation aortic dila-tation (Fig. 3.99). If the coarctation is severe and collateral vessels supplying the descending aorta lie in close proximity to the coarcted segment, then these may be imaged as relatively small vessels in close proximity to the aorta and lying laterally to it. Initial studies which have studied the lumen di-mensions of the aorta in patients with coarctation and which have compared the findings of transeso-phageal imaging, intravascular ultrasound and cine-angiography have confirmed that transesophageal imaging can accurately determine the correct in-ternal lumen dimensions in simple coarctations.

Longitudinal or multiplane imaging have added new information in the assessment of descending aortic coarctations. Whereas the transverse plane technique can identify the minimal lumen diameter, longitudinal or multiplane imaging can determine the length and morphology of the coarctation segment in its longitudinal axis. However, neither imaging approach will allow the correct alignment of the integrated continuous wave Doppler beams to flow across the coarctation and thus coarctation gradient estimation is precluded. Furthermore, it has been our experience that in complex three-dimensional coarctation or aortic interruption even multiplane transesophageal imaging is a less than optimal technique for definition of the coarctation morphology. Both magnetic resonance imaging or biplane angiography are far superior techniques. The role of intravascular imaging in coarctation of the aorta remains to be assessed.

While its diagnostic role may be limited, transesophageal imaging has a useful function as a monitoring technique during balloon dilatation of an aortic recoarctation. This subject is dealt with in Chapter 4.2.

REFERENCES

1. TAAMS MA, GUSSENHOVEN WJ, CORNEL JH, et al. Detection of left coronary artery stenosis by transoesophageal echocardiography. *Eur Heart J* 1988; **9:** 1162–6.

2. GERCKENS U, CATTELAENS N, DRINKOVIC N, et al. Detection of proximal coronary artery stenosis by transesophageal echocardiography (abstract). *Eur Heart J* 1989; **10**(suppl): 121.

3. ILICETO S, MEMMOLA C, DE MARTINO G, RIZZON P. Evaluation of anatomy and flow of the left coronary artery by transesophageal 2D echocardiography (abstract). *Eur Heart J* 1989; **10**(suppl): 121.

4. REICHERT S, VISSER C, KOOLEN J, et al. Transesophageal echocardiographic examination of the left coronary artery with a 7.5 MHz 2D and Doppler transducer (abstract). *Eur Heart J* 1989; **10**(suppl): 122.

5. SAMDARSHI TE, CHANG LK, BALLAL RS, et al. Transesophageal color Doppler echocardiography in assessing proximal coronary artery stenosis (abstract). *J Am Coll Cardiol* 1990; **15:** 93a.

6. KYO S, TAKAMOTO S, MATSUMURA M, et al. Visualization of coronary blood flow by transesophageal Doppler color flow mapping. *J Cardiogr* 1986; **16:** 831–40.

7. ZWICKY P, DANIEL WG, MUGGE A, LICHTLEN PR. Imaging of the coronary arteries by color-coded transesophageal Doppler echocardiography. *Am J Cardiol* 1988; **62:** 639–40.

8. ILICETO S, MARAGELI V, MEMMOLA C, et al. Assessment of coronary flow reserve by transesophageal echo-Doppler (abstract). *J Am Coll Cardiol* 1990; **15:** 62a.

9. LEVIN DC, FELLOWS KE, ABRAMS HL. Hemodynamically significant primary anomalies of the coronary arteries. Angiographic aspects. *Circulation* 1978; **58:** 25–34.

10. ROBERTS WC. *Adult congenital heart disease.* Philadelphia: FA Davis, 1987: 618.

11. GRIFFITHS SP, ELLIS K, HORDOF AJ, et al. Spontaneous complete closure of a congenital coronary artery fistula. *J Am Col Cardiol* 1983; **2:** 1169–73.

12. MARTI V, BAILEN JL, AUGE JM, BORDES R, CREXELLS C. Fistula coronaria a ventriculo derecho en pacientes trasplantados cardiacos como complicacion de biopsias endomiocardicas repetidas. *Rev Esp Cardiol* 1991; **44:** 320–3.

13. FRIEDMAN WF. Congenital heart disease in infancy and childhood. In: Eugene Braunwald (ed), *Heart disease: a textbook of cardiovascular medicine.* Saunders, 1992.

14. VARGAS BARRON J, ATTIE F, SKRONME D, et al. Two-dimensional echocardiography and colour Doppler imaging in patients with systolic-diastolic murmurs. *Am Heart J* 1987; **114:** 1461–6.

15. SHAKUDO M, YOSHIKAWA J, YOSHIDA K, YAMAURA Y. Noninvasive diagnosis of coronary artery fistula by Doppler colour flow mapping. *J Am Col Cardiol* 1989; **13:** 1572–7.

16. VELVIS H, SCHMIDT KG, SILVERMAN NH, TURLEY K. Diagnosis of coronary artery fistula by two dimensional echocardiography, pulsed Doppler ultrasound and colour flow mapping. *J Am Col Cardiol* 1989; **14:** 968–76.

17. SAMDARSHI TE, MAHAM EF, NANDA NC, et al. Transesophageal echocardiography assessment of congenital coronary artery to coronary sinus fistulas in adults. *Am J. Cardiol* 1991; **68:** 263–6.

18. KUO CT, CHIANG CW, FANG BR, et al. Coronary artery fistula: diagnosis by transesophageal two-dimensional and Coppler echocardiography. *Am Heart J* 1992; **123:** 218–20.

19. RUBIN DA, ZAKI AM, ZAGHLOL S, et al. Visualisation of coronary artery fistula with transesophageal echocardiography. *J Am Soc Echocardiogr* 1992; **5:** 173–5.

20. SUNAGA Y, TANIICHI Y, OKUBO N, et al. Biplane transesophageal echocardiographic study of left coronary artery to right atrium fistula. *Am Heart J* 1992; **123:** 1058–60.

21. ARAZOZA EA, BOWSER M, ABEID AI. Coronary artery fistula: diagnosis by biplane transesophageal echocardiography. *J Am Soc Echocardiogr* 1992; **5:** 277–80.

22. CALAFIORE PA, RAYMOND R, SCHIAVONE WA, ROSENKRANZ ER. Precise evaluation of a complex coronary arteriovenous fistula. The utility of transesophageal colour Doppler. *J Am Soc Echocardiogr* 1989; **2:** 337–41.

23. MIYATAKE K, OKAMOTO M, KINOSHITA N, et al. Doppler

echocardiographic features of coronary arteriovenous fistula. *Br Heart J* 1984; **51:** 508–18.

24. SUTHERLAND GR, STÜMPER O, FRASER AG, ROELANDT JRTC. Transoesophageal echocardiographic evaluation of coronary artery fistulae. *JACC* 1992; **19:** 324A.

25. ILICETO S, NANDA NC, RIZZON P, et al. Color Doppler evaluation of aortic dissection. *Circulation* 1987; **75:** 748–55.

26. TAAMS MA, GUSSENHOVEN WJ, SCHIPPERS LA, et al. The value of transosophageal echocardiography for diagnosis of thoracic aorta pathology. *Eur Heart J* 1988; **9:** 1308–16.

27. TAAMS MA, GUSSENHOVEN WJ, BOS E, ROELANDT J. Saccular aneurysm of the transverse thoracic aorta detected by transesophageal echocardiography. *Chest* 1988; **93:** 436–7.

28. KOTTLER MN. Is transesophageal echocardiography the new standard for diagnosing dissecting aortic aneurysms? *J Am Coll Cardiol* 1989; **14:** 1263–5.

29. ERBE R, BÖRNER N, STELLER D, et al. Detection of aortic dissection by transoesophageal echocardiography. *Br Heart J* 1987; **58:** 45–51.

30. ERBEL R, ENGBERDING R, DANIEL W, et al. Echocardiography in diagnosis of aortic dissection. *Lancet* 1989; **i:** 457–61.

31. MÜGGE A, DANIEL WG, LAAS J, et al. False-negative diagnosis of proximal aortic dissection by computed tomography or angiography and possible explanations based on transesophageal echocardiographic findings. *Am J Cardiol* 1990; **65:** 527–9.

32. SHAH PM, OMOTO M, ADACHI H, et al. Diagnostic value of newly developed biplane transesophageal echocardiography in thoracic aortic aneurysms (abstract). *Circulation* 1989; **80:** II-3.

33. MOHR-KAHALY S, ERBEL R, RENNOLETT H, et al. Ambulatory follow-up of aortic dissection by transesophageal two-dimensional and color-coded Doppler echocardiography. *Circulation* 1989; **80:** 24–33.

TEE as a monitoring technique

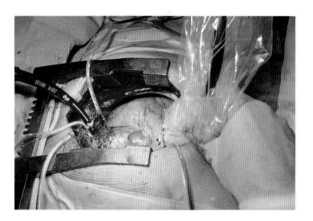

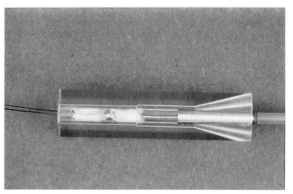

Intraoperative monitoring of surgical repair

O. Stümper

INTRODUCTION

Ultrasound monitoring during surgery for congenital heart disease has been performed for some ten years (1–3). The practice of epicardial cross-sectional imaging combined with contrast echocardiographic studies (4–6) created much initial enthusiasm. However, it soon became evident that these techniques frequently could not answer the range of complex questions which are raised immediately after intracardiac surgical repair of complex congenital heart disease. It was only with the addition of both colour and spectral Doppler facilities, and the development of higher resolution short-focus cross-sectional imaging transducers, that the technique became accepted as an adjunct to routine surgical intraoperative monitoring (8–12).

Direct epicardial imaging was for long the preferred intraoperative ultrasound technique. Use of the intraoperative transesophageal approach to monitor congenital heart surgery was until recently only feasible in the adolescent and adult patient population (12). In 1989 Cyran and associates reported their early experience with intraoperative transesophageal ultrasound in children with more than twenty kilograms of bodyweight (13). In the same year Kyo and colleagues (14) introduced the first dedicated paediatric transesophageal probe that allowed the monitoring of surgical procedures in children as small as some three kilograms of bodyweight. With the increasing availability of such dedicated paediatric probes, the technique finally has been used in a number of centres on a routine basis (15–17).

This chapter will discuss the advantages and limitations of both intraoperative transesophageal and epicardial ultrasound techniques in the monitoring of surgery for congenital heart disease, and will attempt to define their relative roles in this challenging field of paediatric cardiac ultrasound.

GENERAL CONSIDERATIONS

Complex congenital cardiac lesions have been corrected successfully for more than three decades without the use of intraoperative ultrasound techniques. Major advances in both surgical and cardioplegia techniques have permitted correction of the majority of congenital lesions with a low mortality rate. However, residual haemodynamic lesions are a frequent finding in the postoperative follow-up period. Whereas some of these lesions are acquired during the late follow-up period, others are residuae from suboptimal correction. Generally an attempt is made to exclude immediate residual lesions by means of surgical pressure monitoring. (exclusion of valvar regurgitation or stenosis) and oximetry (exclusion of residual shunting). However, there has been only little evidence for the accuracy and sensitivity of such monitoring techniques (18,19).

The aim of intraoperative ultrasound techniques is to provide the surgeon with an additional on-line monitoring technique that allows a detailed assessment of cardiac morphology, function and haemodynamics.

Pre-bypass studies are designed to reassess the intracardiac morphology immediately prior to surgical exploration. In addition, such studies document the haemodynamic features of the lesion with the chest open, while the patient is anesthetised and ventilated. Epicardial cross-sectional pre-bypass imaging studies often provide a more detailed definition of the intracardiac morphology than prior transthoracic studies (10,11). This feasibility to assess complex lesions in the beating heart is often a substantial contribution to subsequent direct surgical inspection in the flaccid heart. This is particularly true of lesions necessitating reconstruction of the atrioventricular valves or involving surgery of the ventricular outflow tracts. The detailed assessment of haemodynamic lesions during the pre-bypass study serves as a baseline value for the interpretation of the subsequent post-bypass study.

Post-bypass ultrasound studies are used to monitor ventricular filling and function while the high risk patient is being weaned from cardiopulmonary bypass. Such studies frequently are an adjunct to pressure recordings for evaluating and adjusting both volume replacement and inotropic support. Combined imaging, colour flow mapping and Doppler studies are performed to document the integrity of the surgical repair and to exclude potential residual lesions. If a lesion is identified then its haemodynamic significance is evaluated to determine whether immediate further repair may be required to improve on a suboptimal immediate surgical result.

The decision to use either the epicardial or transesophageal ultrasound approach should be guided by the relative strengths and weaknesses of each technique in the assessment of individual lesions and the surgical repair (see below).

Epicardial ultrasound studies can be performed in all infants and children undergoing surgical correction of congenital heart disease – there are virtually no restrictions imposed by patient weight. In the infant population the epicardial approach allows a much better image quality than the current generation of paediatric transesophageal probes. We currently use transesophageal studies only in children of more than four kilograms bodyweight (17), although routine studies have been carried out in smaller infants without any complications (15,16). Furthermore we exclude patients with known esophageal or spinal disease, and those with severe coagulation disorders from transesophageal studies.

Potential complications related to the use of epicardial ultrasound studies include the induction of arrhythmias and the theoretical risk of bacterial contamination. Ventricular ectopics are frequently induced when epicardial scan positions near the cardiac apex are used, or when undue pressure is employed in an attempt to maintain good contact with the beating heart. Such arrhythmias, in our experience, are always self-terminating and their recurrence can be avoided by using less pressure and different scan positions. With respect to bacterial infection, it is noteworthy that over a series of some 400 cases we did not experience an increased rate of infection after the introduction of routine epicardial imaging. However, the potential risk of infection cannot be excluded. The potential complications of transesophageal ultrasound studies in the perioperative period include bleeding and trauma to either the hypopharynx or the oesophagus. Such complications so far have not been reported. Thus, transesophageal studies should be considered as a safe monitoring technique.

TECHNICAL CONSIDERATIONS

Intraoperative transesophageal ultrasound studies are performed in exactly the same manner as those carried out for the routine assessment of congenital heart disease. Depending on the operating theatre routine (in particular the method of draping the patient) probe insertion of the probe in the anaesthetic preparation room may have its advantages. In patients who are nasotracheally intubated, transesophageal probe insertion is frequently facilitated by using direct laryngoscopic vision (see Chapter 2). In the majority of children an uncuffed endotracheal tube will be used during anaesthesia. This in turn often requires the use of 'mouth packing' to reduce any resultant air leak. Prior to transesophageal probe insertion such packs have to be removed. Esophageal thermistors may be left in place, but preferably these should be withdrawn to a high esophageal or pharyngeal position in order to guarantee good imaging contact. The same applies to nasogastric tubes. Following completion of the pre-bypass study the transesophageal probe should be advanced to the stomach and can remain positioned there during the entire operation. Using this technique a reinsertion of the probe for the post-bypass study is not required. Adverse effects of leaving the transesophageal probe positioned throughout long operations with complete anticoagulation have not been reported. However, our current preference and practice in children of less than 10 kilograms bodyweight is to leave the probe inserted for only the duration of the studies themselves. This then requires reinsertion of the probe at the end of the procedure, which unfortunately may be cumbersome. Every team embarking on transesophageal echocardiography as a dedicated intraoperative monitoring technique is certain to evolve its own practice, which takes into account both the cardiological and anaesthesiological practice.

Epicardial ultrasound studies are most widely performed using standard precordial ultrasound transducers. The majority of lower frequency transducers (i.e. 3.75 MHz) do not provide adequate image quality in infants and younger children. However, since high-frequency short-focus 5 MHz transducers became widely available some three years ago, excellent image quality can be obtained in virtually every patient. In addition, dedicated intraoperative epicardial transducers have been designed, which further expand on the range of epicardial scan positions (20). The probes are packed in sterile plastic bags containing a small amount of ultrasound gel (Fig. 4.1), and are passed into the operating field where they remain during the entire procedure. Warm saline is poured into the pericardial cradle in order to improve contact with the beating heart and to reduce mechanical irritation, which may cause arrhythmias during direct epicardial scanning (21).

At present, in the majority of centres, transesophageal ultrasound studies are performed by an attending paediatric or adult cardiologist. However, all such intraoperative ultrasound studies are time consuming. Thus, the provision of a regular service in a busy department is a major commitment both in terms of manpower and equipment requirements. One alternative approach has been to train anaesthetists in transesophageal echocardiography. Transesophageal anaesthetic monitoring in adult cardiac surgery has become a well established practice (22–24). Thus, anaesthesiological transesophageal monitoring of routine paediatric cardiac surgery should be considered. Ideally, only studies in complex lesions or complex surgical repairs would be performed by the cardiologist. Similarly, intraoperative epicardial studies should be performed by the surgeon. The cardiologist then would only attend when there are complex questions to be answered or the surgeon is uncertain of the findings. The evolution of such a practice involving the cardiologist, the anaesthetist and the surgeon is time consuming, but in our experience is the only guarantee of providing a routine intraoperative ultrasound service. Almost every surgeon and anaesthetist will be willing to learn and employ these techniques once exposed to their usefulness.

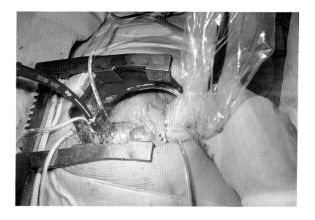

Figure 4.1 *Intraoperative epicardial ultrasound approach in surgery for congenital heart disease. The standard precordial transducer is packed in a long sterile plastic sleeve. Warm saline is poured into the pericardial cradle so as to improve image contact and reduce mechanical irritation of the heart.*

PRE-BYPASS STUDIES

As pointed out above, in cases where transesophageal ultrasound is being used, the probe is best inserted in the anaesthetic preparation room. This allows continuous preoperative monitoring of ventricular function in high risk cases. The intracardiac anatomy should then be reassessed using the techniques discussed in Chapter 3. Such studies should concentrate on the definition of the underlying anatomy of the lesion to be repaired. However, we feel it is essential that complete examinations should be carried out in all patients. In cases who were diagnosed only by transthoracic ultrasound techniques, such studies can contribute additional morphologic and haemodynamic information which is of value in the subsequent surgical repair. Major new insights which may be gained by transesophageal studies into a spectrum of congenital lesions are listed in Table 4.1.

Table 4.1 *Areas of improved insight by pre-bypass transesophageal and epicardial studies when compared with preoperative transthoracic ultrasound studies*

Transesophageal	Epicardial
Pulmonary venous return	Atrioventricular valves
Atrial septal defects	Right and left ventricular outflow tracts
Atrioventricular valves	Ventriculo-arterial connections
Left ventricular outflow tract	Great arteries

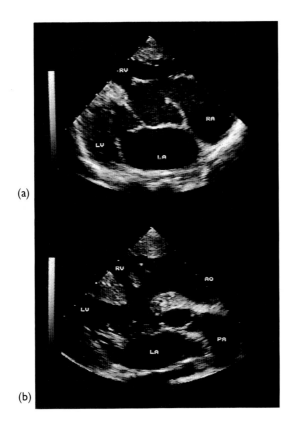

(a)

(b)

Figure 4.2 *Epicardial pre-bypass study in a child with transposition of the great arteries, ventricular septal defect and severe subpulmonary obstruction.* **(a)** *Using modified four-chamber views atrioventricular valve morphology and the pattern of chordal implantation is readily recognised.* **(b)** *Clockwise rotation of the probe demonstrates the ventricular outflow tracts and their relation to the ventricular septal defect. The extent of necessary muscle resection and the orientation of the VSD patch can be judged by the surgeon in the beating heart.*

Pre-bypass colour flow mapping and Doppler ultrasound studies should be carried out, whenever possible, just immediately prior to cannulation for cardiopulmonary bypass. In particular the assessment of right heart lesions, such as tricuspid valve regurgitation, may be significantly influenced by the marked haemodynamic changes which follow the onset of anaesthesia, positive pressure ventilation, and opening of the pericardium. In our experience, establishing of baseline values is crucial for the interpretation of the subsequent post-bypass study, which should ideally be carried out under near similar pressure and loading conditions.

In cases where epicardial ultrasound techniques are used either on their own or in combination with transesophageal ultrasound studies, the pre-bypass studies should be carried out following pericardiotomy. A full epicardial pre-bypass study can be completed routinely within 5 minutes, and frequently in less time than this. Such studies do not prolong the bypass time, although they do prolong the procedure itself, when compared with transesophageal ultrasound studies. However, when pre-bypass studies are specifically used in the ultrasonic surgical inspection of the beating heart (Fig. 4.2), such studies may in fact reduce the amount of time required for the subsequent anatomic inspection of the open heart, and thus save bypass time.

A multitude of epicardial cross-sectional views can be obtained by placing the transducer directly onto the right ventricular epicardium. From a low lateral position near the atrioventricular groove, modified four-chamber views are obtained. This range of views is used for the assessment of the pulmonary veins, the atrial septum, the atrioventricular valves and their subvalvar apparatus and the inlet portion of the interventricular septum. Clockwise transducer rotation from this position will allow demonstration of the right ventricular outflow tract, the pulmonary valve and the proximal pulmonary trunk. In addition, these views are best in evaluating aortic valve morphology. Subsequent gradual angulation of the transducer towards the left ventricular apex will scan both ventricular chambers and the ventricular septum. The true apex and the apical trabecular septum, however, frequently are difficult to visualise using epicardial imaging. This limitation is similar to that encountered using transverse axis transesophageal imaging. The complete range of views which are obtained from standard parasternal scan positions are readily scanned by positioning the transducer on the right ventricular outflow tract. In addition, epicardial views can be obtained from the anterior aspect of the ascending aorta. With the transducer placed on the right atrial surface the systemic venous drainage, the cranial portion of the interatrial septum and the right sided pulmonary veins can be assessed. Apart from these standard views many more additional scan planes can be obtained by slight angulation and rotation of the transducer. The sequence of transducer positions and specific views should be tailored to suit the individual case. Colour flow mapping and Doppler ultrasound studies should complement the initial imaging study. Areas in which direct epicardial scanning is a major benefit in the pre-bypass assessment of congenital lesions are listed in Table 4.2.

POST-BYPASS ASSESSMENT OF VENTRICULAR FILLING AND FUNCTION

The surgical monitoring of ventricular function, volume replacement and dosage of inotropic support immediately after cardiopulmonary bypass is routinely performed by observation of the beating heart, and by assessing both continuous arterial and venous pressure recordings. Although such a practice allows apparently adequate management in the majority of patients, diagnostic and therapeutic difficulties can be encountered in either high risk cases or in instances where these parameters provide ambiguous or conflicting information regarding the status of the patient.

In this situation intraoperative ultrasound techniques offer the unique possibility of continuously monitoring ventricular function by real time cross-sectional imaging combined with M-mode studies (Fig. 4.3). Imaging allows the rapid identification of global or localised ventricular dysfunction and allows an accurate estimation of ventricular volume. In addition, pulsed wave Doppler studies of mitral and tricuspid valve inflow patterns provide a better judgement of diastolic ventricular function and filling.

Although the influence of such studies on individual patient management is difficult to quantitate, it is our experience that the additional on-line information provided by this technique is a most versatile and sensitive adjunct in the management of the immediate post-bypass period. Such studies are essential in defining the cause of failure to come off bypass. Transesophageal ultrasound studies, when compared with epicardial studies, have a definite

advantage in this respect in that they can be performed continuously. In addition, the transesophageal ultrasound approach allows a better alignment of the Doppler beam to the atrioventricular valve inflow patterns. Thus, continuous transesophageal pulsed wave Doppler studies can be used in the early detection of diastolic filling abnormalities and in the assessment of any changes following subsequent anaesthetic or surgical management. Finally, transesophageal studies are not associated with the potential risk of inducing either ventricular arrhythmias or hypotension, as is occasionally encountered during the use of direct epicardial scanning. Interference with anaesthetic management is the only potential limitation of transesophageal studies in the monitoring of the immediate post-bypass situation.

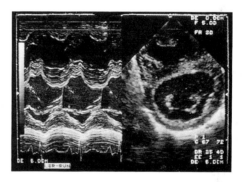

Figure 4.3 *Post-bypass cross-sectional imaging and M-mode study in the assessment of ventricular function in an infant after an arterial switch procedure.*

ASSESSMENT OF THE SURGICAL REPAIR

Post-bypass assessment of the surgical repair ideally is performed when the patient is completely weaned from cardiopulmonary bypass and all cannulae are removed. Cross-sectional imaging should be used to document the post-surgical morphology and the integrity of all suture lines. Colour flow mapping is used to rapidly identify abnormal turbulent flow patterns within the heart or great vessels. However, areas of turbulent flow are a frequent finding immediately following many surgical corrections. For example, following ventricular septal defect closure, turbulent flow patterns may occur by disturbed tricuspid inflow along the right ventricular aspect of the patch. In order to decrease the sensitivity of colour flow maps in the detection of spurious turbulence, the use of high-velocity colour flow maps is strongly advised. Timing of cardiac events during real-time on-line interpretation of colour flow mapping studies is largely facilitated by the use of colour M-mode studies. This is particularly true in infants and young children with rapid heart rates immediately after bypass. As a general rule, occurrence of turbulent flow patterns during only a short period of the cardiac cycle are of little haemodynamic importance. Pulsed and continuous wave Doppler investigations should be considered an essential part in all post-bypass studies in order to define any encountered residual pressure gradients.

Contrast echocardiographic studies often allow a more rapid exclusion and better semi-quantification of residual intracardiac shunts than does colour flow mapping (21). Routinely a small amount of hand-agitated blood and saline is used as the contrast medium. This is prepared by the surgeon by means of two syringes connected via a three way tap. Equal parts of blood and saline are injected under pressure from one syringe into the other until a well agitated solution is obtained. The three way tap is then opened to the patient and the solution is rapidly injected into a cardiac chamber, typically the left atrium. During the injection cross-sectional images of the outlet of the receiving chamber (typically the right ventricular outflow tract) are scanned.

The interpretation of immediate post-bypass ultrasound studies remains complex and difficult. Various degrees of residual haemodynamic lesions will be encountered in about one-third of patients. Only the minority of such lesions are of haemodynamic significance, thus quantification is required to allow appropriate decision making. However, in the face of rapidly changing overall haemodynamic parameters and in view of the inherent limitations of Doppler ultrasound techniques, semi-quantification of residual lesions is frequently the best which can be obtained. Residual interventricular shunting and atrioventricular valve regurgitation can be graded reasonably accurately, and in most cases correlate well with the early postoperative findings. However, the degree of residual ventricular outflow obstruction is difficult to determine and can both be under- or overestimated, when compared with early postoperative data (25). Thus, the immediate post-bypass findings may not represent the early and intermediate term results of the surgical repair. Bearing these limitations in mind, it will be the exception rather than the rule to formulate strict recommendations on which of the encountered residual lesions to operate upon during a second period of bypass. Appropriate decisions on recommencing bypass can only be made when the cardiac surgeon, who knows about the risks and the feasibility of further repair, and the echocardiographer, who knows about the limitations and the pitfalls of the technique, are working in close cooperation. The final decision to revise the repair is, and must be, a surgical one.

Repairs involving the venous return

Following surgical correction of an anomalous pulmonary venous connection, immediate obstructions to either pulmonary or systemic venous return and residual atrial shunting should be excluded. Residual venous obstructions or stenosis at the site of the anastomosis can be assessed by monitoring pull back curves of surgically inserted pressure lines. Using transesophageal echocardiography the anastomoses can be adequately visualised in all patients studied. Unobstructed drainage of all four pulmonary veins can be rapidly documented by combined transesophageal colour flow mapping and pulsed wave Doppler studies (Fig. 4.4). Obstructions are readily identified by the demonstration of continuous turbulent flow patterns within the pulmonary veins. Typically these obstructed flow patterns do not reach baseline during the cardiac cycle (see Chapter 3.1). Subsequent cross-sectional imaging of the site of obstruction allows a detailed assessment of the mechanism of stenosis, and provides information on whether the result could be improved by further patch enlargement. In this respect transesophageal studies are clearly superior to the epicardial approach, which does not allow for

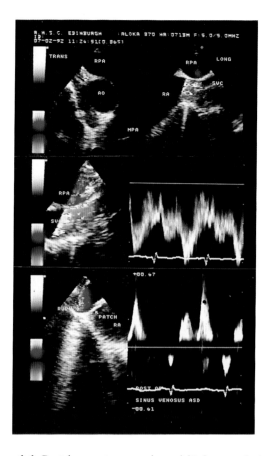

Figure 4.4 *Post-bypass transesophageal biplane study in a child who underwent closure of a sinus venosus atrial septal defect and rerouting of the right sided pulmonary veins by use of a pericardial patch. The morphology and the flow patterns of the superior caval vein can only be evaluated by longitudinal plane imaging (middle). There is mild obstruction at the mid portion caused by a prominent suture line (arrows). The integrity of the patch and the flow patterns of the right pulmonary veins are assessed best using transverse plane imaging (bottom).*

a good Doppler alignment to pulmonary venous return. Obstructions to caval venous return, which may be encountered after patch rerouting of pulmonary veins, are readily identified by epicardial ultrasound studies from the right atrial surface. This is possible by transesophageal imaging only in cases where biplane equipment is used.

Residual atrial shunting following patch repair of anomalous venous return is more readily excluded by transesophageal colour flow mapping studies than by the epicardial approach. Immediate minimal residual shunting may be encountered following both patch and direct surgical closure of any atrial septal defect, and is of little significance. Immediate surgical revision would only be indicated in cases where the post-bypass study shows gross dehiscence of the suture line, which we have never encountered. The routine use of intraoperative ultrasound techniques to monitor the surgical closure of isolated secundum-type atrial septal defects is of little (if any) benefit.

Following the Mustard or the Senning procedure for transposition of the great arteries the major objectives of intraoperative ultrasound studies include, firstly, the exclusion of baffle leakage, secondly, the exclusion of systemic pathway obstruction, and thirdly the exclusion of pulmonary venous pathway obstruction. Transesophageal ultrasound studies will allow a complete evaluation of atrial baffle function (Chapter 5.3). Such studies are clearly superior to the epicardial ultrasound approach. The latter technique remains somewhat cumbersome and limited in the exclusion of residual lesions. Using transesophageal ultrasound techniques, the mechanism and the morphology of any venous pathway obstruction will be readily identified (Fig. 4.5), thus providing invaluable information on which to base any decision to proceed to further surgical revision. Isolated pulmonary venous obstruction, in particular obstruction of the left sided pulmonary veins, are more readily identified by transesophageal studies. Such lesions may result from surgical placement of the left lateral suture line too close to the pulmonary venous orifices. Finally, the entire baffle suture line can be scanned using the transesophageal approach. This allows unequivocal demonstration of the exact site of any baffle leakage (26). The finding of gross baffle dehiscence should lead to immediate revision.

Following Fontan-type procedures for complex congenital cardiac lesions, obstruction of the systemic venous to pulmonary artery anastomosis has to be excluded in every patient studied. Residual atrial shunting should also be excluded. Because of the markedly elevated systemic venous pressures following these procedures, even minimal residual defects inevitably result in persistent arterial desaturation. The monitoring of volume replacement and of ventricular function is a further important aspect of intraoperative ultrasound studies in these high risk patients. Epicardial ultrasound techniques can derive much of this essential information in the im-

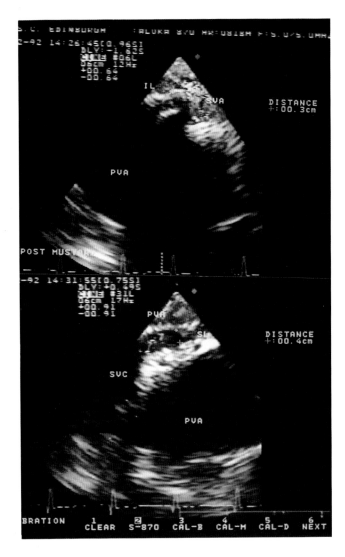

Figure 4.5 *Transesophageal ultrasound study in a patient who underwent Mustard baffle revision for severe systemic pathway obstructions. Both the inferior limb (IL) and the superior limb (SL) of the systemic venous atrium (SVA) are compressed by bulging of the redundant Goretex patch used in the repair. Minimal diameters measure 3 and 4 mm respectively. The pulmonary venous atrium (PVA) was found to be unobstructed.*

mediate post-bypass period of Fontan patients (27). Prior to the introduction of dedicated paediatric transesophageal probes such studies constituted the only technique for intraoperative ultrasound monitoring. The various types of Fontan connections can all be evaluated by epicardial cross-sectional imaging, colour flow mapping and pulsed wave Doppler techniques, thus allowing the rapid exclusion of obstructions (Fig. 4.6). Limitations of the epicardial approach in such patients include a relatively poor alignment of the pulsed wave Doppler beam to flow within the branch pulmonary arteries. Residual atrial shunting can be excluded by detailed colour flow mapping studies in the majority of patients. However, following total cavopulmonary connections (28), with insertion of a large prosthetic patch, epicardial ultrasound studies are frequently limited because of large areas of flow masking behind the patch. To circumvent this problem, we have adopted the routine use of contrast echocardiographic studies to exclude residual shunting after such procedures (27). Contrast material is injected into the 'right atrial' chamber, while scanning a transverse view of the left atrium. Marked contrast appearance in the left atrium, in our opinion, should lead to immediate revision of the suture line. The site of leakage should be clearly documented on subsequent colour flow mapping studies.

With the introduction of dedicated paediatric transesophageal probes, it became feasible to monitor all Fontan-type procedures from within the esophagus. Fyfe and colleagues were the first to report their comparative experience with both transesophageal and epicardial ultrasound techniques, and concluded that the transesophageal approach was clearly superior (29). In particular, following total cavopulmonary connections, the transesophageal technique is not compromised by flow masking artifacts in the exclusion of residual shunting (30). In addition, the evaluation of posterior Fontan connections and bidirectional Glenn shunts is improved, since the transesophageal approach combines excellent visualization of this area and good alignment to flow within the branch pulmonary arteries (Chapter 5.4). However, anterior Fontan connections (in particular right atrial to right ventricular connections) are frequently better evaluated using the epicardial approach.

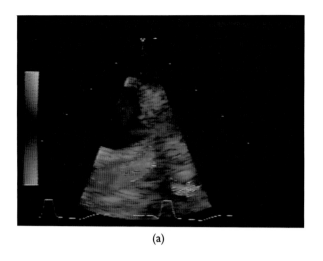

(a)

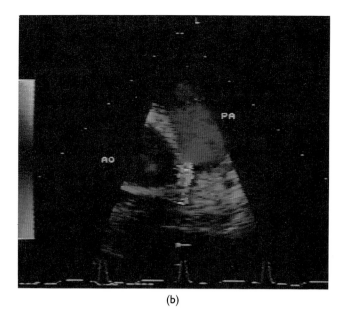

(b)

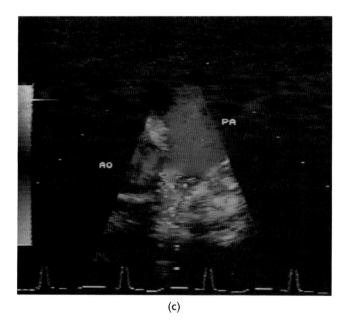

(c)

Figure 4.6 *Sequence of post-bypass colour flow mapping studies in a child after a Fontan procedure (atrio-pulmonary anastomosis)* **(a)** *Immediately after repair there is compression of the left pulmonary artery near the anastomosis.* **(b)** *Lifting up the aorta by means of a pair of forceps results in unobstructed flow patterns.* **(c)** *Following a second period of bypass with patch enlargement of the posterior wall of the anastomosis unobstructed flow towards the left pulmonary artery is established.*

Repairs involving the atrioventricular valves

In the evaluation of reconstructive surgical procedures of either atrioventricular valve, the major objectives of intraoperative ultrasound studies include the exclusion of residual valvar regurgitation, and the exclusion of valvar stenosis. Having identified the presence of such lesions, semi-quantification is required for accurate decision making as to whether the lesion warrants immediate revision. In addition, detailed morphologic studies should provide sufficient information to allow an accurate judgement on whether further surgical repair is likely to improve the result, and which surgical technique might be the most appropriate.

Epicardial ultrasound techniques have been used extensively in this range of lesions (31,32). Scanning an epicardial four-chamber view obtained from the right ventricular epicardium, colour flow mapping studies readily identify residual regurgitation (Fig. 4.7). However, the epicardial approach does not permit the acquisition of high-quality pulsed wave Doppler studies in the evaluation of atrioventricular valve inflow patterns. This is mainly related to the considerable degree of malalignment to the direction of flow. Following concomitant patch closure of a ventricular septal defect, there may be flow masking partially obscuring the left atrial chamber and mitral valve when scanning epicardial four-chamber views. However, subsequent scanning from the roof of the left atrium, with the probe positioned between the ascending aorta and the pulmonary artery, can often circumvent this problem.

Transesophageal ultrasound studies are extremely sensitive in detecting even minor degrees of atrioventricular valve incompetence, and in this respect should be considered superior to direct epicardial imaging (33). Using the transesophageal ultrasound approach the function of either atrioventricular valve can be assessed in detail (Fig. 4.8). The mechanism of valvar regurgitation will be correctly identified in the majority of cases thus enabling the accurate planning of further surgical repair. However, in cases where only single-plane transesophageal imaging is available, a complete assessment of valve morphology may be limited. The transverse axis imaging plane is particularly limited in the assessment of lesions involving the valve closure lines which lie parallel to the scanning plane of the transducer, i.e. the postero-medial commissure of the mitral valve. This limitation is overcome by the use of biplane imaging technology (see Chapter 5.2). Our experience with both single-plane trans-

esophageal and epicardial ultrasound studies in the monitoring of atrioventricular valve repair suggests that the epicardial approach is still superior in the detailed assessment of the underlying morphology of valve dysfunction (17). Only biplane transesophageal imaging would appear to give comparable accuracy.

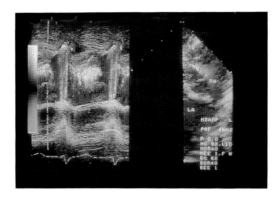

Figure 4.7 *Intraoperative epicardial detection of moderate to severe tricuspid regurgitation. The lesion is readily identified although there is considerable malalignment to the flow patterns.*

Quantification of atrioventricular valve regurgitation remains one of the most complicated aspects of intraoperative ultrasound studies, irrespective of the technique employed. A widely used quantification technique is measurement of the jet area during colour flow mapping studies, and its correlation with the dimension of the atrial chamber (34). However, regurgitant jet area is largely dependent on the equipment and settings used during the individual studies, and is poorly reproducible. In addition, the area of regurgitant jets which adhere to either the atrial surface of the valve leaflets, or the interatrial septum, will frequently be underestimated. Moreover, in face of the rapidly changing haemodynamics which occur immediately after bypass, the severity of valvar regurgitation may vary greatly

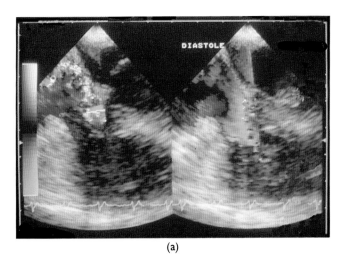

(a)

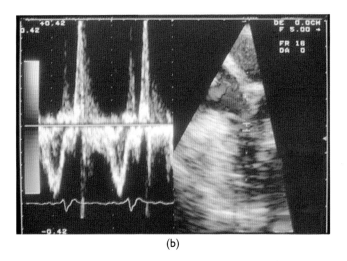

(b)

Figure 4.8 *Transesophageal echocardiographic evaluation of tricuspid valve function in a patient after repair of Ebstein's anomaly of the tricuspid valve.* **(a)** *Colour flow mapping studies demonstrate residual mild tricuspid regurgitation, and exclude any significant obstruction to right ventricular inflow.* **(b)** *Corresponding pulsed wave Doppler study in the same patient.*

over a short time interval. When compared with both early postoperative ultrasound studies and intermediate term results, the degree of atrioventricular valve regurgitation, as assessed by intraoperative ultrasound studies, may be both under- and overestimated (25). Thus, the effect of varying haemodynamic parameters on the degree of valvar regurgitation should be assessed.

Our current approach to the quantification of valvar regurgitation tries to account for these limitations and difficulties. Regurgitation occurring only during early systole is judged to be mild and should not promote revision. Pansystolic regurgitant jets with a jet area of up to one-third of the atrial cavity represent moderate valvar regurgitation. The underlying mechanism of the regurgitation should

be cleary defined so as to enable the surgeon to decide whether further repair is feasible. Studies are repeated after a short time interval, and the effects of different loading conditions and inotropic support on the severity of the regurgitation are assessed. In cases where jet dimensions do not change with these manipulations, and where there appears to be a suitable anatomy for further surgical correction, the decision to go back onto bypass is taken. Severe atrioventricular valve regurgitation is assumed in cases where the jet area exceeds one-half of the atrial cavity dimension, and is not influenced by different loading conditions or inotropic states. Whenever possible, further reconstructive surgery should be attempted in these cases. Further criteria, which may help in the decision whether residual regurgitation is severe, include the pulsed wave Doppler assessment of pulmonary venous flow patterns for evaluation of the mitral-valve (35), and caval venous flow patterns for the tricuspid valve. In cases where systolic retrograde flow is encountered in these vessels, the degree of regurgitation should be considered to be severe.

Obstruction to ventricular inflow is rarely encountered following surgical repair of congenital atrioventricular valve lesions. Occasionally this lesion may result from excessive surgical closure of the so-called cleft of the mitral valve in patients with atrioventricular septal defects. Epicardial imaging will readily identify the restrictive pattern of valve movement, and colour flow mapping studies will demonstrate turbulent ventricular inflow patterns. However, because of a generally poor alignment to ventricular inflow patterns when using epicardial scanning, it will be the exception that epicardial Doppler studies can quantitate the pressure gradient. In contrast, by using transesophageal studies, this can be achieved with ease. Again, it is the feasibility of further reconstructive repair and the influence of different loading conditions, that will allow appropriate decision making concerning immediate revision.

Repairs involving the ventricular chambers

Residual shunting following ventricular septal defect closure and residual right ventricular outflow tract obstruction are among the most frequently encountered lesions that are amenable to and may warrant immediate revision during a second period of bypass. The exclusion of such lesions is one of the major objectives of intraoperative ultrasound studies. In addition the evaluation of surgical relief of left ventricular outflow tract obstruction will be discussed in this section.

VENTRICULAR SEPTAL DEFECTS

Currently, closure of ventricular septal defects is most commonly effected by the use of a prosthetic patch. When assessing the integrity of such repairs by intraoperative ultrasound techniques, there is invariably marked ultrasound attenuation posterior to the patch. When using the epicardial approach, this results in ultrasound shadowing and flow masking of the left ventricular and left atrial cavity. Thus, in this condition the recognition of coexisting mitral regurgitation may be limited using the epicardial approach. However, when using the transeso-

phageal approach the ultrasound attenuation partially obscures the right ventricular cavity and the right ventricular outflow tract (Fig. 4.9). Thus, the recognition of residual left-to-right shunts on transesophageal colour flow mapping studies is limited (17). The routine use of biplane imaging equipment does not circumvent this problem (Fig. 4.10). Although some investigators have reported good results with transesophageal techniques in the monitoring of ventricular septal defect closure (15,16,36,), in our experience the epicardial technique remains the more accurate approach (21).

Following prosthetic patch closure of ventricular septal defects, minimal residual shunting across the suture line of the patch is found in a large proportion of patients studied. Such trivial leaks are of no haemodynamic significance and are likely to close during the early postoperative period. Grading of moderate and significant residual shunts on the basis of colour flow mapping studies uses visual assessment of the depicted flow areas in relation to right ventricular cavity dimensions (Table 4.2). However, as might be expected, there is a wide degree of overlap and observer variability when using these semi-quantitative techniques. Further difficulties in interpreting the colour flow maps occur when there is a combination of a residual ventricular septal defect and residual right ventricular outflow obstruction, both of which produce turbulent systolic flow patterns within the right ventricular outflow tract. In our experience, more reproducible results can be obtained when contrast echocardiographic studies are used for grading residual shunting. Contrast medium is injected into a left atrial line, while scanning a view which demonstrates both the left ventricular cavity and the right ventricular outflow tract. Such a view is readily obtained from an epicardial scan position near the right atrioventricular groove. In cases where transesophageal imaging is performed, contrast studies should be used, while scanning a view that demonstrates both the ascending aorta and the main pulmonary artery (Fig. 4.11). In cases where these techniques suggest a moderate or significant shunt, a repeat colour flow mapping study should be conducted, in order to identify the exact site of shunting. This, in our experience, can be better performed by epicardial imaging as outlined above. It will be the exception that gross patch dehiscence is identified as the underlying cause. Such a finding should inevitably lead to an immediate revision during a second period of bypass. In addition all cases with significant shunting, as assessed by the techniques detailed above, should be considered for immediate patch revision. However, when analysing the immediate and early follow-up

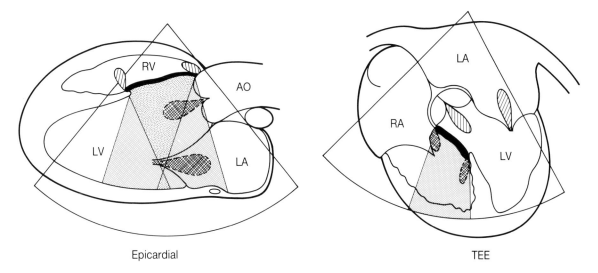

Epicardial   TEE

Figure 4.9 *Diagram of the areas of flow masking after ventricular septal defect patch closure during epicardial and transesophageal studies in the exclusion of residual shunting. (Compare Fig. 5.16 on page 230).*

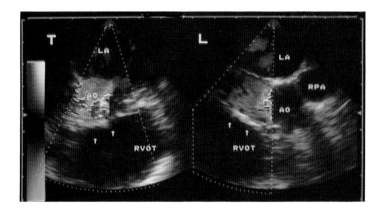

Figure 4.10 *Transesophageal biplane colour flow mapping study in a child with tetralogy of Fallot after prosthetic patch closure of the ventricular septal defect. Note the large area of flow masking within the right ventricle produced by the patch, precluding the definite exclusion of residual shunting.*

Table 4.2 *Grading of residual ventricular shunting by intraoperative ultrasound techniques*

	Mild	Moderate	Significant
CFM	Flame-like jet	Broad, short jet	Broad, expanding jet
CE	<25%	<50%	>50%

CFM = Colour flow mapping; CE = contrast echocardiography [assessment of the relative contrast densities in right and left heart chambers].

results of patients who are identified of having an immediate moderate residual shunt, it becomes apparent that such defects may still close spontaneously. On the other hand, such defects may also become larger over the course of time. Thus, the decision for immediate revision should be based on the individual case. If doubt persists, repeat studies should be performed after five to ten minutes.

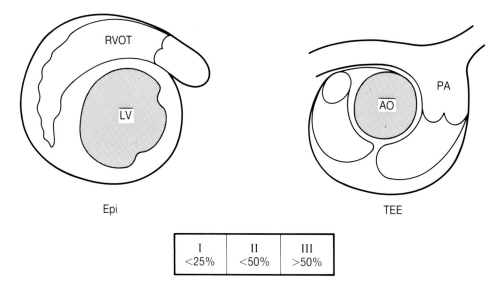

I <25%	II <50%	III >50%

Figure 4.11 *Optimal scan positions for epicardial and transesophageal contrast echocardiographic studies in the exclusion of residual ventricular shunting following VSD closure.*

RIGHT VENTRICULAR OUTFLOW TRACT OBSTRUCTION

As outlined in Chapter 3.8. the single-plane transesophageal evaluation of lesions producing right ventricular outflow tract obstruction is limited. Although the existence of obstruction can be documented by the finding of turbulent flow within the right ventricular outflow tract (37), a detailed assessment of the underlying cause generally is not obtainable by transverse axis transesophageal imaging. The use of transgastric imaging for visualisation of the right ventricular outflow tract (see Chapter 3.8) is limited during surgery. Most often entrapped air in the pericardial cradle will preclude adequate imaging from the stomach. The addition of longitudinal plane imaging has largely overcome these shortcomings, but the technique does not allow the acquisition of high-quality Doppler information. This in turn precludes estimation of the resulting gradient across any encountered obstruction. In addition, following ventricular septal defect closure a large area of the right ventricular outflow tract frequently will be found obscured, making the transesophageal evaluation a virtual impossibility. Thus, in our experience the epicardial ultrasound approach will remain the technique of choice in assessing this spectrum of lesions. Not only does the technique allow detailed definition of the post-surgical morphology, but also, by the use of continuous wave Doppler techniques, it is possible to determine the residual gradient. This contribution of intraoperative epicardial studies obviates the need for routine surgical pressure recordings which are generally obtained by transventricular puncture – a technique which is both traumatic and time consuming. Furthermore, surgical pressure recordings do not allow differentiation between dynamic and organic forms of obstructions, nor do they provide any insight into the underlying morphology.

Estimation of the haemodynamic significance of residual right ventricular outflow obstruction remains difficult, and no clear-cut guidelines on when to intervene can be formulated. The finding of a moderate or severe organic, fixed obstruction which could easily be resected would favour immediate revision. On the other hand, dynamic obstructions are likely to partially or completely resolve during the early postoperative period. It is rather the overall condition, the response to changes in inotropic support and the repeat study after a short time interval, that will allow for optimal decision making.

LEFT VENTRICULAR OUTFLOW OBSTRUCTION

Unlike the many limitations that are experienced in the assessment of right ventricular outflow tract obstruction, the transesophageal evaluation of obstructive lesions of the left ventricular outflow tract provides an excellent insight into the underlying morphology (see Chapter 3.7). However, because of considerable malalignment to the direction of blood flow, both the transverse and the longitudinal imaging approach are limited in the acquisition of reliable Doppler gradients. In the post-bypass exclusion of residual left ventricular outflow obstruction, transesophageal imaging studies can provide rapid detection of remnants of fibromuscular membranes (Fig. 4.12) or residual muscular hypertrophy following resection in patients with hypertrophic obstructive cardiomyopathy (38). In addition, the technique allows unequivocal identification of other causes of left ventricular outflow obstruction, for example marked systolic anterior motion of the mitral valve. In general, the epicardial approach does not provide additional morphologic insights (39), and, in fact, it may be limited following closure of an associated ventricular septal defect. However, it is only the epicardial technique that permits acquisition of high-quality continuous wave Doppler signals (Fig. 4.13).

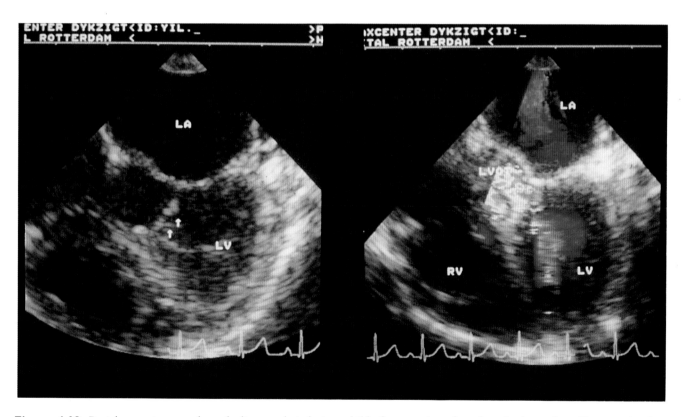

Figure 4.12 *Post-bypass transesophageal ultrasound study in a child after resection of a subaortic obstruction. Cross-sectional imaging discloses the presence of a prominent remnant of the fibromuscular membrane and colour flow mapping reveals the presence and the exact level of the obstruction. Considerable malalignment precludes definition of the resulting pressure gradient.*

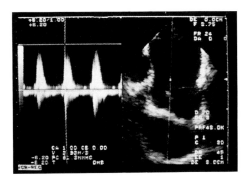

Figure 4.13 *Epicardial continuous wave Doppler study in the evaluation of surgical valvotomy for valvar aortic stenosis. The probe is positioned directly onto the distal ascending aorta and the aortic valve is scanned from above. There is a residual gradient but no regurgitation.*

Repairs involving the great arteries

Following surgical relief of stenoses of the main or the branch pulmonary arteries, residual obstructions should be excluded. The same applies for patients who have undergone an arterial switch procedure for transposition of the great arteries and for those who underwent the placement of right ventricular to pulmonary artery conduits. Using transverse axis transesophageal imaging, only the main and the right pulmonary artery can be adequately visualised, whereas the left pulmonary artery in most cases will be obscured by the interposed left main bronchus (Chapter 3.8). Epicardial imaging on the other hand provides an unimpaired view of the entire central pulmonary arterial system using a series of short axis cuts. Epicardial Doppler ultrasound studies will readily identify any residual obstruction either within the main pulmonary artery or at the level of the bifurcation. Furthermore, assessment of the function of right heart conduits and the exclusion of obstructions at the site of the distal anastomosis with the pulmonary arteries is better performed by epicardial imaging. In the Doppler assessment of more peripheral obstructions the transesophageal approach is likely to yield the better results.

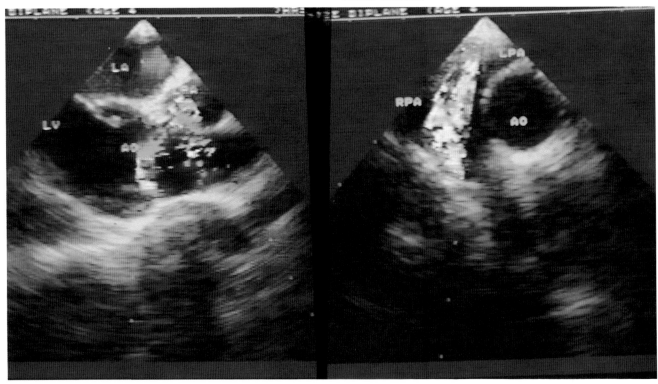

Figure 4.14 *Biplane transesophageal study following an arterial switch procedure for transposition of the great arteries. The longitudinal plane image demonstrates best the anastomosis of the ascending aorta, whereas the pulmonary artery bifurcation, in this case, is better evaluated using the transverse plane.*

Obstructions at the site of the great artery anastomoses following an arterial switch procedure are a relatively infrequent finding in the immediate post-bypass period. Such obstructions more often involve the pulmonary artery anastomosis, particularly when a Lecompte procedure has been performed. In our experience, such obstructions are readily excluded using intraoperative epicardial ultrasound techniques (40). In contrast, in the few neonates that were evaluated by transesophageal ultrasound studies, our results were rather disappointing. Using transverse axis imaging planes we were unable to define accurately the relative dimensions of the great arteries proximal and distal to the site of anastomosis. Only peripheral segments of the pulmonary arteries could be visualised, and coronary artery anastomoses could be demonstrated in only the minority. Interestingly, Zahn and colleagues reported their results on ten consecutive patients following an arterial switch procedure, stating that the great artery anastomoses could be visualised in all patients. Both coronary artery anastomoses were visualised in 5 of 10 patients (41). We were unable to obtain similar results and continue to use the epicardial ultrasound approach in these patients. With the recent advent of paediatric longitudinal and biplane imaging equipment, evaluation of these lesions may be largely improved (Fig. 4.14), but it is unlikely that the above mentioned limitations will be completely overcome.

Transesophageal Ultrasound in the Postoperative Period

The transthoracic ultrasound evaluation of patients in the immediate postoperative period is most often limited. Entrapped air within the pericardium reduces the parasternal ultrasound windows to a minimum. Chest drains and drapings largely restrict subcostal and suprasternal windows. Thus, in the majority of cases, no adequate ultrasound information can be obtained in the early postoperative period. In contrast, transesophageal ultrasound studies are not compromised. Thus, the technique is increasingly often being used in the critically ill patient in whom major lesions are suspected. In view of the generally poor quality of transthoracic ultrasound studies, the indications for transesophageal studies are relatively broad. Advantages and limitations of the technique in the assessment of specific lesions have been detailed elsewhere in this book.

Studies in the intubated and ventilated child can be performed with ease. We currently use local anaesthetic and diamorphine for sedation. Recently, dedicated neonatal transesophageal probes have been developed. The maximal shaft diameter measures about 4 mm. Such probes can be left positioned within the esophagus for a long time period without any potential complications. This offers the unique possibility for continuous monitoring in the critically ill infant throughout the early postoperative period (Fig. 4.15).

In patients in whom the chest has been left open after the initial correction transesophageal ultrasound studies should be considered to be the technique of choice to assess the haemodynamic situation prior to subsequent chest closure.

Summary

Intraoperative transesophageal and epicardial ultrasound studies provide the surgeon with detailed morphologic and haemodynamic information. In addition, such studies proved to be a most versatile adjunct in the anaesthetic monitoring of high risk patients. They are complementary rather than exclusive techniques. The selection of one or the other technique should be based on the individual case and the surgical procedure planned. Moreover, the team experience with one or the other technique will be a major determinant. Our current practices and preferences, are listed in Table 4.3.

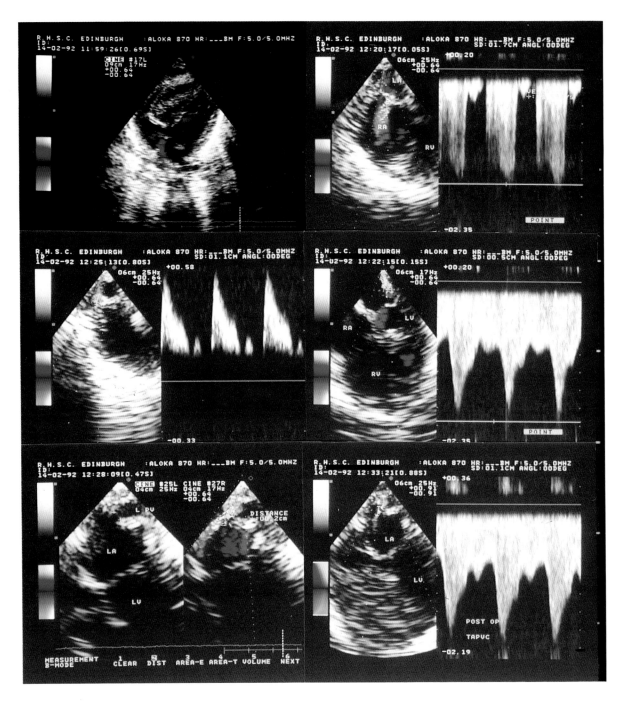

Figure 4.15 *Comparison between transthoracic and transesophageal ultrasound studies in the early postoperative evaluation of a newborn who underwent correction of total anomalous pulmonary venous drainage. The subcostal image (top left) suggested mild obstruction of a left sided pulmonary vein. The distal portion of the vein is seen dilated and there are increased flow velocities documented on pulsed wave Doppler studies. The subsequent transeosophageal study demonstrated mild to moderate residual shunting with a maximal Doppler velocity of 1.6 m/s (top right). The right lower pulmonary venous return was found to be unobstructed (mid left). Both the left upper (mid right) and the left lower pulmonary veins (bottom) were found to obstructed at the site of anastomosis.*

Table 4.3 *Comparison of intraoperative epicardial and single-plane transesophageal echocardiography in the assessment of intracardiac morphology and function in surgery for congenital heart disease*

	Epicardial morphology	Function	Transesophageal morphology	Function
Systemic venous return	++	++	++	+
Pulmonary venous return	+	+	+++	+++
Atrial septum	++	++	+++	+++
Tricuspid valve	++	++	+	++
Mitral valve	+++	++	++	+++
Ventricular septum	+++	+++	+	+[1]
Ventricular chambers	+++	++	+	+++
LVOT	+++	+++	+++	+
RVOT	+++	+++	− (+)[2]	−
Thoracic aorta	++	++	+	−
Pulmonary arteries	++	++	+[2]	+[2]
Fontan procedure	++	+	+++	+++
Mustard procedure	+	−	+++	+++
Arterial switch procedure	+++	+++	+	−

− = inadequate; + = adequate; ++ = good; +++ = excellent;
LVOT = left ventricular outflow tract; RVOT = right ventricular outflow tract;
[1] = inadequate after prosthetic patch closure of ventricular septal defects;
[2] = largely dependent on the size of the acoustic window.

REFERENCES

1. SPOTNITZ HM, MALM JR, KING DL, POOLEY RW, BOWMAN FO, BERGMAN D, EDIE RN, REEMSMA K, KRONGRAD E, HOFFMAN BF. Outflow tract obstruction in tetralogy of Fallot. Intraoperative analysis by echocardiography. *NY State J Med* 1978; **78:** 1100–3.
2. SYRACUSE DC, GAUDIANI VA, KASH DG, HENRY WL, MORROW AG. Intraoperative intracardiac echocardiography during left ventriculomyotomy and myectomy for hypertrophic subaortic stenosis. *Circulation* 1978; **58**(suppl I): 23–7.
3. SPOTNITZ HM, MALM JR. Two-dimensional ultrasound and cardiac operations. *J Thorac Cardiovasc Surg* 1982; **83:** 43–51.
4. REID CL, KAWANISHI DT, MCKAY CR, ELKAYAM U, RAHIMTOOLA SH, CHANDRARATNA PAN. Accuracy of evaluation of the presence and severity of aortic and mitral regurgitation by contrast two-dimensional echocardiography. *Am J Cardiol* 1983; **52:** 519–24.
5. HERWERDEN LA, GUSSENHOVEN WJ, ROELANDT J, BOS E, LIGTVOET CM, HAALEBOS MM, MOCHTAR B, LEICHER F, WITSENBURG M. Intraoperative epicardial two-dimensional echocardiography. *Eur Heart J* 1986; **7:** 386–95.
6. GUSSENHOVEN EJ, VAN HERWERDEN LA, ROELANDT J, LIGTVOET KM, BOS E, WITSENBURG M. Intraoperative two-dimensional echocardiography in congenital heart disease. *J Am Coll Cardiol* 1987; **9:** 565–72.
8. TAKAMOTO S, KYO S, ADACHI H, MATSUMURA M, YOKOTE Y, OMOTO R. Intraoperative color flow mapping by real-time two-dimensional Doppler echocardiography for evaluation of valvular and congenital heart disease and vascular disease. *J Thorac Cardiovasc Surg* 1985; **90:** 802–12.
9. HAGLER DJ, TAJIK AJ, SEWARD JB, SCHAFF HV, DANIELSON GK, PUGA FJ. Intraoperative two-dimensional Doppler echocardiography. *J Thorac Cardiovasc Surg* 1988; **95:** 516–22.

10. UNGERLEIDER RM, GREELEY WJ, SHEIKH KH, KERN FH, KISSLO JA, SABISTON DC. The use of intraoperative echo with doppler color flow imaging to predict outcome after repair of congenital cardiac defects. *Ann Surg* 1989; **210:** 526–34.

11. STÜMPER O, VAN DAELE M, SREERAM N, KAULITZ R, FRASER AG, HESS J, BOS E, QUAEGEBEUR J, SUTHERLAND GR. Intraoperative epicardial Doppler ultrasound in surgery for congenital heart disease. *Eur Heart J* 1990; **11:** 135 (abstract).

12. SUTHERLAND GR, VAN DAELE MERM, STÜMPER O, HESS J, QUAEGEBEUR J. Epicardial and transoesophageal echocardiography during surgery for congenital heart disease. *Int J Cardiac Imag* 1989; **4:** 37–40.

13. CYRAN SE, KIMBALL TR, MEYER RA, BAILEY WW, LOWE E, BALISTERI WF, KAPLAN S. Efficacy of intraoperative transesophageal echocardiography in children with congenital heart disease. *Am J Cardiol* 1989; **63:** 594–8.

14. KYO S, KOIKE K, TAKANAWA E, et al. Impact of transoesophageal Doppler echocardiography of pediatric cardiac surgery. *Int J Card Imag* 1989; **4:** 41–2.

15. RITTER SB, HILLEL Z, NARANG J, LEWIS D, THYS D. Transesophageal real time Doppler flow imaging in congenital heart disease: experience with the new pediatric transducer probe. *Dynam Cardiovasc Imag* 1989; **2:** 92–6.

16. SAHN DJ, MOISES V, CALI G, VALDEZ-CRUZ LM, MAZZEI W, MITCHELL M. Important roles of transesophageal color Doppler flow mapping studies in infants with congenital heart disease. *J Am Coll Cardiol* 1990; **15:** 1204A (abstract).

17. STÜMPER O, KAULITZ R, SREERAM N, FRASER AG, HESS J, SUTHERLAND GR. Intraoperative transesophageal versus epicardial echocardiography in surgery for congenital heart disease. *J Am Soc Echo* 1990; **3:** 392–401.

18. MAVROUDIS C, REES A, SOLINGER R, ELBL F. The prognostic value of intraoperative pressure gradients in patients with congenital aortic stenosis. *Ann Thor Surg* 1984; **38:** 237–41.

19. VALDEZ-CRUZ LM, PIERONI DR, ROLAND JM, SHEMATEK JP. Recognition of residual postoperative shunts by contrast ecocardiographic techniques. *Circulation* 1977; **55:** 148–52.

20. SMYLLIE J, VAN HERWERDEN L, BROMMERSMA P, et al. Intraoperative epicardial echocardiography: early experience with a newly developed small surgical transducer. *J Am Soc Echo* 1991; **4:** 147–54.

21. STÜMPER O, FRASER AG, ELZENGA NJ, et al. Asssment of ventricular septal defect closure by intraoperative epicardial ultrasound. *J Am Coll Cardiol* 1990; **16:** 1672–9.

22. BEAUPRE PN, KREMER PF, CAHALAN MK, LURZ FW, SCHILLER NB, HAMILTON WK. Intraoperative detection of changes in left ventricular segmental wall motion by transoesophageal two-dimensional echocardiography. *Am Heart J* 1984; **107:** 1021–3.

23. DE BRUIJN NP, CLEMENS FM, KISSLO JA. Intraoperative transesophageal color flow mapping: initial experience. *Anesth Analg* 1987; **66:** 386–90.

24. ABEL MD, NISHIMURA RA, CALLAHAN MJ, REHDER K, ILSTRUP DM, TAJIK AJ. Evaluation of intraoperative transoesophageal two-dimensional echocardiography. *Anesthesiology* 1987; **66:** 64–8.

25. SREERAM N, KAULITZ R, STÜMPER O, HESS J, QUAEGEBEUR J, SUTHERLAND GR. The comparative roles of intraoperative epicardial and early postoperative precordial echocardiography in the assessment of surgical repair for congenital heart disease. *J Am Coll Cardiol* 1990; **16:** 913–20.

26. KAULITZ R, STÜMPER O, GEUSKENS R, et al. The comparative values of precordial and transesophageal echocardiography in the assessment of atrial correction procedures for transposition of the great arteries. *J Am Coll Cardiol* 1990; **16:** 686–94.

27. STÜMPER O, SUTHERLAND GR, SREERAM N, et al. The role of intraoperative ultrasound in patients undergoing a Fontan-type procedures. *Br Heart J* 1991; **65:** 204–210.

28. DELEVAL MR, KILNER P, GEWILLIG M, BULL C. Total cavopulmonary connection: a logical alternative to atriopulmonary connection for complex Fontan operations. Experimental studies and early clinical experience. *J Thorac Cardiovasc Surg* 1988; **96:** 682–95.

29. FYFE DA, KLINE CH, SADE RM, CRAWFORD FA, BRAHEN NH, HOLLON M, ALPERT C, GILLETTE PC. Comparison of transesophageal and epicardial echocardiography in infants and small children during heart surgery. *Echocardiography* 1990; **7:** 353 (abstract).

30. STÜMPER O, SUTHERLAND GR, GEUSKENS R, ROELANDT JRTC, BOS E, HESS J. Transesophageal echocardiography in the evaluation of management of the Fontan circulation. *J Am Coll Cardiol* 1991; **17:** 1152–60.

31. UNGERLEIDER RM, KISSLO JA, GREELEY WJ, VAN TRIGT P, SABISTON DC. Intraoperative prebypass and postbypass epicardial color flow imaging in the repair of atrioventricular septal defects. *J Thorac Cardiovasc Surg* 1989; **98:** 90–100.

32. CANTER CE, SEBARSKI DC, MARTIN TC, GUITERREZ FR, SPRAY TL. Intraoperative evaluation of atrioventricular septal defect repair by color flow mapping echocardiography. *Ann Thorac Surg* 1989; **48:** 544–50.

33. ROBERSON DA, MUHIUDEEN IA, SILVERMAN NH, TURLEY K, HASS GS, CAHALAN MK. Intraoperative transesophageal echocardiography of atrioventricular septal defects. *J Am Coll Cardiol* 1991; **18:** 537–45.

34. MIYATAKE K, IZUMI S, OKAMOTO M, et al. Semiquantitative grading of severity of mitral regurgitation by real-time two-dimensional Doppler flow imaging technique. *J Am Coll Cardiol* 1986; **7:** 79–83.

35. KLEIN AL, COHEN GI, DAVISON MB, et al. Importance of sampling both pulmonary veins in the transesophageal assessment of severity of mitral regurgitation. *J Am Coll Cardiol* 1991; **17:** 199A (abstract).

36. MUHIUDEEN IA, ROBERSON DA, SILVERMAN NH, TURLEY K, CAHALAN MK. Intraoperative transesophageal echocardiography in infants and children with congenital cardiac shunt lesions: transesophageal versus epicardial. *J Am Coll Cardiol* 1990; **16:** 1687–95.

37. ELKADI T, SAHN DJ, RITTER S, GOLEBIOVSKI P, MOISES V, CHAO K. Importance of color flow Doppler imaging of the right ventricular outflow tract and pulmonary arteries by transesophageal echocardiography during surgery for congenital heart disease. *Circulation* 1990; **82**(III): 438 (abstract).

38. STÜMPER O, ELZENGA NJ, SUTHERLAND GR. Obstruction of the left ventricular outflow tract in childhood – improved diagnosis by transesophageal echocardiography. *Int J Cardiol* 1990; **28:** 107–9.

39. SREERAM N, SUTHERLAND GR, BOGERS AJJC, STÜMPER O, HESS J, BOS E, QUAEGEBEUR JM. Subaortic obstruction: intraoperative echocardiography as an adjunct to operation. *Ann Thorac Surg* 1990; **50:** 579–85.

40. VAN DAELE M, SUTHERLAND GR, SREERAM N, STÜMPER O, HESS J, QUAEGEBEUR JM. Intraoperative ultrasound assessment of the arterial switch operation. *Eur Heart J* 1990; **11**(suppl): 346 (abstract).

41. ZAHN E, MUSEWE N, DYCK J, et al. Transesophageal echocardiographic evaluation of the arterial switch in the early post-operative period. *Circulation* 1990; **82**(III): 439 (abstract).

Monitoring of interventional cardiac catheterisation

O. Stümper and J. Hess

INTRODUCTION

Interventional cardiac catheterisation techniques have largely influenced the therapeutic approach to a wide spectrum of congenital cardiac lesions (1,2). Balloon atrial septostomy has dramatically changed the management of transposition of the great arteries (3). Pulmonary valvuloplasty has become the treatment of first choice for valvar pulmonary stenosis (4). Many more interventional catheterisation techniques have become established in the modern practice of paediatric cardiology, and several other techniques are under evaluation, such as transcatheter atrial septal defect occlusion (5).

The monitoring of interventional cardiac catheterisation routinely includes a combination of fluoroscopy, angiography and pressure recordings. Transthoracic ultrasound has been used to monitor selected interventional procedures, such as balloon atrial septostomy, and has been reported to be a valuable adjunct to conventional monitoring techniques (6). However, because of a multitude of limitations and difficulties, transthoracic ultrasound studies have failed to attain an established role in monitoring a wider range of interventional procedures. The major limitation of the transthoracic technique lies in its interference with the procedure, which precludes continuous simultaneous echocardiographic and radiographic monitoring of the intervention. In addition, with the patient lying in a supine position, transthoracic ultrasound frequently will not provide adequate imaging or Doppler information of sufficient quality in the older child.

The use of transesophageal ultrasound techniques in the monitoring of interventional cardiac catheterisation potentially offers a new and highly versatile monitoring and diagnostic approach. The technique does not interfere with the procedure, yet is able to provide real-time cross-sectional imaging and a wide range of haemodynamic information by the use of colour flow mapping and Doppler ultrasound studies. Initial reports on the usefulness of the technique in selected interventional procedures originated from experiences obtained in the adult cardiology catheterisation laboratory. The role of the technique in monitoring mitral valvuloplasty (7,8), and in the assessment of left ventricular function during coronary angioplasty (9), have been reported. However, to date, little is known about the value and the potential impact of transesophageal monitoring in the wide range of interventional cardiac catheterisation procedures which are performed in the treatment of congenital heart disease (10).

This chapter will discuss mainly the experience with transesophageal monitoring of balloon dilatation procedures. Chapter 4.3 covers the monitoring of transcatheter occlusion techniques of both atrial and ventricular septal defects.

GENERAL CONSIDERATIONS

The use of transesophageal ultrasound studies in the monitoring of interventional cardiac catheterisation in children makes anaesthesia a necessity. Optimally, this should include endotracheal intubation. Although such studies could be carried out in the sedated but awake adult patient, it remains our practice to use general anaesthesia also in this group of patients. At our institutions, the vast majority of all diagnostic and interventional cardiac catheterisations in children are performed under general anaesthesia, thus transesophageal studies do not require additional anaesthesia time. When carried out in such a fashion, transesophageal studies do not increase the risk of cardiac catheterisation.

As with intraoperative ultrasound studies, provision of a routine ultrasound service to monitor interventional procedures imposes considerable demands both in terms of manpower and equipment. However, because of the range of information that can be obtained from such studies, and because of their potential value in individual patient management, we believe that the provision of this service is a valuable investment. Finally, the experience gained with some of the newer interventional techniques, such as atrial septal defect closure (see Chapter 4.3), has suggested that transesophageal monitoring is a prerequisite for a high success rate (11).

In order to obtain the maximal benefit from such studies, there should be an excellent understanding between the echocardiographer and the interventionalist. The echocardiographer has to be aware of the information that is sought at any given stage during the procedure, and has to master the skills to provide this information rapidly. The catheteriser, on the other hand, has to have a detailed understanding of transesophageal imaging and Doppler techniques. In particular, the anatomic basis of transesophageal cross-sectional imaging should be fully appreciated by the catheteriser, so as to be able to take advantage of this real-time imaging information during catheter manipulation. This should help to reduce screening times and contrast agent requirements in these procedures.

The ultrasound machine should be positioned at the head end of the patient, preferably opposite the catheteriser. It is useful to plan the required radiographic projections in advance so that adjustments of the lateral radiographic tube, in particular, will not require repositioning of the ultrasound machine. Ideally, there should be two monitors connected to the ultrasound machine: one would be the standard monitor of the machine, which should be positioned in such a way that both parties have easy visualisation, and the second monitor should be placed preferably beside the routine angiographic and fluoroscopy monitors. Using such a set-up the catheteriser then can readily appreciate and integrate the information provided by both the radiographic and the transesophageal studies, and a dialogue can be maintained between the echocardiographer and the catheteriser without interruption of the procedure.

In the following sections the contributions and the limitations of transesophageal monitoring of individual interventional catheterisation procedures will be discussed. This information reflects our current clinical practice and the results of ongoing investigations.

ATRIAL SEPTOSTOMY PROCEDURES

Balloon atrial septostomy is routinely performed in all neonates who depend on adequate mixing of systemic and pulmonary venous blood at atrial level. Fluoroscopic monitoring of this procedure is usually effective and allows the imaging of safe balloon inflation after demonstrating the correct positioning of the catheter tip near the orifice of a left sided pulmonary vein. Allan and associates have documented that balloon septostomy can equally well be performed using transthoracic echocardiographic monitoring (6). The adequacy of the septostomy can be assessed by combined imaging and Doppler ultrasound studies using a subcostal approach. Thus, during this procedure there is usually no need for transesophageal monitoring. However, in those patients in whom transthoracic imaging does not provide adequate image quality, or in those with a suspected or proven abnormal orientation of the atrial septum, it may be beneficial to use transesophageal imaging. It is for patients with juxtaposed atrial appendages that the technique is likely to be of most benefit. In such cases the atrial septum is orientated in a more frontal plane, and the atrial septal defect is often positioned relatively superiorly (see Chapter 3.2). Passage of the catheter across such defects using only fluoroscopic control may be difficult (12). Precordial imaging frequently fails to delineate this abnormality (13). Our current preference is to proceed with a transesophageal study in all cases where difficulties during balloon septostomy are encountered (Fig. 4.16). The technique can readily delineate atrial septal morphology and thus is of value in directing catheter manipulation and in the documentation of the adequacy of the procedure.

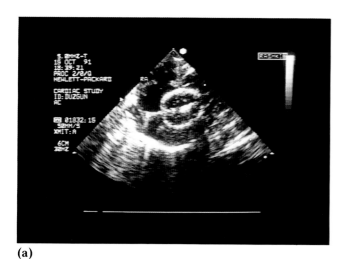

(a)

(b)

Figure 4.16 *Transesophageal imaging during a Rashkind balloon septostomy in a child with complex congenital heart disease, in whom difficulties were encountered in passing the catheter into the left atrium using fluoroscopy.* **(a)** *Cross-sectional image showing the inflated balloon across the atrial septum just prior to the pull-through.* **(b)** *Subsequent colour flow mapping study documenting the result of the procedure.*

In children older than two months, the tissue of the atrial septum markedly thickens and frequently precludes adequate tearing by the balloon septostomy technique. In such cases blade atrial septostomy is the preferred technique (14). Although

good immediate and long-term results together with a low complication rate have been reported (15,16), these procedures can be hazardous in less experienced hands. Using transesophageal monitoring during blade atrial septostomies should allow a detailed assessment of the atrial septal morphology, and thus define the most appropriate plane of blade orientation. In addition, malorientation of the blade catheter should be readily identifiable, thus limiting the risks of a hazardous outcome (e.g. perforation of the atrial free wall, pulmonary veins, or the aortic root). Such studies should improve on the safety and efficacy of these procedures.

Balloon dilatation has been proposed as an alternative to blade septostomy for the relief of a restrictive atrial communication (17,18). The major potential complication that may be experienced would appear to be a widespread tearing of the atrial septum with extension into the surrounding structures or eventual penetration of the atrial free wall. Transesophageal monitoring during such procedures should be able to identify immediately any of these complications, and thus may be expected to be of benefit in judging the safety of progressive dilatations until a perfect result is obtained.

DILATATION OF VENOUS OBSTRUCTIONS

Balloon dilatation of idiopathic, congenital or postoperative venous channel obstructions has been reported by Lock and colleagues (19). Although this technique has been proven to be of value in a subset of patients failure to relieve venous obstructions adequately is a well recognised problem (20–22).

Recently, the use of endovascular stents has been suggested in the treatment of rare congenital pulmonary venous obstruction (23), however initial results have been disappointing. The use of transesophageal ultrasound to monitor balloon dilatation of such lesions would seem to offer significant advantages. Firstly, by visualising the distal segments of the pulmonary veins and their junction with the left atrial cavity, the pre- and post-dilatation morphology can be assessed in detail. This should also be of value in monitoring guidewire and balloon catheter placement. Secondly, the immediate haemodynamic changes can be assessed by transesophageal pulsed wave Doppler studies. Residual obstruction is readily identified by persistence of continuous turbulent flow patterns throughout the cardiac cycle (Chapter 3.1), whereas a return to phasic flow patterns, with flow velocities approximating zero following atrial contraction, is a good indicator of successful gradient relief. This information should obviate the need for repeat pulmonary angiography and pulmonary wedge pressure measurements during the procedure. When used during the placement of endovascular stents, the technique should allow the visualisation of correct stent position and the degree of stent expansion.

Obstructions to the systemic venous return are frequently encountered following a Mustard procedure for transposition of the great arteries. As detailed in Chapter 5.3. the transesophageal ultrasound approach allows a complete evaluation of the systemic venous pathways in such patients. In particular, both obstructions of the superior limb of the baffle and baffle leakage are better defined by this technique than by either precordial ultrasound or cardiac catheterisation (24). Thus, not surprisingly, transesophageal monitoring of balloon baffle dilatation is a most valuable technique. Using cross-sectional imaging, the site and the precise morphology of the obstruction can be clearly documented. Whereas shelf-like obstructions (produced by a remnant of the atrial septum) are likely to be much improved by means of baffle dilatation, the finding of longer segment calcific obstructions is often associated with an unsatisfactory outcome. Real-time transesophageal imaging can also allow improved guidewire and catheter manipulation in cases where the obstruction is subtotal, leaving only a pinhole opening. In the absence of proximal baffle leakage, colour flow mapping and pulsed wave Doppler studies readily identify the persistence of obstruction by the finding of continuous turbulent flow patterns. These obstructions may persist even following the disappearance of waisting of an adequate sized balloon on fluoroscopy. In such cases subsequent further dilatations using a bigger balloon are required. In contrast, disappearance of turbulent flow patterns documents adequate gradient relief (Fig. 4.17). Although transesophageal Doppler ultrasound studies would appear to be a most sensitive indicator for the detection of even minor baffle obstructions, the technique, in our experience, does not permit calculation of the resulting pressure gradients across venous obstructions. This is related to, firstly, a considerable degree of malalignment of the Doppler beam to the flow through the stenotic segment and, secondly, the limited applicability of the Bernouilli equation for venous flow patterns. Thus, the use of transesophageal ultrasound studies in the monitoring of these procedures does not replace the acquisition of pre- and post-intervention pressure measurements.

In patients with a significant baffle leakage proximal to the obstruction, direct visualisation and measurement of the minimal diameter of the narrowing would appear to be the most valuable indicator in an estimation of the severity of obstruction (Fig. 4.18). Because of the proximal run-off through the leak, continuous flow patterns across the obstruction will not be recorded. In these cases catheter derived pressure gradients are misleading. The post-dilatation morphology is readily documented on the final transesophageal imaging study. In rare cases, intimal dissection or calcific plaque protrusion into the systemic venous atrium may be noted (Fig. 4.19). Such lesions, in our experience, are not visualised on angiographic films.

The last group of lesions to be considered under this heading are obstructions within the Fontan circulation. There are three potential sites for residual or acquired stenoses: firstly, the site of anastomosis between the right atrial chamber and the pulmonary artery system; secondly, within any incorporated conduit; and thirdly, within the branch pulmonary arteries (particularly in patients who had previous palliative shunt procedures). Balloon dilatation of such obstructions have been attempted, although their clinical value is not yet established (22,25). Transesophageal ultrasound evaluation of Fontan procedures provides detailed morphologic and haemodynamic insights (Chapter 5.4). Cross-sectional imaging appears to be the most sensitive technique in the detection of atrial thrombus formation, which is frequently associated with the presence of significant obstruction. The presence of thrombi has to preclude any attempt at subsequent balloon dilatation, in order to prevent embolisation into the pulmonary artery. Following balloon dilatation repeat imaging studies should exclude the presence of fresh thrombus within the atrial cavity. Fontan pathway obstructions at the site of posterior anastomoses or within the right pulmonary artery are clearly identified by transesophageal imaging (26). This should make transesophageal ultrasound studies a powerful monitoring tool during balloon dilatation of such lesions. The haemodynamic evaluation of the immediate results is enhanced by the use of transesophageal pulsed wave Doppler studies, demonstrating a normalisation of both the flow patterns within the pulmonary arteries and within the corresponding pulmonary veins (see Chapter 5.4).

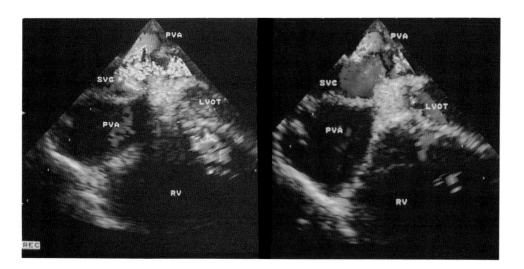

Figure 4.17 *Transesophageal colour flow mapping studies during balloon dilatation of a systemic venous pathway obstruction following the Mustard procedure. Prior to dilatation (left) the morphology of the stenosis within the superior limb of the systemic venous atrium at the site of the former atrial septum is clearly visualised. There are continuous turbulent flow patterns across this area. Following balloon dilatation (right) there is a marked increase in the internal dimensions of the superior limb of the baffle, and there is only minimal turbulence noted on colour flow mapping studies.*

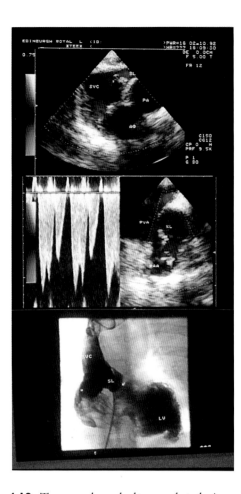

Figure 4.18 *Transesophageal ultrasound study in a child with superior baffle limb obstruction and proximal baffle leakage. The morphology of the obstruction is clearly documented on imaging, but there are no turbulent flow patterns across that site noted on colour flow mapping studies (top). Longitudinal plane imaging demonstrated best the site of baffle leakage at the antero-lateral suture line of the baffle (middle). The corresponding subsequent angiographic frame is shown at the bottom. SL = superior limb of the systemic venous atrium.*

VALVULOPLASTY OF ATRIOVENTRICULAR VALVES

Transcatheter balloon dilatation of stenotic atrioventricular valves offers an alternative to surgical commissurotomy in selected patients (27,28). The majority of such procedures are performed in patients with rheumatic mitral valve stenosis, although cases with congenital mitral or tricuspid valve stenosis have been dilated. Transthoracic ultrasound techniques are widely used in the selection of patients (29), and patients with heavily calcified, immobile valves that show involvement of the subvalvar apparatus are generally excluded from balloon valvuloplasty. Recently, the additional use of transesophageal ultrasound studies prior to mitral valvuloplasty has been recommended in order to exclude atrial thrombi (30). Both transthoracic and transesophageal ultrasound studies have been reported to be of value in the monitoring of such procedures (7,8,31). Transthoracic ultrasound studies allow evaluation of the changes in valve mobility, exclusion of valvar regurgitation and, by using continuous wave Doppler, evaluation of the resulting haemodynamic changes. The merits of transesophageal monitoring in this setting include, firstly, the real-time guidance of trans-septal puncture (32), guidewire and balloon catheter placement, and secondly, continuous monitoring of valvar function and ventricular function between subsequent inflations (Fig. 4.20). Undoubtedly, such studies add a degree of safety to these procedures and, in addition, help to reduce radiation exposure. However, in the absence of continuous wave Doppler facilities, complete haemodynamic evaluation is limited. Whereas routine transesophageal monitoring has not achieved an established role in the monitoring of mitral valvuloplasty in the adult patient population, it is felt that it should prove to be a most valuable contribution in the younger patient population because of the inherently more difficult and potentially traumatic catheter manipulations which make continuous monitoring a necessity.

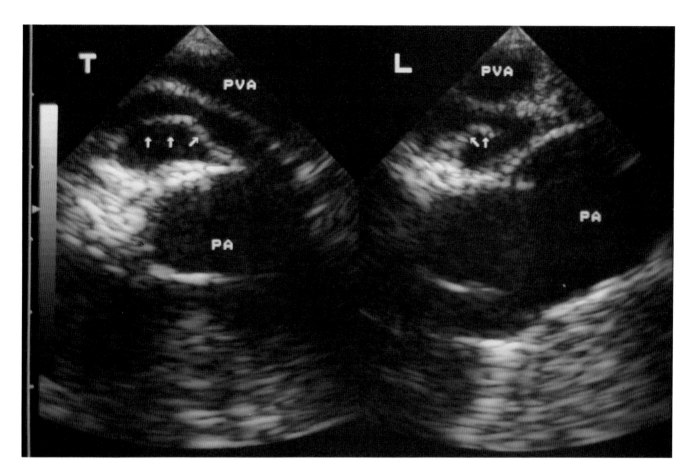

Figure 4.19 *Biplane transesophageal imaging study immediately after balloon dilatation of superior limb obstruction in a Mustard patient. There is a rather extensive intimal flap protruding into the lumen of the superior limb of the systemic venous atrium. Doppler evaluation excluded the presence of residual obstruction. This lesion was not demonstrated on the final angiogram.*

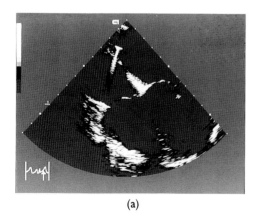

(a)

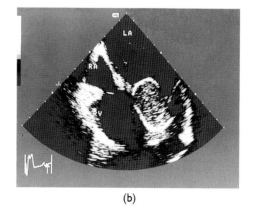

(b)

Figure 4.20 *Transverse axis monitoring during balloon mitral valvuloplasty.* **(a)** *Four-chamber views define the optimal site for trans-septal puncture.* **(b)** *Optimal balloon positioning during inflation.*

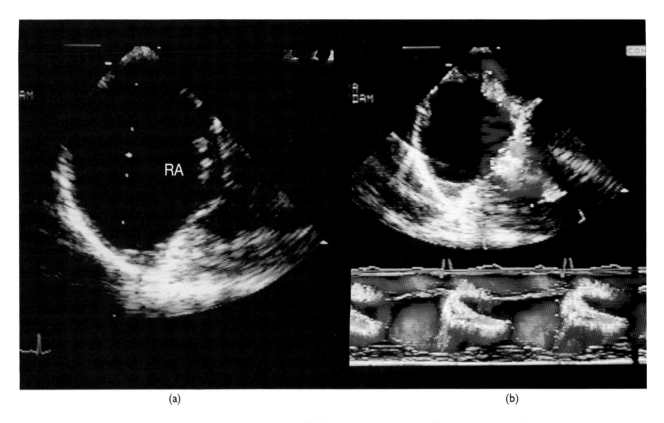

(a)   (b)

Figure 4.21 *Post-pulmonary valvuloplasty study in a child who experienced moderate tricuspid valve regurgitation during the procedure.* **(a)** *The cross-sectional imaging study clearly defines partial rupture of the chordae of the anterior leaflet of the tricuspid valve to be the underlying mechanism for tricuspid regurgitation.* **(b)** *Corresponding colour flow mapping and colour M-mode study.*

VALVULOPLASTY OF ARTERIAL VALVES

After its introduction in 1982 by Kan (33), pulmonary valvuloplasty has become the treatment of choice for valvar pulmonary stenosis. The technique combines excellent immediate and longterm results with a low incidence of complications (4,34). Taking these facts into account, there would appear to be only limited value in the transesophageal monitoring of such procedures. However, in our experience, transesophageal real-time imaging can be advantageous especially in monitoring guidewire and balloon catheter placement across the tricuspid valve. When using this technique routinely, it becomes apparent that the valvuloplasty catheter frequently passes through the subvalvar tricuspid valve apparatus, especially in cases where the guidewire has not been placed by means of a balloon endhole catheter (which should be the preferred technique). If the balloon is inflated in such a position, there is a potential risk of damage to the chordal apparatus with resultant tricuspid valve regurgitation (Fig. 4.21). Although this is a rare complication, the potential for tricuspid valve damage is readily diagnosed on transesophageal studies, and repositioning of the balloon catheter should then be performed prior to inflation. Furthermore, in small children and infants, because of the relative length of the balloon compared with right heart chamber dimensions, the proximal end of the balloon is frequently found to be within the tricuspid valve orifice (Fig. 4.22). Although this would not appear to cause damage to the tricuspid valve, it is our preference to advance the balloon further and to proceed to full inflation only when the entire balloon is beyond the tricuspid valve. In comparison, both the exact catheter course and the position of the balloon relative to the tricuspid valve apparatus are virtually impossible to ascertain on fluoroscopy. In terms of evaluation of both the immediate morphologic and the haemodynamic changes following pulmonary valvuloplasty, transverse axis transesophageal ultrasound is strictly limited. Neither the pulmonary valve morphology nor the residual gradient can be assessed from within the esophagus. Better results are obtained when using transgastric imaging planes (Chapter 3.8). It is likely that biplane transesophageal imaging will contribute more detailed information on the immediate changes in valve morphology, but residual pressure gradients cannot be determined.

Balloon dilatation of congenitally stenotic aortic valves is a highly effective interventional procedure (35) that compares favourably with surgical results (36,37). Potential complications include the development of aortic valve regurgitation, which can be caused by various mechanisms, including avulsion of an aortic valve leaflet or leaflet perforation. Transesophageal monitoring of these procedures provides a detailed insight into the pre- and post-dilatation anatomy of the stenotic aortic valve. The location and the extent of commissural fusion can be documented as well as the immediate changes in valve morphology following gradient relief. The dimensions of the aortic root can be accurately assessed, thus providing further information for selection of the appropriate balloon diameter (Fig. 4.23). In addition, there is recent evidence that transesophageal cross-sectional imaging, especially biplane imaging, can reliably assess the effective valve area (38), thus providing objective data for evaluating these procedures. As with the experience gained in monitoring of pulmonary valvuloplasties, transesophageal real-time imaging would appear to be the technique of choice in documenting the optimal balloon catheter course and position. In a minority of cases the guidewire will be found to pass through the chordal apparatus of the mitral valve rather than along the ventricular septum (Fig. 4.24). Such a finding should lead to guidewire repositioning, so as to prevent subsequent balloon inflation with potential risk of damage to the mitral valve apparatus. The most important contribution of transesophageal ultrasound in the monitoring of aortic valvuloplasties is the immediate exclusion of aortic regurgitation prior to any further balloon inflation. The sensitivity of transesophageal colour flow mapping studies in the detection of even minimal regurgitation is excellent (Fig. 4.23 (c)). In combination with cross-sectional imaging, the technique also allows exact localisation and determination of the underlying mechanism of the regurgitation. The information thus provided is extremely helpful in deciding whether to proceed with further inflations, and certainly adds a considerable degree of overall safety to these procedures. Finally, the transesophageal exclusion of aortic regurgitation immediately after the procedure should obviate the need for a final aortogram. The residual gradient across the aortic valve, however, cannot be determined by transverse plane transesophageal Doppler techniques because of the generally poor alignment to flow. The use of the transgastric approach to image the left ventricular outflow tract is likely to overcome this problem. Moreover, using longitudinal imaging planes, good results in the definition of the residual gradient can be obtained in a subset of patients.

Pulsed wave Doppler recordings of atrioventricular valve and pulmonary venous flow patterns were obtained in all patients undergoing pulmonary

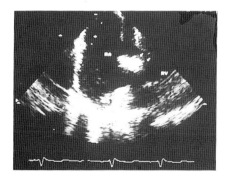

Figure 4.22 *Transesophageal imaging of the tricuspid valve apparatus during pulmonary valvuloplasty. Trial inflation of the dilatation balloon documents balloon position well within the tricuspid valve. The balloon catheter was subsequently repositioned.*

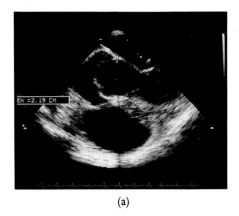

(a)

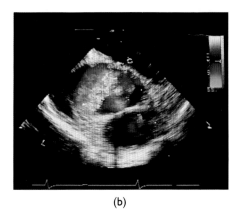

(b)

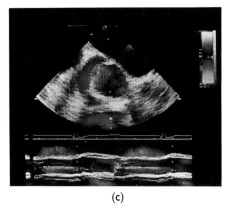

(c)

Figure 4.23 *Sequence of transverse axis transesophageal images in a child undergoing aortic valvuloplasty.* **(a)** *The pre-dilatation study defines aortic valve morphology and aortic annulus size.* **(b)** *Colour flow mapping defines jet morphology and excludes regurgitation prior to dilatation.* **(c)***. Post-dilatation study defining trivial central aortic regurgitation.*

or aortic valvuloplasty at our institutions. Analysis of these flow profiles confirmed the observation that successful gradient relief of an arterial valve is not followed by immediate changes of the diastolic filling properties of the underlying ventricle (39,40). However, following successful gradient relief of severe pulmonary valve stenosis, improved early diastolic filling of the left ventricle can be observed in a subset of patients (10). This is most likely to be related to an immediate improvement of left ventricular systolic function, with an improved descent of the mitral valve annulus which has as a consequence an increase in systolic pulmonary venous return (Fig. 4.25). However, there was no correlation between the absolute value of gradient relief and the occurrence of this finding.

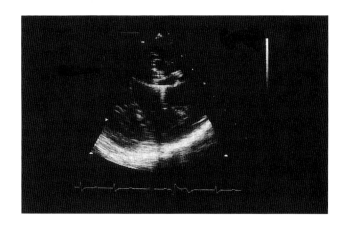

Figure 4.24 *Transesophageal echocardiographic demonstration of entrapment of the exchange guidewire used for aortic valvuloplasty within the chordal apparatus of the mitral valve. The guidewire was subsequently repositioned under combined fluoroscopic and transesophageal control.*

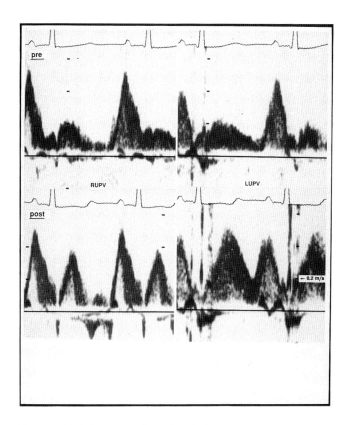

Figure 4.25 *Transesophageal pulsed wave Doppler evaluation of pulmonary venous flow patterns pre (top) and post (bottom) pulmonary valvuloplasty. There is a marked increase in the time velocity integrals of systolic forward flow, suggesting improved left ventricular systolic function.*

BALLOON ANGIOPLASTY

Catheter dilatation of aortic recoarctation is an established procedure (41,42), whereas the role of the technique in the management of native aortic coarctation remains controversial (43). The purpose of transesophageal studies during these procedures is to identify immediate changes in aortic wall morphology, i.e. the exclusion of either intimal tears or aneurysm formation. However, following surgical repair, the image quality which can be obtained by transesophageal imaging of the stenosed segment is frequently inadequate to definitively rule out such immediate complications. This limitation is particularly pronounced in patients with a tortuous course of the descending aorta. In cases in whom adequate imaging can be obtained, transverse axis scanning can accurately assess changes in wall morphology and changes in minimal vessel dimensions following dilatation. However, it is only the longitudinal axis plane that allows adequate

demonstration of the length of the obstruction. Although we currently have no experience with intravascular ultrasound techniques in the assessment of these lesions, it is felt that the intravascular monitoring approach can potentially provide a wider range of information in the monitoring of this procedure (44).

Pulmonary angioplasty of branch pulmonary artery stenoses offers an alternative to surgical correction. In cases with obstructions peripheral to the hila, balloon angioplasty may be the only therapeutic approach. However, at present, both the immediate and long-term follow-up results of either technique are disappointing (45). As outlined in Chapter 3.8, transesophageal ultrasound evaluation of the central pulmonary arterial system is somewhat limited. Whereas the main and right pulmonary arteries can be visualised in detail in all patients studied, this proves to be difficult for the left pulmonary artery. Its proximal segment is most often hidden by the interposed left main bronchus. A distal segment of the left pulmonary artery routinely can be visualised lying anterior to the descending aorta. The assessment of lesions involving the lobar arteries is not feasible using transesophageal techniques. Despite these limitations, transesophageal cross-sectional imaging of the pulmonary arteries combines high image quality, allowing assessment of the immediate changes of stenotic lesions, with detailed Doppler evaluation, allowing assessment of the immediate haemodynamic changes (10,46). The alignment to flow within the main or either branch pulmonary artery is excellent, thus allowing calculation of the residual pressure gradient following dilatation (Fig. 4.26). In addition, immediate changes in the patterns of pulmonary venous return allow a semiquantitive assessment of changes in perfusion of the affected lung (Chapter 3.8). Finally, the technique allows the immediate exclusion of intimal tears or aneurysm formation. Recently, balloon dilatation with subsequent stent implantation has become the preferred therapeutic approach in the management of patients with this range of lesions (23). Although our current experience with the transesophageal monitoring of these procedures is limited, it is felt that it will be of additional value both in stent placement as well as in the evaluation of the immediate results.

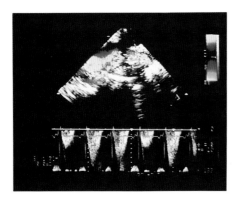

Figure 4.26 *Transverse axis study following balloon dilatation of a left pulmonary artery stenosis distal to a previous left Blalock Taussig shunt with marked reduction in the Doppler derived gradient. There were no intimal tears noted on imaging studies*

Miscellaneous procedures

Recently the use of balloon dilatation techniques has been expanded to the management of obstructive lesions within both the right and the left ventricular outflow tract, and of stenosed conduits. None of these procedures is currently performed in our institutions, because we consider such lesions to be approached more efficiently by surgical techniques. In patients in whom transesophageal monitoring may be considered it has to be remembered that only the morphology of the left ventricular outflow tract can be assessed in detail using transverse axis technology. For evaluation of procedures within the right ventricular outflow tract or right ventricular to pulmonary artery conduits, the use of biplane technology appears to be mandatory.

Coil embolisation of fistulae or collateral vessels is a further newer interventional procedure which has been shown to be effective in selected patients. We currently do not have any experience with transesophageal ultrasound in the monitoring of such procedures. However, such studies would appear to be particularly rewarding in the monitoring of embolisation of coronary artery fistulae. As pointed out in Chapter 3.10, both the entrance and exit sites of these vessels are clearly documented on transesophageal ultrasound studies. Thus, the real-time assessment of coil positioning and colour flow evaluation of the resultant flow patterns should be extremely helpful, and is likely to reduce the requirements for repeat angiography. In contrast, the transesophageal monitoring of coil embolisation of both arterio-venous fistulae or aorto-pulmonary collaterals does not appear to be rewarding because of the generally poor evaluation of such structures from within the esophagus.

Summary

Transesophageal echocardiography is a valuable additional monitoring technique during interventional cardiac catheterisation in patients with congenital heart disease. Close cooperation between the interventionalist and the echocardiographer is required to obtain maximal value from such studies. In our initial experience the technique allowed for a real-time assessment of cardiac morphology, providing valuable information on the nature of the individual lesion and in the guidance of catheter manipulations. Moreover, the use of transesophageal Doppler techniques allows an assessment of the immediate haemodynamic results and the exclusion of immediate complications.

References

1. RASHKIND WJ. Interventional cardiac catheterization in congenital heart disease. *Int J Cardiol* 1985; **7:** 1–11.
2. BULL C. Interventional catheterization in infants and children. *Br Heart J* 1986; **56:** 197–200.
3. NECHES WH, MULLINS CE, McNAMARA DG. The infant with transposition of the great arteries. II. Results of balloon atrial septostomy. *Am Heart J* 1972; **84:** 603–9.
4. STANGER P, CASSIDY SC, GIROD DA, KAN JS, LABABIDI Z, SHAPIRO SR. Balloon pulmonary valvuloplasty: results of the valvuloplasty and angioplasty for congenital anomalies registry. *Am J Cardiol* 1990; **65:** 775–83.
5. BRIDGES WD, NEWBURGER JW, MAYER JE, LOCK JE. Transcatheter closure of secundum ASD in pediatric patients: the first year's experience. *Am J Cardiol* 1990; **66:** 522 (abstract).

6. ALLAN LD, LEANAGE R, WAINWRIGHT R, JOSEPH MC, TYNAN M. Balloon atrial septostomy under two-dimensional echocardiographic control. *Br Heart J* 1982; **47:** 41–3.

7. JAARSMA W, VISSER CA, SUTTORP MJ, HAAGEN FDH, ERNST SMPG. Transesophageal echocardiography during percutaneous balloon mitral valvuloplasty. *J Am Soc Echo* 1990; **3:** 384–91.

8. DEN HEIJER P, HAMER J, PIEPER E, VAN DIJK R, LIE K. Percutaneous mitral balloon valvotomy guided by biplane transesophageal echocardiography. *Eur Heart J* 1991; **12**(suppl): 47 (abstract).

9. VISSER CA, KOOLEN JJ, DAVID GK, DUNNING AJ. Cumulative left ventricular dysfunction may occur during coronary angioplasty. *Eur Heart J* 1991; **12**(suppl): 335 (abstract).

10. STÜMPER O, WITSENBURG M, SUTHERLAND GR, CROMMER A, GODMAN MJ, HESS J. Monitoring of interventional cardiac catheterization by pediatric transesophageal echocardiography. *J Am Coll Cardiol* 1991; **18:** 1504–12.

11. HELLENBRAND WE, FAHEY JT, MCGOWAN FX, WELTIN GG, KLEINMAN CS. Transesophageal echocardiographic guidance of transcatheter closure of atrial septal defect. *Am J Cardiol* 1990; **66:** 207–13.

12. TYRELL MJ, MOES CAF. Congenital levoposition of the right atrial appendage: its relevance to balloon septostomy. *Am J Dis Child* 1971; **121:** 508–10.

13. STÜMPER O, RIJLAARSDAM M, VARGAS-BARRON J, ROMERO A, HESS J, SUTHERLAND GR. The assessment of juxtaposed atrial appendages by transoesophageal echocardiography. *Int J Cardiol* 1990; **29:** 365–71.

14. PARK SC, ZUBERBUHLER JR, NECHES WH, et al. A new atrial septostomy technique. *Cathet Cardiovasc Diagn* 1975; **1:** 195–201.

15. PARK SC, ZUBERBUHLER JR, NECHES WH, et al. A new atrial septostomy technique. *Cathet Cardiovasc Diagn* 1975; **1:** 195–201.

16. PLOWDEN JS, MULLINS CE, NIHILL MR, et al. Blade and balloon atrial septostomy: results and follow-up in 131 patients. *J Am Coll Cardiol* 1991; **17:** 135A (abstract).

17. MITCHELL SE, KAN JS, ANDERSON JH, WHITE RI, SWINDLE MM. Atrial septostomy: stationary angioplasty balloon technique. *Pediatr Res* 1986; **20:** 173A (abstract).

18. WEBBER SA, CULHAM JAG, SANDOR GGS, PATTERSON MWH. Balloon dilatation of restrictive interatrial communications in congenital heart disease. *Br Heart J* 1991; **65:** 346–8.

19. LOCK JE, BASS JL, CASTANEDA-ZUNIGA W, FUHRMAN BP, RASHKIND WJ, LUCAS RV. Dilation angioplasty of congenital or operative narrowings of venous channels. *Circulation* 1984; **70:** 457–64.

20. WALDMAN JD, WALDMAN J, JONES MC. Failure of balloon dilation in mid-cavity obstruction of the systemic venous atrium after Mustard operation. *Pediatr Cardiol* 1983; **4:** 151–4.

21. DISCROLL DJ, HESSLEIN PS, MULLINS CE. Congenital stenosis of individual pulmonary veins: clinical spectrum and unsuccessful treatment by transvenous balloon dilation. *Am J Cardiol* 1982; **49:** 1767–72.

22. MULLINS CE, LATSON LA, NECHES WH, COLVIN EV, KAN J. Balloon dilation of miscellaneous lesions: results of valvuloplasty and angioplasty of congenital anomalies registry. *Am J Cardiol* 1990; **65:** 802–3.

23. O'LAUGHLIN MP, PERRY SB, LOCK JE, MULLINS CE. Use of endovascular stents in congenital heart disease. *Circulation* 1991; **83:** 1923–39.

24. KAULITZ R, STÜMPER O, GEUSKENS R, et al. The comparative values of the precordial and transeosophageal approaches in the ultrasound evaluation of atrial baffle function following atrial correction procedures. *J Am Coll Cardiol* 1990; **16:** 686–94.

25. PELIKAN P, FRENCH WJ, RUIZ C, LAKS H, CRILEY JM. Percutaneous double-balloon angioplasty of a stenotic modified fontan aortic homograft conduit. *Cathet Cardiovasc Diagn* 1988; **15:** 47–51.

26. STÜMPER O, SUTHERLAND GR, GEUSKENS R, ROELANDT JRTC, BOS E, HESS J. Transesophageal echocardiography in the evaluation and management of the Fontan circulation. *J Am Coll Cardiol* 1991; **17:** 1152–60.

27. AL-ZAIBAG M, RIBEIRO PA, AL-KASSAB S, AL-FAGIH MR. Percutaneous double balloon mitral valvotomy for rheumatic mitral valve stenosis. *Lancet* 1986; **1:** 757–61.

28. INOUE K, OKAWI T, NAKAMURA T, KITAMURA F, MIYAMOTO N. Clinical application of transvenous mitral commisurotomy by a new balloon catheter. *J Thorac Cardiovasc Surg* 1984; **87:** 394–402.

29. WILKINS GT, WEYMAN AE, ABASCAL VM, BLOCK PC, PALACIOS IF. Percutaneous balloon dilatation of the mitral valve: an analysis of echocardiographic variables related to outcome and the mechanism of dilatation. *Br Heart J* 1988; **60:** 299–308.

30. THOMAS MR, MONAGHAN MJ, SMYTH DW, METCALFE J, JEWITT DE. The comparative value of transoesophageal and transthoracic echo prior to mitral valvuloplasty. *Eur Heart J* 1991; **12**(suppl): 234 (abstract).

31. PANDIAN NG, ISUER JM, HOUGEN TJ, DESNOYERS MR, MCINERNEY K, SALEM DV. Percutaneous balloon valvuloplasty of mitral stenosis aided by cardiac ultrasound. *Am J Cardiol* 1987; **59:** 380–2.

32. OFILI EO, CASTELLO R, DELIGONUL U, LENZEN PM, KERN MJ, LABOVITZ AJ. Usefulness of transesophageal echocardiography during invasive intracardiac procedures. *J Am Coll Cardiol* 1991; **17:** 315A (abstract).

33. KAN JS, WHITE RI, MITCHELL SE, et al. Percutaneous balloon valvuloplasty: a new method for treating congenital pulmonary valve stenosis. *N Eng J Med* 1982; **307:** 540–2.

34. KVESCLIS DA, ROCCHINI AP, SNIDER AR, ROSENTHAL A, CROWLEY DC, DICK M. Results of balloon valvuloplasty in the treatment of congenital valvar pulmonary stenosis in children. *Am J Cardiol* 1985; **56:** 527–31.

35. LABADIDI Z, WU RJ, WALLS TJ. Percutaneous balloon aortic valvuloplasty: results in 23 patients. *Am J Cardiol* 1984; **53:** 194–7.

36. SULLIVAN ID, WREN C, BAIN H, et al. Balloon dilatation

of the aortic valve for congenital aortic stenosis in childhood. *Br Heart J* 1989; **61:** 186–91.

37. ROCCHINI AP, BEEKMAN RH, BEN SHACHAR G, BENSON L, SCHWARTZ D, KAN JS. Balloon Aortic Valvuloplasty: Results of the valvuloplasty and angioplasty of congenital anomalies registry. *Am J Cardiol* 1990; **65:** 784–9.

38. CHANDRASEKARAN K, FOLEY R, WEITRAUB A, et al. Evidence that TEE can reliably and directly measure the aortic valve area in patients with aortic stenosis. *J Am Coll Cardiol* 1991; **17:** 20A (abstract).

39. STODDARD MF, VANDORMAEL MG, PEARSON AC, et al. Immediate and short-term effects of aortic balloon valvuloplasty on left ventricular diastolic function and filling in humans. *J Am Coll Cardiol* 1989; **14:** 1218–28.

40. VERMILION RP, SNIDER AR, MELIONES JN, PETERS J, MERIDA-ASMUS L. Pulsed doppler evaluation of diastolic filling in children with pulmonary valve stenosis before and after balloon valvuloplasty. *Am J Cardiol* 1990; **66:** 79–84.

41. HESS J, MOOYART EL, BUSCH HJ, BERGSTRA A, LANDSMAN MLJ. Percutaneous transluminal balloon angioplasty in restenosis of coarctation of the aorta. *Br Heart J* 1986; **55:** 459–61.

42. HELLENBRAND WE, ALLEN HD, GOLINKO RJ, HAGLER DJ, LUTIN W, KAN J. Balloon Angioplasty for aortic recoarctation: Results of the valvuloplasty and angioplasty of congenital anomalies registry. *Am J Cardiol* 1990; **65:** 793–7.

43. TYNAN M, FINLAY JP, FONTES V, HESS J, KAN J. Balloon Angioplasty for the treatment of native coarctation: Results of the valvuloplasty and angioplasty of congenital anomalies registry. *Am J Cardiol* 1990; **65:** 790–2.

44. HARRISON K, SHEIK KH, DAVIDSON CJ, et al. Balloon angioplasty of coarctation of the aorta evaluated with intravascular ultrasound imaging. *J Am Coll Cardiol* 1990; **15:** 906–9.

45. ROTHAN A, PERRY SB, KEANE JF, LOCK JE. Early results and follow-up of balloon angioplasty for branch pulmonary artery stenoses. *J Am Coll Cardiol* 1990: **16:** 1109–17.

46. TODT M, ERBEL R, POP T, BEDNARCZYK I, DREXLER M, MEYER J. Dilatation einer supravalvulären Pulmonalisstenose bei transösophagealem echokardiographishem Monitoring – Kissing Balloon Technique. *Z Kardiol* 1988; **77:** 385–8.

Transcatheter occlusion of atrial and ventricular septal defects

A. Ludomirsky

INTRODUCTION

The last decade has seen a dramatic change in the management of congenital heart defects. The introduction and development of echocardiography and colour modalities has enabled the definitive diagnosis of many congenital lesions without cardiac catheterisation. At the same time, new therapeutic procedures for congenital defects using the catheter as a channel for different procedures have been developed. These catheter-based therapeutic procedures have replaced cardiac surgery in many types of defects. Rashkind, Mullins and Lock were the pioneers in developing the concept of intracardiac therapy (1). While the early experience and emphasis was on the area of balloon techniques for the dilation of stenotic valves or narrowed vessels, there was simultaneous development and studies on devices for closing or occluding abnormal openings. It was Dr Rashkind who developed and designed the double-umbrella device for closing of a patent ductus arteriosus. This device has been used successfully in over 500 patients in the United States and in at least an equal number in other countries around the world where it has already been accepted as the preferable therapy for the patent ductus arteriosus (2). The enormous success of the patent ductus arteriosus device stimulated Dr James Lock from Boston and Dr Charles Mullins from Houston to develop a modified double umbrella device for other defects, especially in secundum ASD and in some selected cases of intraventricular septal defect.

The new developments in echocardiography and Doppler modalities can provide accurate imaging and visualisation of the transcatheter closing devices and have brought the interventional cardiologist and the echocardiographer into a close marriage. The use of echocardiography and Doppler in the catheterisation laboratory has been a must, especially when used in atrial and ventricular septal defect closure. Pre-, intra- and post-monitoring and evaluation of the procedure can be performed simultaneously in the catheterisation laboratory.

Transesophageal echocardiography has opened a new window for cardiac imaging. The proximity of the oesophagus to the left atrium facilitates the imaging of the posterior structures of the heart and provides an accurate visualisation of all parts of the atrial septum (3). In patients with poor precordial windows, the transesophageal approach is the only method for accurate visualisation of posterior structures; i.e. atrial septum, coronary sinus, pulmonary veins, left atrial appendage and the right atrium. This advantage of transesophageal echocardiography accelerated the close co-operation between the cardiac catheteriser and cardiac echocardiographer in order to guide and monitor therapeutic procedures. In this chapter, we will detail the role of transesophageal echocardiography in transcatheter closure of ASD and VSD.

CLOSURE OF ATRIAL SEPTAL DEFECTS

Atrial septal defects represent approximately 10% of all congenital cardiac lesions and their presence, even in patients without symptoms, represents an indication for closure. The surgical closure of an atrial septal defect is a relatively safe procedure, but carries the inherent physical discomfort of surgery, the risk of general anaesthesia, thoracotomy, an added risk of cardiopulmonary bypass and the morbidity and mortality of surgery (4). A catheter-positioned occluder device implanted during standard cardiac catheterisation precludes the need for this surgery, eliminates the risk of surgery and reduces the recovery and convalescence time associated with correction of the defect to one day. The device used today is of the double-umbrella type which attaches to the septum by means of two opposing umbrellas held against opposite sides of the septum by an inherent spring mechanism. It is totally retrievable after deployment and testing until the actual release of the delivery wire. The device was given the trade name of Clamshell ASD Occluding Device (Figure.4.27). It comes in multiple sizes, the largest capable of consistently closing defects up to a stretched diameter of 20–21 mm (5). The technique is based on the initial delivery of a sheath which is introduced percutaneously over a dilator into a vein in the groin. Using fluoroscopy, the sheath is manoeuvered to the right atrium and from there through the defect into the left atrium. The folded device in its delivery catheter is introduced into the previously positioned sheath and advanced into the left atrium. This sheath is very carefully and precisely withdrawn from the device until only the distal umbrellas spring to the open position within the cavity of the left atrium. The entire system, sheath, catheter and umbrella, are then slowly withdrawn together until the open umbrella is seen on fluoroscopy to catch and flex against the septal wall as it nears the defect. When the operator is satisfied with the position and the catching of the umbrella against the septum, the sheath alone is withdrawn further from the still partially folded device (Fig. 4.28). This allows the proximal umbrella to spring open on the right side of the atrial septum (6). This particular catheterisation procedure has demonstrated the necessity of a marriage between echocardiography and catheter therapeutic techniques. Although the occluder device can be seen by fluoroscopy, neither the ASD nor the atrial

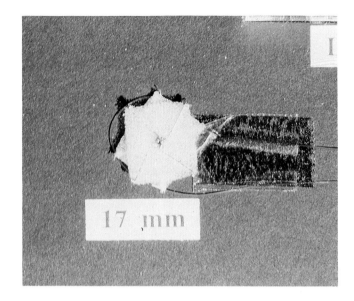

Figure 4.27 *A double-umbrella Clamshell ASD occluding device with attachments to each side.*

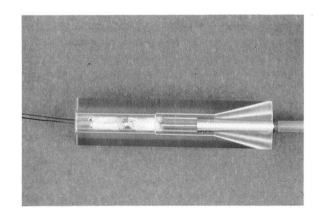

Figure 4.28 *The ASD occluding device shown inside its sheath.*

septum itself and the upper and lower rim can be seen on fluoroscopy (Fig. 4.29). The features of the defect which must be determined by transesophageal studies are listed in Table 4.4.

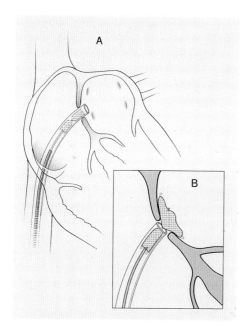

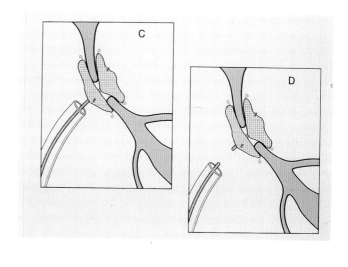

Figure 4.29 (a) *The sheath across the atrial septum into the left atrium.* **(b)** *The distal legs of the device are open in the left side of the septum and are withdrawn toward the atrial septal defect.* **(c)** *The proximal legs are open. The device is still attached to the release mechanism.* **(d)** *The device is released from the catheter and the sheath. Both are withdrawn toward the inferior vena cava.*

Table 4.4 *The role of transesophageal echo in ASD device closure*

ASD sizing and visualisation of upper and lower rim
Assessment of ASD size during balloon stretch technique measurements
Detection of leaks around the balloon by pulsed and colour flow Doppler
Device location; left atrium/right atrium, atrial appendages
Proximity of the device through the mitral valve and tricuspid valve
Identification of a fenestrated ASD
Guidance of the release of the device
Assessment of leaks across the device immediately after implantation

ASD sizing and visualisation of upper and lower rim

One of the most difficult parts of transcatheter occlusion device closure of an ASD is the accurate determination of which defects will or will not be suitable for closure. The Clamshell ASD device is usable for most centrally located ASDs <21 mm in diameter in patients over 10–15 kg in weight and of any age. The current ASD device (diagonal length) must be twice the stretched size of the ASD. Since the largest device now available is 40 mm, defects larger than 20 mm are generally unsuitable for transcatheter closure. Transesophageal echocardiography has proven to be extremely useful, if not essential, in the imaging of the atrial septum for ASD dimension measurements (7,8). ASDs with unusually high or low position may require further evaluation. The atrial septum must be of normal proportions and with an adequate upper rim and lower rim that will accommodate the total diameter of the device. The atrial septum is anatomically a concave convex structure. For that reason, the imaging beam can cut the defect in different planes and not reflect the true size of the ASD. In the evaluation of atrial size, one should be aware of this limitation and try to document the largest diameter of the ASD by manipulating the probe anteriorly or posteriorly as well as medially and laterally (Fig. 4.30). Adequate upper and lower rims are crucial for successful implantation of the ASD device. If the lower rim of the defect is minimal, the centre of the device will be lower in the atrial septum and potentially closer to the atrioventricular valve leaflet tissue (Fig. 4.31). Atrioventricular valve regurgitation (either right or left) could result from a device positioned caudally on the atrial septum in patients with an inadequate inferior rim of the septum. A case of a very small upper rim or a very high secundum ASD could result in an inadequate release of the distal legs and implantation in the roof of the left atrium. In our institutions (9), we have established echocardiographic criteria for patient selection for transcatheter occlusion of ASD as (1): echocardiographic ASD size of <20 mm (2); presence of an adequate superior and inferior rim of septum (3); ASD to total atrial septal ratio = 0.46.

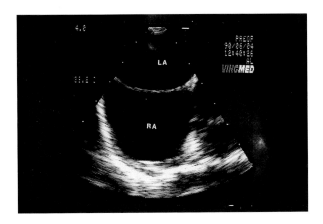

Figure 4.30 *Transesophageal echocardiography of the atrial septum. The total atrial septum length can be evaluated from this view.*

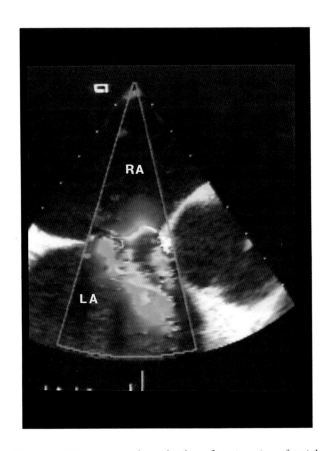

Figure 4.31 *Transesophageal colour flow imaging of atrial septal defect using the transesophageal approach.*

Balloon stretching technique for ASD sizing

Atrial septal defect size should be measured during cardiac catheterisation by the use of a balloon stretching sizing technique in all patients. A balloon septostomy catheter or a 9 fr balloon ASD occlusion catheter are used to size the ASD. Prior to introduction into the patient, the balloon catheter diameter when inflated with a specific amount of dilute contrast is calibrated and the volume of contrast required to produce a certain balloon diameter is recorded. The smallest balloon which is caught by the atrial septum as it is slowly withdrawn from the left atrium to right atrium is defined as the stretched ASD size (Fig. 4.32). This technique does not incorporate the measurement of a waist in the sizing balloon and therefore avoids over distend in the atrial septum. Once the diameter of the defect is established, sizing of the balloon is performed by direct visualisation using transesophageal echocardiography. Caudal and coronal diameters are measured and the location of the balloon within the centre of the ASD is established. Only if the balloon diameter and the echocardiographic measurements are similar, is the procedure continued. The balloon is well seen using fluoroscopy, but the catheteriser does not have tools to evaluate the location of the balloon within the atrial septum and visualise the upper and lower rims (Fig. 4.33).

Detecting residual leaks around the balloon

Even though the balloon is 'caught' by the atrial septum as it is withdrawn slowly from the left atrium to the right atrium, residual shunts around the balloon can exist and can mislead as to the real size of the desirable device. The only way to determine this using fluoroscopy is to perform either a left atrial or left upper pulmonary vein angiogram to document whether there are residual leaks around the balloon. Using colour flow Doppler, the site(s) and degree of any residual trans-septal shunting can rapidly be determined. This serves as a very sensitive modality for the detection of leaks across the sizing balloon (Fig. 4.34). Colour flow Doppler maps which enhance low velocities are recommended for this purpose as the pressure gradient between the atria is usually low and thus flow velocities across the atrial septum are very low. When a residual leak across the balloon is documented, the catheteriser is requested to further inflate the balloon to a diameter at which no residual leaks are visualised.

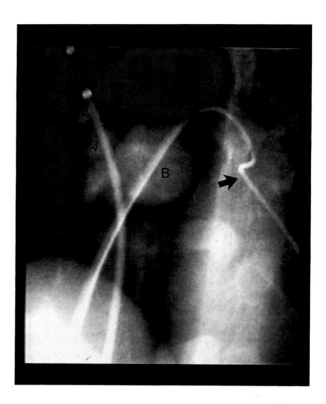

Figure 4.32 *A balloon ASD occlusion catheter (arrow) is placed across the atrial septal defect. The balloon (B) is inflated to a previously known diameter. Note that the atrial septum itself and the upper and lower rims cannot be seen by fluoroscopy.*

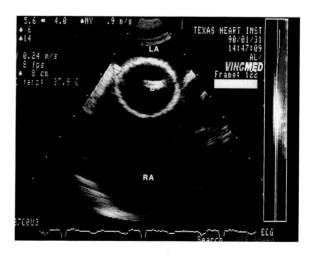

Figure 4.33 *Transesophageal echocardiography display of the balloon catheter across the atrial septum. The balloon (B) occupies all of the atrial septum to cause the atrial septal defect to stretch.*

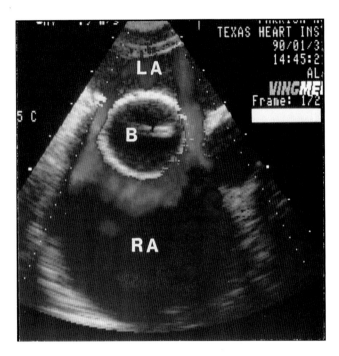

Figure 4.34 *The balloon catheter across the atrial septal defect with colour flow mapping. Note the slow velocity flow from left atrium to right atrium surrounding the balloon. The balloon is not inflated enough to occlude the total length of the atrial septal defect.*

Localisation of the device

After the ASD size is determined and an appropriate device is selected, a sheath and a catheter are introduced into the inferior vena cava and then through the right atrium across the ASD into the left atrium. Transesophageal echocardiography is of help in localisation of the tip of the sheath and/or catheter before the release of the device. Such monitoring prevents opening of the device in the pulmonary veins and/or left atrial appendage. During this manoeuvre, it is crucial to visualise all pulmonary veins, especially the left upper and lower, as well as the atrial appendage. As was mentioned before, the sheath is then withdrawn and the distal limbs are opened. Accurate visualisation of the atrial appendage to exclude localisation of the tip of the sheath in this area is crucial for subsequent successful implantation, as opening the device in the appendage can trap the legs within its walls thus destroying the symmetric configuration of the device.

Problems can arise in transcatheter occlusion of patent foramen ovale. Because of the existence of the relatively rigid septum primum, the catheter sometimes pushes the secundum septum toward the left atrium. This can result in deployment of the device on the right side of the atrial septum. Transesophageal echocardiography should exclude this by visualising the tip of the sheath and should confirm its course across the patent foramen ovale and into the left atrium. Until tip localisation within the left atrium has been established, deployment of the distal legs should not be performed.

Proximity to the atrioventricular valves

In cases where there is a relatively short lower rim to the defect, it is possible to deploy the lower legs of the device (distal and proximal) into the right and left atrioventricular valve. Releasing the device in this position close to the mitral or tricuspid valve can result in atrioventricular valve regurgitation of differing degrees. This should be assessed immediately by direct visualisation of the device and by evaluating atrioventricular valve flow using colour flow Doppler. In cases of device-induced mitral regurgitation, the anterolateral leaflet is involved, whereas in cases of tricuspid regurgitation the septal leaflet is the affected one. Immediate evaluation and assessment of the regurgitant is crucial and should be established immediately before the release of the device. The catheteriser then has the capability of relocating the device within the atria as long as it was not released. After relocation of the ASD Clamshell device, further evaluation of atrioventricular valve function and definition of the new location of the lower legs of the device are easily obtained by directing the transesophageal probe more posteriorly. It is important to visualise *all* 8 legs of the device. This task is sometimes very difficult because the legs are lying in different planes. Flexion and antiflexion, lateral and medial movement of the tip of the endoscope should be used to enable visualisation of the legs. Biplane imaging facilitates imaging of the whole device.

Fenestrated ASD

Transthoracic echocardiographic imaging of the atrial septum is often limited by poor image resolution. The presence of fenestrated ASDs are a major problem for transcatheter occluding procedures. If the fenestrations are not picked-up by either transthoracic echocardiography or angiography, the balloon sizing technique could underestimate the actual size of the ASD as the balloon will be trapped within the fenestrations. In such cases, the only practical method to use to create an intact atrial septum is to choose a device that will cover the whole of the fenestrations. We have found that transesophageal echocardiography provides a superb modality for the visualisation of fenestrated defects. It is not only imaging alone, but colour flow Doppler studies too which will easily demonstrate multiple defects within the septum or multiple adjacent areas of abnormal trans-septal flow, thus confirming the presence of a fenestrated atrial septal defect.

Guidance of the release of the device

As previously discussed, the release of the device is divided into three major steps (1): deploying the distal legs in the left atrium (2), withdrawing the centre of the device into the ASD and deploying the distal legs of the device, and (3) releasing the device itself. Transesophageal echocardiography is essential in monitoring and helping to guide the catheteriser in each of these stages. When the distal legs are opened in the left atrium, visualisation of the four legs, the proximity to the atrial appendage and to the mitral valve is depicted. After the distal legs are opened, the echocardiographer should inform the catheteriser about the exact location of the device, and the distance between the centre of the device and the lower and upper rims. Once this information is established, the catheteriser will withdraw the sheath and the device toward the centre of the ASD until the legs are opposing the left side of the septum. Once at this point, slight pressure is transmitted to the centre of the device before releasing the proximal legs (Fig. 4.35). After establishing the relationship between the distal legs and the left side of the septum, the catheteriser then opens the proximal legs of the device which is now centred within the ASD. At this point, the release mechanism is still hooked to the device and complete retrieval is possible. Transesophageal echocardiography at this point should assess the true deployment of the proximal and distal legs, the proximity to the left and right AV valve, possible mitral and/or tricuspid regurgitation and detection defecting devices, i.e. one or more legs are not in the normal position or angle toward the atrial septum. If any of these occurr, relocation of the device is necessary. When the catheteriser and the echocardiographer are satisfied with the localisation of the device within the ASD, the catheteriser will

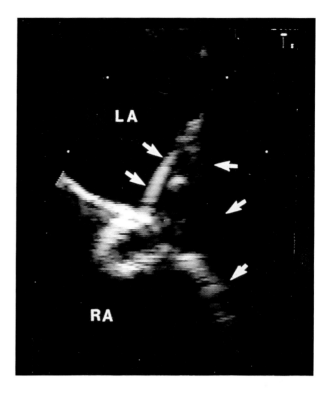

Figure 4.35 *Transesophageal echocardiography of the opening of the proximal legs of the device (arrows). Note that the legs are open in the left atrial side and the device is withdrawn toward the atrial septal defect.*

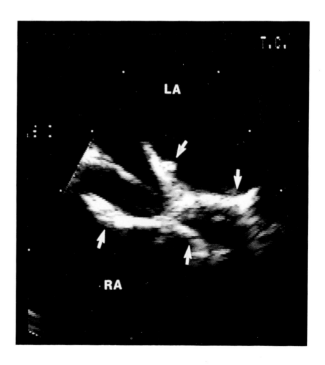

Figure 4.36 *Transesophageal echocardiography of the atrial septal defect device in place post-release. Note that two pair of legs are well seen in the left side of the septum and two pair of legs are well seen in the right side of the septum (arrows). The device is located centrally within the atrial septal defect.*

release the device under direct visualisation by fluoroscopy and transesophageal echocardiography (Fig. 4.36). Continuous monitoring by echocardiography is of value in preventing excess radiation exposure. Immediate dislodgement of the device is well documented by echocardiography and, for this reason, continuous monitoring is desirable.

Residual leaks across the device

Colour flow Doppler is very sensitive in the detection of residual leaks across ASD devices. An immediate post-implantation evaluation, and then further examinations at five, ten and fifteen minutes are required. Small residual leaks are commonly seen immediately after device implantation, but in most a complete haemodynamic closure will be obtained within fifteen minutes. If a residual leak is demonstrated, its location (i.e. around the lower, middle or upper part of the device) should be established. It is important to ascertain the exact location of the residual leak in order to plan further follow-up evaluations using both transthoracic and transesophageal echocardiography. If a large leak is present, the placement of a second device in the future is an option (Fig. 4.37).

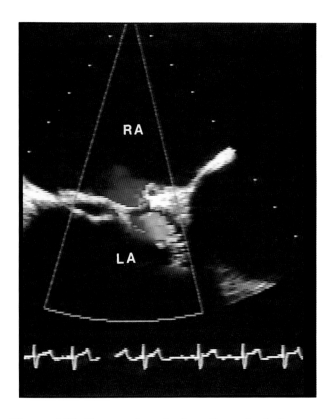

Figure 4.37 *Transesophageal echocardiography depicts a small residual leak post-implantation of the atrial septal defect device. Note the origin of the leak is near the lower legs of the device.*

VENTRICULAR SEPTAL DEFECT

An isolated defect in the intraventricular septum is the most common congenital cardiac malformation (bicuspid aortic valve and mitral valve prolapse excluded). A ventricular septal defect (VSD) occurring as a solitary lesion comprises approximately 20% of all congenital heart disease. The incidence of VSD is reported to be 1.5–3.8 per 1000 live births. In addition, VSDs are an integral part of tetralogy of Fallot and double-outlet right ventricle and occur as well in association with transposition of the great arteries, pulmonary atresia and coarctation of the aorta(10). There are four anatomical types of VSD. This subdivision is based on the relative location of the defect in the septum: (1) perimembranous VSD, (2) supracristal VSD, (3) inlet VSD, and (4) muscular VSD. Muscular VSDs may be single or multiple and occur anywhere in the trabecular septum. These account for 5–20% of all VSDs. Perimembranous and muscular VSDs may become smaller with time or undergo spontaneous closure. The chances of spontaneous closure are greatest in the first year of life and with small defects.

Another population of patients in whom VSDs are seen are adults who have sustained rupture of the intraventricular septum secondary to myocardial infarction. This complication is estimated to occur in 1–3% of acute myocardial infarctions and accounts for roughly 5% of infarction death(11). Many of these patients present in cardiogenic shock and require repair of the VSD. Without VSD closure, most of these patients will die. Unfortunately, surgical repair of these lesions is associated with a higher than 50% mortality. If the patient does not present in cardiogenic shock, the mortality of the surgical repair decreases to 18–27%. Until recently, all haemodynamically significant VSDs required closure by surgical means. The repair of a muscular VSD presents additional problems. One is the inaccessibility of the defect through the right atrium or ventricle because of heavy trabeculation(12). This necessitates an approach via a left ventriculotomy. The surgical repair of a muscular VSD is associated with a significant increase in morbidity or mortality when compared with repair of other types of VSDs(13). Furthermore, because of difficulty in visualisation of these defects, they are often missed at the time of surgical repair. These patients frequently require reoperation for this, which substantially increases the risk for long-term ventricular dysfunction and mortality. Recently, Lock and O'Laughlin have reported the use of a Rashkind umbrella to close VSDs in patients with post-myocardial infarction and congenital VSD(14,15). Muscular defects in the trabecular septum are the preferred site for occlusion device insertion. However, the proximity of the VSD to atrioventricular valve tissue in the perimembranous or inlet septum make device insertion difficult and may interfere with valve function.

Technique

The occlusion device is delivered via a sheath passed through the defect from the venous side(16). The delivery route of the occlusion device depends upon the location of the defect; mid-trabecular and apical muscular defects are approached from the right jugular vein, whereas outflow, anterior and posterior perimembranous defects can be accessed from the femoral approach. As an initial step in the procedure, the VSD is crossed from the left ventricle. Either from the trans-septal or retrograde femoral approach, an end-hole balloon catheter is directed through the VSD into the right ventricle and then to the right atrium. This balloon catheter also serves as the sizing catheter used to determine the size of the defect. An exchange wire is advanced through the catheter into the right ventricle and then to the right atrium. The wire is snared and withdrawn through either the jugular or femoral sheath. Another sheath and dilator are advanced over the exchange wire from the venous side and the tip of the sheath is passed through the VSD into the left ventricle. The occlusion umbrella and its loading catheter is then advanced through the long sheath until the distal legs open within the left ventricle. The sheath and device are withdrawn as a single unit until the distal legs impinge upon the left ventricular endocardium. The sheath is pulled back until the proximal legs are opened. With the device firmly in place, it will then be released (Fig. 4.38).

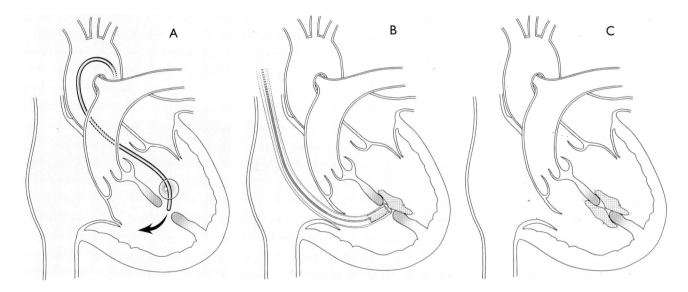

Figure 4.38 (a) *A balloon catheter is directed across the ventricular septal defect in order to estimate defect size.* **(b)** *The sheath and catheter when the device is introduced from the right side across the ventricular septal defect into the left side with the distal legs opened.* **(c)** *The sheath and catheter are withdrawn toward the right ventricle. The proximal legs are open and the device is released.*

Echocardiographic monitoring

Transesophageal echocardiography has a major role in the definition of VSD morphology and in the monitoring and guidance of its closure by the device. Every patient should be carefully evaluated by transthoracic echocardiography before entering the catheterisation laboratory. With apical muscular VSDs, echocardiographic visualisation of the cardiac apex is normally better effected using the transthoracic approach rather than the transesophageal one. Visualisation of the apex of the heart in most cases is much easier using the apical precordial four-chamber or subcostal long and short axis view than the transgastric transesophageal view(3). The main benefits of transesophageal echocardiography during transcatheter closure of VSD are listed in Table 4.5

Localisation and sizing of the VSD

Transesophageal echocardiography using transgastric and esophageal four-chamber views will normally enable visualisation of the VSD. It is crucial to measure the size of the defect itself on both its left and right septal aspects. In addition, most of the muscular VSDs have a tunnel-type morphology and it is important to provide the catheteriser with information about the length of the tunnel. In cases of multiple muscular VSD, the exact positioning of the various defects, with regard to the septal length and to landmarks like the moderator band, is helpful in guiding the procedure. In cases of multiple VSDs consisting of a combination of perimembranous and muscular defects, definition of the borders of the different defects, and the distance between them, are important for accurate deployment and release of the device (Fig. 4.39).

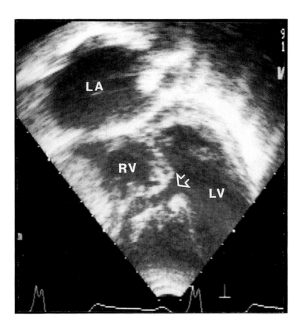

Figure 4.39 *Echocardiographic examination revealed a ventricular septal defect (tunnel type). Note the total length of the ventricular septal defect. The arrow shows the origin of the ventricular septal defect from the left side.*

Table 4.5

Localisation and sizing of the VSD

Guiding different stages of the procedures, including catheter and wire insertion through the VSD

Assessment of device location within the left ventricle/right ventricle

Guidance of release of the device

Assessing proximity of the device to the atrioventricular valves

Detection of residual leaks

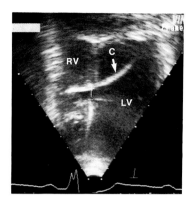

Figure 4.40 *Echocardiography showing the catheter (C) when placed across the ventricular septal defect from the left side.*

Guidance of the end-hole balloon catheter and the wire across the VSD

As described above, an end-hole balloon catheter is introduced from the left side into the right side followed by a wire. Usually if there is a significant left-to-right shunt, a balloon catheter will be flow-directed into the VSD and across the defect. Transesophageal echocardiography is of help in guiding the catheteriser in his manipulations of the tip of the catheter and balloon toward the VSD. Using a combination of esophageal four-chamber and transgastric approaches, the echocardiographer can guide the catheteriser by providing accurate information on the spacial localisation of the catheter. Continuous flexion and extension of the transesophageal transducer tip will provide two-dimensional spacial localisation of the catheter, and once the tip is near the orifice of the VSD, transesophageal echocardiography can further guide the 'fishing' process.

Once the balloon catheter is across the VSD, the sizing of the defect by the balloon stretching technique (described previously in the ASD closure section) is performed. The ventricular septum is a more rigid structure than the atrial septum and smaller balloons are used. The smallest balloon passing across the VSD will serve as the VSD size for determining the device selection. Once the balloon catheter is across the VSD, a wire is advanced through the catheter into the right ventricle and then to the right atrium. This wire is snared and withdrawn through the jugular or femoral sheath. This snaring procedure can use echocardiography and fluoroscopy as a complementary imaging technique in order to grasp the wire and advance it from the internal jugular vein and pull it back and out the venous sheath to complete an intracardiac loop (Fig. 4.40). When this stage of the procedure is performed, echocardiographic visualisation of right ventricle, tricuspid valve, right atrium and SVC right atrial junction are important. The basal and four-chamber view are used and sheath and catheter are visualised during this procedure. In cases of combined perimembranous muscular VSD, echocardiography will be the first modality to assure the catheteriser that the end-hole catheter, as well as the wire, went through the septum in the muscular defect and not in the perimembranous one.

Introduction of the device

Once the intracardiac loop is complete, a sheath is introduced into the left ventricle. The occlusion device on top of its designated catheter is then introduced through the sheath into the left ventricle. Transesophageal echocardiography will visualise the tip of the sheath in the left ventricle. It is important to be sure that the sheath is directed toward the mid-cavity and is not trapped in the apex or located close to the left AV valve. Once the device reaches the tip of the sheath in the left ventricle, the sheath and the catheter are withdrawn. This results in deployment of the distal legs. Even when the distal legs are opened, the catheteriser still has complete control of the device. Under echocardiography guidance, the device is brought as close as possible to the VSD until it opposes the left side of the ventricular septum. Once in this position, it is important to detect any abnormal relationship between the legs of the device and the AV valve, including any trapping of the legs on a false tendon, or an incomplete opening of the distal springs. The catheter with the device is then withdrawn toward the mouth of the VSD on the left side of the septum

(Fig. 4.41). If the VSD has a tunnel-type configuration, the extent of the device into the tunnel should be evaluated before the release of the distal legs. Once the distal legs are released, the proximity to the tricuspid valve as well as trapping of the legs of the device on the right-sided trabeculation should be evaluated. Only after the echocardiographer and the catheteriser are satisfied with the location of the device within the intraventricular septum, a colour flow Doppler examination and a left ventricular angiogram will be performed to evaluate possible residual leaks. The device is then released under continuous fluoroscopy and echocardiographic monitoring, and the final configuration of the device is evaluated; namely the extension of the arms, their angle and any evidence of collapse. Continuous monitoring of the device should be performed for up to 15 minutes after the release in order to demonstrate any possible dislodgement (Fig. 4.42).

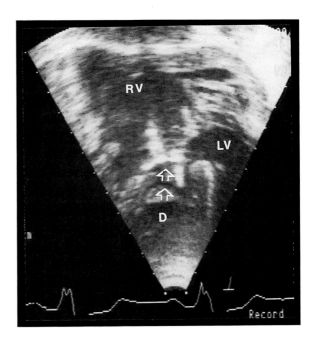

Figure 4.42 *The device (D) is completely opened on both sides. Note the four pairs of legs on the left and right side in the ventricular septum.*

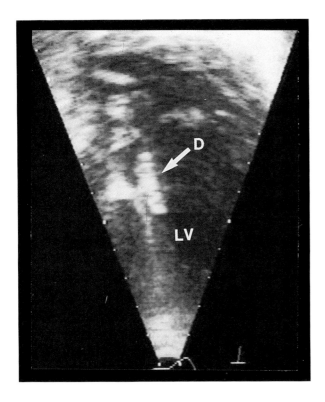

Figure 4.41 *The distal legs of the device (D) are open on the left side very close to the origin of the ventricular septal defect in the septum.*

Evaluation post-implantation

Transesophageal echocardiography with Doppler and colour flow imaging has been found to be very useful in the evaluation of residual leaks. Complete or partial occlusion is easily documented and the exact localisation of residual leaks is easily visualised. Usually the flow across residual leaks will be of high velocity and a turbulent flow is depicted with the colour flow Doppler modality. High pulse repetition frequency or continuous wave Doppler enables assessment of the left ventricular to right ventricular gradient across the defect. The appearance of atrioventricular valve incompetence (either right or left) due to an encroachment of one of the cuffs, should be evaluated and a complete Doppler study across both atrioventricular valves should be performed before the transesophageal study is complete.

In conclusion, therapeutic catheter closure of VSDs, especially muscular ones, is becoming more and more attractive as the preferable modality of treatment for this lesion. Transesophageal echocardiography provides the catheteriser with an immediate, on-line, accurate, spacial localisation of the device, the catheters and the wires. With the continuous improvement in transesophageal transducers (i.e. miniaturisation, high resolution, lower frequencies and biplane and multiplane modalities), we envisage an era of more and more co-operation between cardiac catheterisation and echocardiography. Using biplane and/or multiplane modalities will enable visualisation of the devices in each plane and the possibility of three-dimensional real time reconstruction. This technology, together with the development of transluminal imaging, will bring echocardiography as a major participant in any interventional cardiac procedure in the future.

REFERENCES

1. MULLINS CE. Therapeutic cardiac catheterisation. In: Garson A, Bricker JT, McNamara DG (eds), *The science and practice of pediatric cardiology*. Philadelphia: Lea and Febiger, 1990: 2183–209.
2. ALI KHAN MA, MULLINS CE, NIHILL MR, YOUSEF SA, et al. Percutaneous catheter closure of the ductus arteriosus in children and young adults. *Am J Cardiol* 1989; **64:** 218–21.
3. MATSUZAKI M, TOMA Y, KUSUKAWA R. Clinical applications of transoesophageal echocardiography. *Circulation* 1990; **82:** 709–21.
4. VICK GW, TITUS J. Defects of the atrial septum including the atrioventricular canal. In: Garson A, Bricker JT, McNamara DG (eds), *The science and practice of pediatric cardiology*. Philadelphia: Lea and Febiger, 1990: 1023–54.
5. LOCK JE, ROME JJ, DAVIS R, VAN PRAAGH S, PERRY SB, VAN PRAAGH R, KEANE JF. Transcatheter closure of atrial septal defects: Experimental studies. *Circulation* 1989; **79:** 1091–9.
6. BRIDGES ND, NEWBURGER JW, MAYER JE, LOCK JE. Transcatheter closure of secundum ASD in pediatric patients. The first year's experience (abstract). *Am J Cardiol* 1990; **66:** 522(18).
7. HELLENBRAND WE, FAHEY JT, McGOWEN FX, WELTIN GE, KLEINMAN CS. Transoesophageal echocardiographic guidance of transcatheter closure of atrial septal defect. *Am J Cardiol* 1990; **66:** 207–13.
8. MORIMOTO K, MATSUZAKI M, TACHMA Y, ONO S, TANAKA N, MICHISHIGE H, MURATA K, ANNO Y, KUSUKAWAR ?. Diagnosis and quantitative evaluation of secundum-type atrial septal defect by transoesophageal Doppler echocardiography. *Am J Cardiol* 1990; **66:** 85–91.
9. CABALKA AK, LUDOMIRSKY A, VICK GW, O'LAUGHLIN MP, PIGNATELLI R, MULLINS CE. Patient selection for transcatheter occlusion of atrial septal defect: 2-D echocardiographic criteria. *Circulation* 1993 (in press).
10. COOLEY DA, GARRETT HE, HOWARD HS. The surgical treatment of ventricular septal defect: An analysis of 300 consecutive surgical cases. *Prog Cardiovasc Dis* 1967; **4:** 312.
11. GUILIANI ER, DANIELSON GK, PLUTH JR, ODYNIECK NA, WALLACE RB. Postinfarction ventricular septal rupture. *Circulation* 1974; **49:** 455–9.
12. KIRKLIN JK, CASTENEDA AR, KEANE JF, FELLOWS KE, NORWOOD WI. Surgical management of multiple ventricular septal defects. *J Thorac Cardiovasc Surg* 1980; **80:** 485–93.
13. GRIFFITHS SP, TURI GK, KRONGRUD E, SWIFT LH, GERSONY WM, et al. Muscular ventricular septal defects repaired with left ventriculotomy. *Am J Cardiol* 1981; **48**(5): 877–86.
14. LOCK JE, BLOCK PC, McKAY RC, BAIM DS, KEANE JF. Transcatheter closure of ventricular septal defects. *Circulation* 1988; **78**(2): 361–8.
15. O'LAUGHLIN MP, MULLINS CE. Transcatheter occlusion of ventricular septal defect. *Cathet Cardiovasc Diagn* 1989; **17:** 175–9.
16. LOCK JE, COCKERHAM JT, KEANE JF, FINLEY JP, WAKELY PE, FELLOWS KE. Transcatheter umbrella closure of congenital heart defects. *Circulation* 1987; **73**(3): 593–9.

The follow-up of congenital heart disease

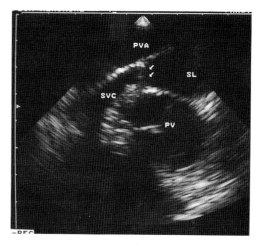

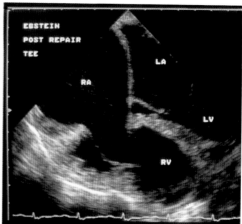

Atrioventricular valve repair

A. G. Fraser

INTRODUCTION

Mitral valve reconstruction is now the commonest indication for intraoperative echocardiography in adults. Repair or replacement of an atrioventricular valve is required much less often in children, but when it is, intraoperative echocardiography is also extremely useful. Before bypass, transesophageal and epicardial imaging provide detailed information about the morphological basis of any valve lesion, and after bypass, colour flow mapping and other Doppler techniques reveal the function of the repaired valve under relatively physiological loading conditions. Determining the outcome of surgery before the chest is closed enables the surgeon to revise the repair immediately, if the result appears unsatisfactory. Obviously, valve replacement should be avoided in children whenever possible; intraoperative echocardiography helps the paediatric cardiac surgeon to achieve this goal by allowing him or her to attempt ambitious repairs.

The principles of using echocardiography to assess the structure and function of the atrioventricular valves are similar in children and adults, although the spectrum of disease varies. When investigating patients of any age, a sound understanding of the anatomy of the mitral and tricuspid valves is required, if their different components are to be imaged logically. The assessment of valvar function with Doppler techniques is similar in congenital and acquired disease.

ECHOCARDIOGRAPHIC ANATOMY OF THE ATRIOVENTRICULAR VALVES

The mitral and tricuspid valves are large structures relative to the size of the heart, and complete assessment is possible only if they are studied in multiple imaging planes. In a patient being considered for surgery, the aim of echocardiographic imaging is to identify the precise site(s) and mechanism of the valve fault. Competence of any valve depends on normal, intact coaptation of its leaflets. In patients with mitral or tricuspid regurgitation, the pattern of closure of the edges of the leaflets should therefore be studied in detail, along the whole length of each zone of coaptation including the commissures. Misleading information may be obtained unless the plane of imaging remains orientated at right angles to the bodies and edges of the leaflets; this can be achieved successfully only if the anatomy of the orifice is known.

When an abnormal pattern of opening or closure of the mitral or tricuspid leaflets is detected, its mechanism should be investigated by studying the structure and function of the other components of the valve. These include the tendinous cords (chordae tendineae), the papillary muscles, adjacent segments of ventricular myocardium, and the atrioventricular junctions (mitral and tricuspid annuli). Additional imaging planes, such as transgastric longitudinal scans, are required to study these structures.

The mitral valve

The normal mitral valve has two leaflets. The anterior or aortic leaflet is relatively broad, and it is attached along approximately one-third of the circumference of the left atrioventricular junction. Superiorly the aortic leaflet of the mitral valve is contiguous with the posterior aortic root. The posterior or mural leaflet of the mitral valve has a much longer attachment, to the lateral as well as to the inferior or 'posterior' portion of the atrioventricular junction, which explains why the name 'mural' leaflet is preferred. The body of the mural leaflet is relatively narrow, and it is divided into a variable number of scallops (usually three). The commissures of the mitral valve are located anterolaterally, just inferior to the orifice of the left atrial appendage, and posteromedially, inferior to the subaortic diverticulum of the left ventricle and on the opposite side of the ventricular septum from the orifice of the coronary sinus. Between these limits, the orientation of the zone of coaptation of the mitral leaflets rotates through 90 degrees. The relationships of the leaflets and commissures of the mitral valve to the standard transesophageal imaging planes are shown in Fig. 5.1.

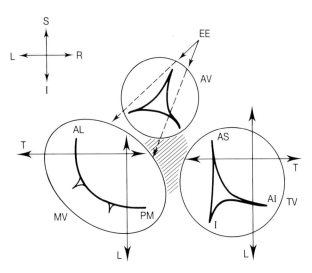

Figure 5.1 *Drawing of the atrioventricular junctions, as viewed from the posterior (esophageal) aspect of the heart. The shaded area represents the central fibrous body. The leaflets of the valves are depicted in their true anatomical orientations (see compass), and the superimposed lines represent the orientation of standard transesophageal imaging planes (T = transverse, L = longitudinal), and also the planes used to study the mitral valve on epicardial echocardiography (EE). S = superior, I = inferior, R = right, L = left. AV = aortic valve. MV = mitral valve, with anterolateral (AL) and posteromedial (PM) commissures. TV = tricuspid valve, with anterosuperior (AS), inferior (I), and anteroinferior (AI) commissures.*

Transesophageal imaging in the transverse axis (for example using a single-plane probe) is ideal for demonstrating the mitral leaflets adjacent to the anterolateral commissure, and the lateral third of the orifice. In contrast, the posteromedial commissure and the medial thirds of the mitral leaflets are demonstrated clearly during transesophageal echocardiography only by imaging in longitudinal planes (i.e. with a biplane probe) (1). A transverse scan of the medial part of the mitral valve may fail completely to show the pattern of closure of the leaflets at this site, since the plane of imaging runs along the orifice of the valve rather than, as required, at right angles to it. Conversely, transesophageal imaging in the longitudinal axis near to the anterolateral commissure is unhelpful, or even misleading if the clefts between the scallops of the mural leaflet are misinterpreted as the orifice of the valve. The centre of the mitral orifice is shown well in both transverse and longitudinal planes, which traverse large segments of the aortic leaflet tangentially, and small segments of the mural leaflet. Thus, biplane imaging is required to localise disease of the mitral leaflets (2). Transverse and longitudinal images of a particular valve may be very different (Fig. 5.2).

The commonest causes of congenital mitral regurgitation are atrioventricular septal defect and cleft mitral valve. The so-called cleft in patients with a partial atrioventricular septal defect is not a true cleft at all, but the space between the conjoined anterior and posterior leaflets which is orientated towards the ventricular septum. In patients with a complete atrioventricular septal defect, the anatomy of the orifice is even more different from normal (3). Usually, there are four leaflets – anterosuperior, posteroinferior, and two lateral leaflets (4). The anterosuperior leaflet has two separate components, which are sometimes called the right and left anterior leaflets (5). The standard transesophageal imaging planes are not ideally aligned to study the four commissures between the central and lateral leaflets, but the middle of the orifice is shown well in longitudinal planes (Fig. 5.3(a)). In complete atrioventricular septal defect, the space between the bridging leaflets functions as a commissure rather than a cleft (6), while in partial defects it is a common site of regurgitation.

In patients with an isolated cleft of the mitral valve, the anatomy of the aortic and mural leaflets is relatively normal. A 'true' cleft in the aortic leaflet of the mitral valve is orientated towards the left ventricular outflow tract (7,8), midway between the longitudinal and transverse axes. Regurgitation through a cleft is shown by either a transverse or a longitudinal transducer (Fig. 5.3(b)), especially if

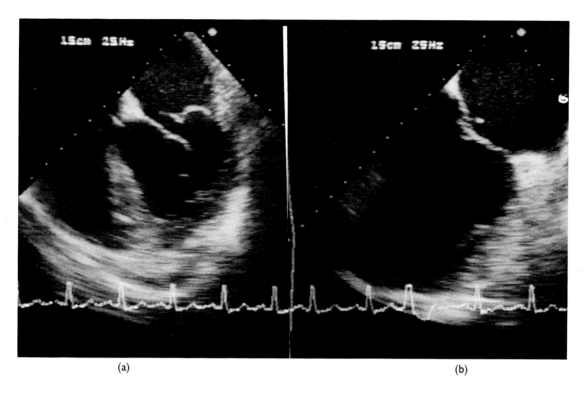

(a)   (b)

Figure 5.2 (a) *Transverse and* **(b)** *longitudinal transesophageal images in a patient with mitral regurgitation due to a ruptured tendinous cord to the mural mitral leaflet. The transverse image demonstrates a regurgitant orifice, with the ruptured cord trailing from the prolapsing edge of the leaflet. There is also slight 'prolapse' of the body of the mural leaflet. In the longitudinal image coaptation appears normal and there is no evidence of 'prolapse'. The additional echo observed on the atrial side of the closure line of the valve is caused by the ruptured cord. Together, these images demonstrate that the valvar pathology is located in the lateral (anatomical left) third of the zone of coaptation, towards but not including the anterolateral commissure.*

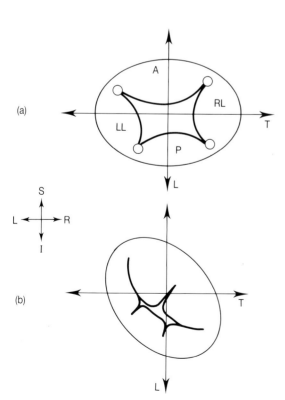

Figure 5.3 *Orientation of the leaflets of the atrioventricular valves to standard transesophageal imaging planes (T = transverse, L = longitudinal) in congenital heart disease.* **(a)** *Complete atrioventricular septal defect with a common atrioventricular valve. The circles represent the sites of the papillary muscles. The leaflets are anterosuperior (A), posteroinferior (P), left lateral (LL) and right lateral (RL). Adapted from Arisawa et al.(4).* **(b)** *Isolated cleft mitral valve.*

the tip of the probe is tilted, but diastolic separation of the thickened edges of the leaflets at the cleft (the diagnostic hallmark on precordial imaging) can be very difficult to show on transesophageal echocardiography (see Fig. 5.14). Unless a clear short-axis image of the mitral orifice is obtained from a transgastric approach, it may be necessary to perform epicardial studies, if pre-bypass images are required to plan surgery.

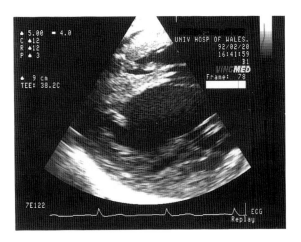

Figure 5.4 *Transgastric longitudinal image of the papillary muscles and subvalvar apparatus of the mitral valve, obtained with a multiplane probe. The subtle variation of imaging planes possible with this probe allows accurate alignment to the subvalvar apparatus. In this patient, there are three heads of the posteromedial papillary muscle, and numerous cords are displayed separately.*

The anterolateral and posteromedial papillary muscles of the normal mitral valve insert into the free wall of the left ventricle, opposite the commissures. The papillary muscles cannot be displayed in a single transverse scan from the oesophagus, but they are demonstrated well in transgastric images. Using the longitudinal transducer, it is usually possible to depict both papillary muscles and some of their tendinous cords in a single plane. It may be easier to study the subvalvar apparatus of the mitral valve using a multiplane probe, because it gives a greater choice of imaging planes (Fig. 5.4). Both papillary muscles supply cords to both leaflets, inserting into the bodies of the leaflets (secondary cords) as well as into their edges (primary cords).

Transgastric images of the subvalvar apparatus are particularly important in patients with congenital mitral stenosis, which is caused more often by abnormalities of the papillary muscles and cords than by disease of the bodies of the leaflets. On precordial echocardiography, it may be difficult to distinguish between different abnormalities of the subvalvar apparatus, such as cordal fusion and fibrosis (9). In short-axis planes, a single papillary muscle may be seen in patients with a parachute mitral valve, and abnormalites of the cords may be seen in patients with an anomalous mitral arcade, in which the papillary muscles extend right up to the leaflets, or a hammock mitral valve in which shortened cords are attached to enlarged papillary muscles (10). Transgastric imaging is also the best transesophageal technique for studying global or regional function of the left ventricle. This may be important in patients with mitral regurgitation related to myocardial ischaemia and congenital abnormalities of the coronary arteries.

Mitral valve prolapse

Traditionally, echocardiographic analysis of a regurgitant mitral valve has concentrated on the detection of mitral valve prolapse, defined as systolic displacement of part of a leaflet towards the left atrium beyond the level of the annulus. However, this particular criterion is relatively unimportant for 'surgical echocardiography' of the mitral valve. Abnormal motion of the *body* of a mitral leaflet does not matter *per se*, unless it also causes abnormal motion of the *edge* of the leaflet. 'Prolapse' of the bodies of both leaflets may be present in a valve which functions normally if its leaflets still coapt, and it is abnormal closure of the edges of the leaflets which the surgeon aims to correct. In practice, problems of interpretation will arise only if the location of the annulus is used as a reference point for identifying mild prolapse in a patient in whom no other morphological basis for regurgitation is found, and if this information is then used to select the surgical technique.

Mitral valve prolapse should be identified on transesophageal echocardiography only if the orientation of the imaging plane to the annulus is appreciated. The annulus of the mitral valve is saddle-shaped, with 'high' points lying anteriorly (adjacent to the aortic root) and posteriorly, and 'low' points, which are closer to the left ventricular apex, lying laterally and medially (11). Using single-plane transesophageal echocardiography, transverse four-chamber planes (which pass near to the 'low' points of the annulus) will tend to exaggerate prolapse (12). Longitudinal planes are more accurate (see Fig. 5.2). This situation is exactly analogous to the higher incidence of prolapse found when imaging the mitral valve from the precordium in apical four-chamber planes (equivalent to transesophageal transverse planes) rather than in parasternal long-axis ones (equivalent to transesophageal longitudinal planes). For example, Warth *et al.* found a prevalence of mitral valve prolapse in 10–18-year-old subjects of 35%, when imaging from the apex, but this fell to only 1% when positive parasternal studies were also required for the diagnosis (13). Transverse-plane transesophageal imaging in adults will also give a high false positive rate. For example, Zenker *et al.* found prolapse in 17% of normal controls (14). In adults, the mean deviation of the annulus from a central reference plane is about 5 mm, while the maximum deviation from non-planarity (that is, the distance between parallel planes passing respectively through the low points and the high points of the annulus) is as much as 1.4 cm (11). These data were obtained in 15 adults aged 18–41 years; corresponding allowances should be made in children.

The tricuspid valve

The three leaflets of the tricuspid valve are the anterosuperior, septal and inferior leaflets (see Fig. 5.1). Between these, there are two zones of coaptation. In precordial four-chamber views, and in the standard transesophageal (transverse) four-chamber image, the zone of coaptation which is demonstrated clearly is that between the septal and anterosuperior leaflets. The zone of coaptation between the anterosuperior and inferior leaflets is shown well by imaging in longitudinal planes. In patients with tricuspid regurgitation caused by enlargement of the right atrioventricular junction, the regurgitant jet tends to arise in the centre of the tricuspid orifice at the junction of all three leaflets, and so it can usually be identified clearly while using either a transverse or a longitudinal transducer. The subvalvar apparatus of the tricuspid valve can be demonstrated on transgastric imaging, but much manipulation of the probe is required to identify all structures. Multiplane probes may be particularly useful for studying the tricuspid valve (Fig. 5.5).

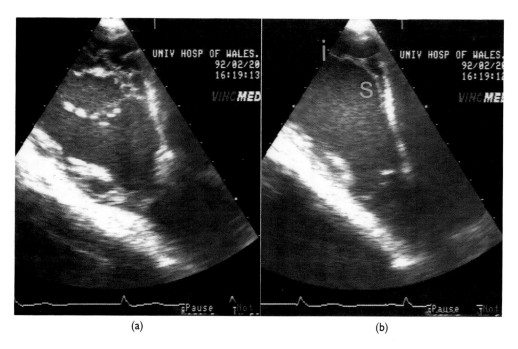

(a) (b)

Figure 5.5 *Transgastric transesophageal images of the tricuspid valve in* **(a)** *systole and* **(b)** *diastole obtained with a multiplane probe. The systolic image shows the subvalvar apparatus (mostly the tendinous cords) in short axis. In the diastolic image, sections of the septal (s) and inferior (i) leaflets) are displayed around the perimeter of the inlet of the right ventricle.*

Epicardial imaging

If a biplane or multiplane transesophageal probe is not available, it may be impossible to study the mitral and tricuspid valves fully from the oesophagus. However, an additional epicardial echocardiographic study can provide detailed images of the morphology of both valves. A standard precordial transducer is inserted into a sterile plastic sleeve and then placed directly on the epicardium, usually over the right ventricular outflow tract (15). In small children, good quality images are obtained with a 5 MHz transducer, but the 3.5 MHz transducer may be required for colour flow mapping. When scanning along the anatomical long axis of the heart, with the probe directed to the right, the anterosuperior and inferior leaflets of the tricuspid valve together with the right ventricular inlet are observed in a long-axis image. The transducer can then be directed towards the mitral valve, tilting the beam of ultrasound towards both mitral commissures in turn, while maintaining planes of imaging which are orthogonal to the edges of the mitral leaflets (see Fig. 5.1). The orifices of the mitral and tricuspid valves can also be imaged in short-axis views.

The value of epicardial echocardiography during surgery for congenital heart disease has been well documented. After bypass, transesophageal echocardiography has advantages when assessing residual atrioventricular valvar regurgitation (16). Thus the two techniques should be considered as complementary rather than alternative approaches to intraoperative diagnosis.

SURGERY FOR MITRAL STENOSIS IN CHILDHOOD

Obstruction to left ventricular inflow may be caused by a wide variety of congenital abnormalities, ranging from cor triatriatum and supravalvar mitral ring to a hypoplastic or imperforate mitral valve. Carpentier *et al.* describe four main causes of congenital mitral stenosis, namely commissural fusion in a dysplastic valve, hammock lesion, parachute deformity, and a funnel-shaped valve (10). Common conditions involving the subvalvar apparatus are associated with shortened, tethered, fused or absent cords or papillary muscles (17). Double-orifice mitral valve may be associated with either stenosis or regurgitation.

The diagnosis is established by cross-sectional imaging and Doppler studies from the precordium (9). However, it may be difficult to demonstrate the tendinous cords clearly from the precordium, and some patients may have more than one cause of mitral stenosis (for example, supravalvar ring co-existing with a parachute mitral valve) (9). Without surgery, the prognosis of congenital mitral stenosis is poor, with less than 40% of patients surviving for 10 years (18). Fortunately, a large proportion of patients can be treated successfully by mitral valve repair, with good results (10,19). In some series a substantial minority of patients have required late reoperation, sometimes for a fault persisting from the first operation. Thus, intraoperative echocardiography has two functions in these patients – it can guide the surgical approach to reconstruction, and it may reduce the need for late reoperation.

In young patients with rheumatic mitral stenosis, the leaflets remain relatively pliable and mobile while the commissures become fused. Such valves are ideal for surgical or balloon valvotomy. These procedures can be monitored by transesophageal echocardiography (20) but it may be difficult to justify the added expense and complexity involved, particularly in those countries in which rheumatic mitral stenosis is still common. Nonetheless, if the immediate result is poor, echocardiography may be used to identify the site, mechanism and significance of induced regurgitation before the patient is subjected to further surgery. Echocardiography is more useful in selecting patients who are suitable for balloon valvotomy, as the likelihood of a successful outcome can be predicted fairly well by assessing the thickness and mobility of the leaflets, the amount of calcification, and the degree of subvalvar involvement (21). Transesophageal echocardiography is also used prior to the procedure to check that there is no thrombus within the left atrium.

MECHANISMS OF MITRAL REGURGITATION

The surgeon tries to restore competence to a leaking atrioventricular valve, by aligning the edges of its leaflets so that they coapt as normally as possible. Thus, the information which the surgeon requires is related primarily to the pattern of closure of the leaflets at their edges. This is defined in terms of coaptation and apposition. *Coaptation* occurs when the mitral leaflets remain in contact throughout systole; *apposition* is normal if the leaflets are symmetrically aligned opposite each other throughout systole, so that the whole of their rough zones are in contact. Analysing valve closure by studying these functions is useful because abnormalities can then be related logically to the type of repair which is appropriate (22).

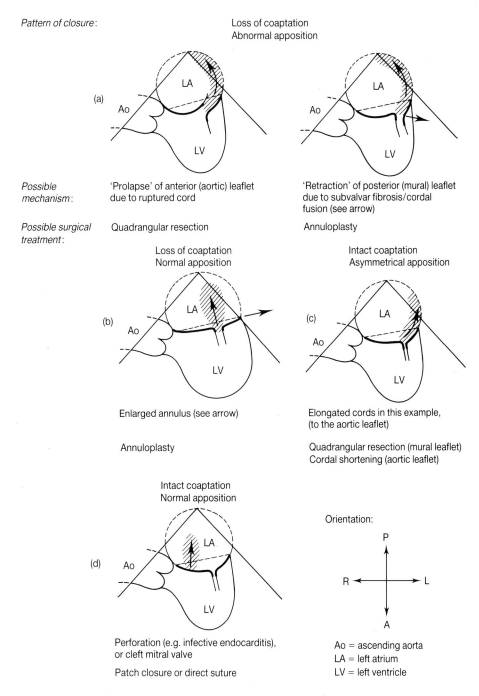

Pattern of closure:

Loss of coaptation
Abnormal apposition

(a)

Possible mechanism:

'Prolapse' of anterior (aortic) leaflet due to ruptured cord

'Retraction' of posterior (mural) leaflet due to subvalvar fibrosis/cordal fusion (see arrow)

Possible surgical treatment:

Quadrangular resection

Annuloplasty

Loss of coaptation
Normal apposition

(b)

Enlarged annulus (see arrow)

Annuloplasty

Intact coaptation
Asymmetrical apposition

(c)

Elongated cords in this example, (to the aortic leaflet)

Quadrangular resection (mural leaflet)
Cordal shortening (aortic leaflet)

Intact coaptation
Normal apposition

(d)

Perforation (e.g. infective endocarditis), or cleft mitral valve

Patch closure or direct suture

Orientation:

P

R — L

A

Ao = ascending aorta
LA = left atrium
LV = left ventricle

Figure 5.6 *The mitral valve in mitral regurgitation. The drawings illustrate different patterns of closure of the mitral leaflets which may be observed on transesophageal echocardiography in transverse planes.*

The commonest mechanism of regurgitation is loss of coaptation. This produces a systolic regurgitant orifice which is identified on cross-sectional imaging as well as on colour flow mapping. If apposition is also abnormal (that is, the leaflets at the regurgitant orifice are asymmetrical), (Fig. 5.6(a)), then the regurgitation is caused by systolic displacement (or 'prolapse') of the edge of one leaflet (Fig. 5.7), or by retraction of the edge of the other one. In both instances, the regurgitant jet will be eccentric (23). If the prolapse is caused by elongated or ruptured tendinous cords (24), competence may be restored by shortening or transferring cords, or by resecting the flail segment of the leaflet. Rupture of

a commissural cord causes prolapse of both leaflets at that commissure. Loss of coaptation due to retraction or restricted motion of a leaflet occurs in congenital abnormalities of the subvalvar apparatus, acquired rheumatic damage to the subvalvar apparatus, or other unusual pathology (Fig. 5.8). In adults the commonest cause is basal infarction of the left ventricle, producing localised dyskinesis and increased systolic tension on the cords to the mural leaflet. Mitral regurgitation associated with outflow tract obstruction may be caused by retraction of the anterior leaflet at the site of attachment of a membrane, or by haemodynamic factors in hypertrophic cardiomyopathy (25).

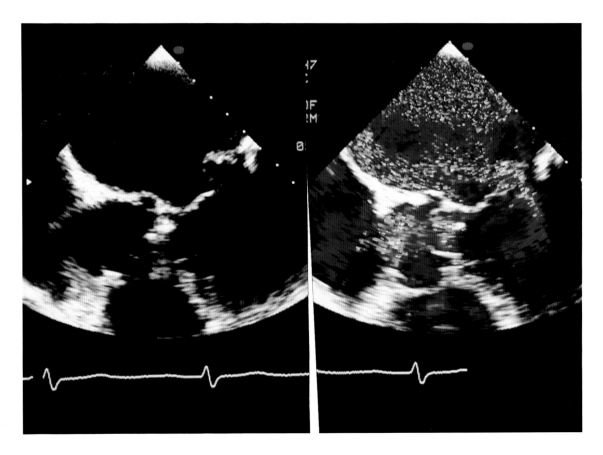

Figure 5.7 *Transverse axis images in a patient with severe mitral regurgitation due to elongation of the cords to the mural leaflet. This prolapses, causing a large regurgitant orifice. The broad turbulent jet is very eccentric, being directed medially and then coursing along the posterior wall of the left atrium.*

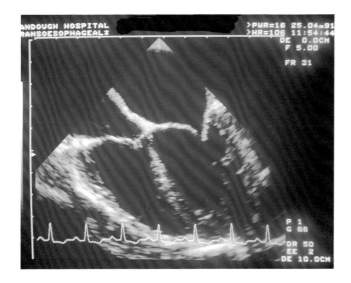

Figure 5.8 *Cross-sectional image obtained in an 11 year old boy who presented with pulmonary oedema due to severe mitral regurgitation. The transverse image shows a regurgitant orifice, with loss of coaptation and abnormal apposition. This was caused by immobility and restriction of the mural (posterior) leaflet, and not by any disease of the aortic (anterior) leaflet. This patient had previously undergone radiotherapy to the left chest following excision of a rib for Ewing's sarcoma.*

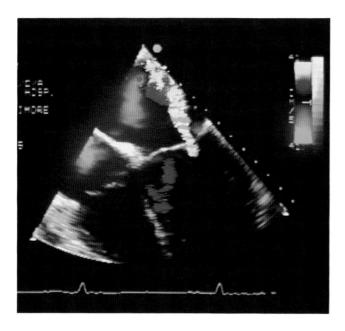

Figure 5.9 *Central regurgitant jet caused by enlargement of the left atrioventricular junction (mitral annulus). In systole, both leaflets appear 'flat' in relation to the plane of the annulus but even with this displacement they are still unable to achieve coaptation in the middle of the orifice of the valve.*

When coaptation is absent but the mitral leaflets are aligned symmetrically (Fig. 5.6(b)), the commonest cause is enlargement of the atrioventricular junction (annulus). The regurgitant jet is central and directed into the middle of the left atrium (Fig. 5.9). Such valves may be treated successfully by narrowing the atrioventricular junction, using annuloplasty as the only operative procedure. Unfortunately, it is hard to find published reference values for normal dimensions (rather than areas) of the atrioventricular junction in children. In patients with a partial or complete atrioventricular septal defect, it may be necessary to restore coaptation by suturing the medial edges of the anterior and posterior leaflets together, or to obliterate the space between the ventricular components of the bridging leaflets.

Some patients have significant mitral regurgitation even when the leaflets remain in contact with each other throughout systole (that is, there is intact coaptation), because apposition of the leaflets is abnormal (Fig. 5.6(c)). If the edges and rough zones of the leaflets are aligned assymetrically, a regurgitant jet may arise from under the free edge of the leaflet which is displaced towards the left atrium (Fig. 5.10). Studies of adult hearts have shown that overlap of as little as 3 mm may be sufficient to cause regurgitation (26). Regurgitation due to abnormal apposition causes an eccentric jet, and may be treated by techniques similar to those required for the combination of abnormal apposition and loss of coaptation. The same mechanism is probably the cause of mitral regurgitation in patients with secundum atrial septal defects, in whom the anterior leaflet bulges towards the left atrium in the region of the posteromedial commissure (27). If the subtle finding of abnormal apposition cannot be recognised, then colour flow mapping is very helpful. The orientation of the convergence zone on the ventricular surface of the mitral valve, and the direction of the jet within the left atrium, both provide strong clues to the underlying abnormality (28).

Occasionally, mitral regurgitation may occur even when coaptation and apposition of the leaflets in the zone of coaptation are normal (Fig. 5.6(d)). In these circumstances, unusual sites and mechanisms of regurgitation should be considered. These may be suggested on colour flow mapping by finding a convergence zone on the ventricular surface of one of the mitral leaflets at a site distant from the orifice. Congenital causes include a cleft in the aortic leaflet, and acquired causes include perforation of a leaflet due to infective endocarditis (Fig. 5.11) (29). There may be a communication between the left ventricular outflow tract and the left atrium

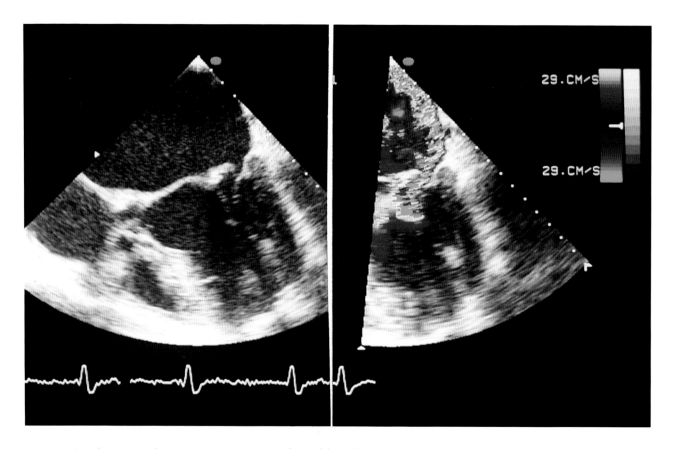

Figure 5.10 *This patient has eccentric regurgitation directed laterally around the left atrium, related to abnormal apposition of the leaflets. There is contact between the edges of the leaflets in systole (i.e. coaptation is present), but the overlap of the edge of the aortic leaflet (0.8 cm), allows regurgitation from under its edge. Compare with Fig 5.8 which shows a similar regurgitant jet – but the aetiologies and surgical treatment of these patients are very different.*

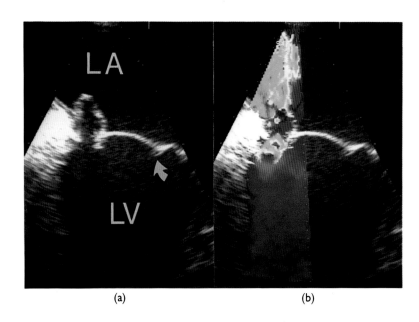

(a)   (b)

Figure 5.11 (a) *Transesophageal image and* **(b)** *colour flow map obtained in an oblique transverse plane, using a multiplane probe, in a patient with mitral regurgitation complicating infective endocarditis. Coaptation and apposition of the leaflets are normal (arrow), but there is a perforation of the aortic leaflet medially, adjacent to the atrioventricular junction.*

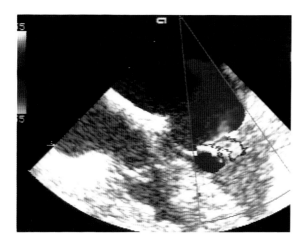

Figure 5.12 *The transesophageal pre-bypass study in this young child with congenital mitral stenosis confirmed that there was restricted movement of the mitral leaflets, and colour flow mapping and pulsed Doppler demonstrated high velocities of flow within the orifice (as seen in this transverse four-chamber view). No more detailed morphological information could be obtained.*

caused by rupture of the intervalvular fibrosa (30). Repair may be achieved by suturing a cleft or, after excising any vegetations, by suturing or patching a perforation.

All of these patterns of mitral regurgitation occur in children (10). Some additional congenital causes include hypoplastic leaflets, and absent tendinous cords (31).

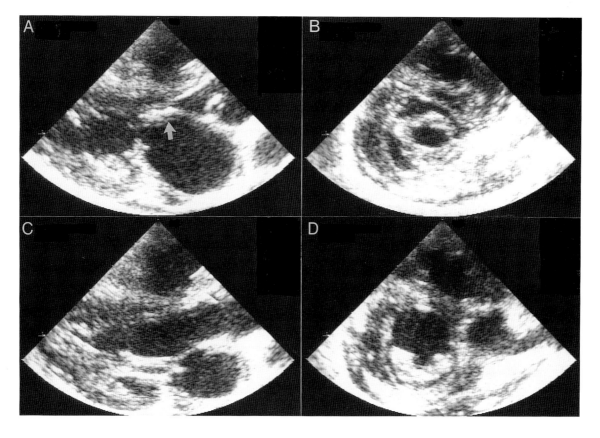

Figure 5.13 *Epicardial echocardiographic images obtained in the same patient as Fig. 5.12. In the long-axis image in diastole* **(a)**, *doming of the aortic leaflet of the mitral valve (arrow) and narrowing of the mitral orifice are observed. There was little movement of the mural leaflet between diastole* **(a)** *and systole* **(c)**, *and bright echoes were obtained from its subvalvar apparatus. Short axis images in diastole* **(b)** *and systole* **(d)** *also demonstrated movement of the aortic leaflet, but absent movement of the mural leaflet with marked thickening, fusion and shortening of its cords.*

Mitral valve repair

Pre-bypass study

The diagnosis of *mitral stenosis* is always established before surgery, usually by precordial rather than by transesophageal echocardiography. Intraoperative pre-bypass imaging may add relatively little further information to that obtained on direct inspection of the valve. If images are required by the surgeon, transesophageal studies with a single plane probe may be uninformative (Fig. 5.12) when compared with epicardial imaging (Fig. 5.13).

During the pre-bypass study in a patient undergoing valve repair for *mitral regurgitation*, the orifice of the valve should be imaged carefully from one commissure to the other, as already discussed, in order to establish the patterns of coaptation and apposition. If a biplane probe is available, the lateral part of the mitral orifice should be studied with the transverse transducer and the medial part with the longitudinal one. If a single-plane (transverse) probe is being used, the lateral part of the orifice will be seen well but epicardial imaging may be needed to demonstrate the leaflets adjacent to the posteromedial commissure (32). It is important to assess whether or not valvar pathology extends into the commissures since this adds considerably to the complexity of repair which is required. Transgastric imaging of the mitral orifice with a transverse transducer can also be used to localise the site(s) of regurgitation, particularly when colour flow mapping is employed. Several sites of regurgitation may be found in a single patient, for example with an atrioventricular septal defect, sometimes indicating the need for several operative procedures. For example, a perforation may coexist with regurgitation from the central orifice of the valve caused by abnormal apposition.

Combined transesophageal and epicardial echocardiography may be needed in patients with an isolated cleft (Fig. 5.14) or with regurgitation associated with an atrioventricular septal defect. It is important to identify if there is cordal straddling through the ventricular septal defect (33), since this determines whether or not a biventricular repair can be performed. A short-axis image through the atrioventricular valves is particularly useful for planning surgery (34).

The severity of mitral regurgitation is assessed with colour flow mapping, although this is notoriously unreliable for quantitation since turbulence is influenced by many factors in addition to regurg-

itant volume (35,36). It is not unusual to find that regurgitation related to left ventricular dysfunction appears less severe on intraoperative echocardiography than it was at cardiac catheterisation (37), and the day-to-day variability of mitral regurgitant jets is such that a change in severity cannot be diagnosed with confidence unless the area of the jet has altered by = 30% (38). In general, the size of a turbulent jet correlates with the severity of regurgitation estimated by preoperative angiography (39), especially if the jet is directed into the centre of the atrium. However, angiographic findings correlate poorly with regurgitant volume and they are not predictive of haemodynamic dysfunction (40). Using precordial colour flow mapping, the most accurate estimates have been obtained by studying three orthogonal planes (apical four-chamber, and parasternal long- and short-axis views) in order to select the one which shows the largest jet. Then, the maximal jet area, expressed as a percentage of the area of the left atrium, correlates well with angiography (> 40% representing severe regurgitation) (41). Since transesophageal echocardiography cannot display the whole of the atrium in one image, a simpler measurement is used. A jet which does not extend beyond the plane of the mitral annulus is deemed trivial (+), and mild, moderate or severe (or +, ++ and +++) regurgitation is diagnosed when the jet extends to within one-third or two-thirds of the depth of the left atrium, or when it reaches the posterior wall of the atrium, respectively (39). Colour flow maps obtained on intraoperative transesophageal echocardiography correlate closely with those obtained on epicardial echocardiography (42).

A major disadvantage of using colour flow mapping to grade mitral regurgitation is that it greatly underestimates the severity of eccentric jets. A jet which impinges on the atrial wall tends to flatten out over its surface, so that colour flow maps which are obtained in planes at right angles to the wall give an area of turbulence which is only 40% of the area produced by a freestanding jet with the same regurgitant fraction (43). Eccentric regurgitation is very common in patients undergoing mitral valve repair, and so additional echocardiographic criteria should also be used. Colour M-mode echocardiography measures the duration of regurgitation, and continuous wave Doppler may show early attenuation of the velocity of regurgitation in patients with high left atrial pressure. Further useful evidence is obtained by studying the pattern of flow within the pulmonary veins, using transesophageal pulsed Doppler echocardiography. In normal patients, blood flows into the left atrium during

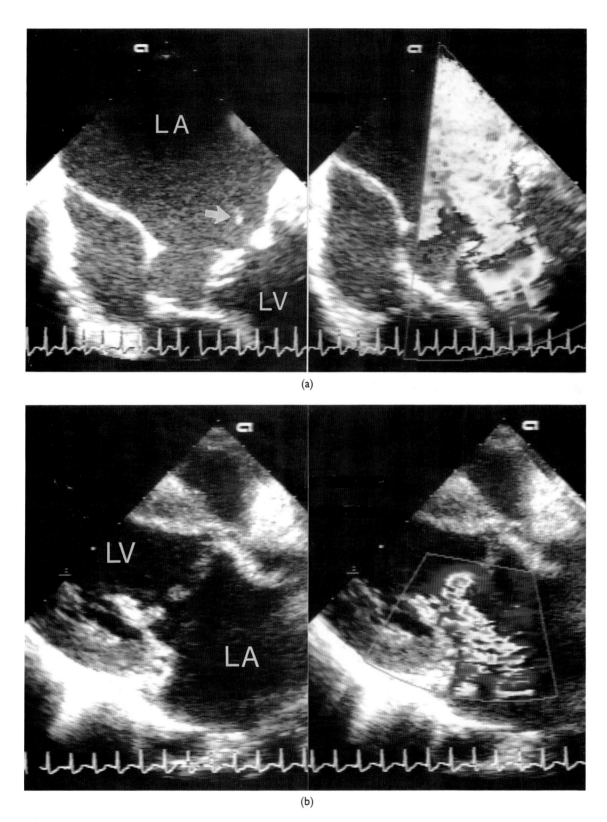

(a)

(b)

Figure 5.14 (a) *Pre-bypass transesophageal study performed using a single-plane probe in a 5 year old boy with severe mitral regurgitation. Imaging demonstrates a ruptured tendinous cord (arrow) and also a small central regurgitant orifice. Colour flow mapping shows severe regurgitation. This patient also has anomalous drainage of the coronary sinus into the left atrium (asterisk).* **(b)** *Epicardial study in the same patient, using a modified four-chamber view obtained with the transducer near the acute margin of the right ventricle. In addition to absent coaptation of the edges of the leaflets, a second defect is observed within the aortic leaflet. Colour flow mapping shows separate regurgitant jets arising from both of these sites.*

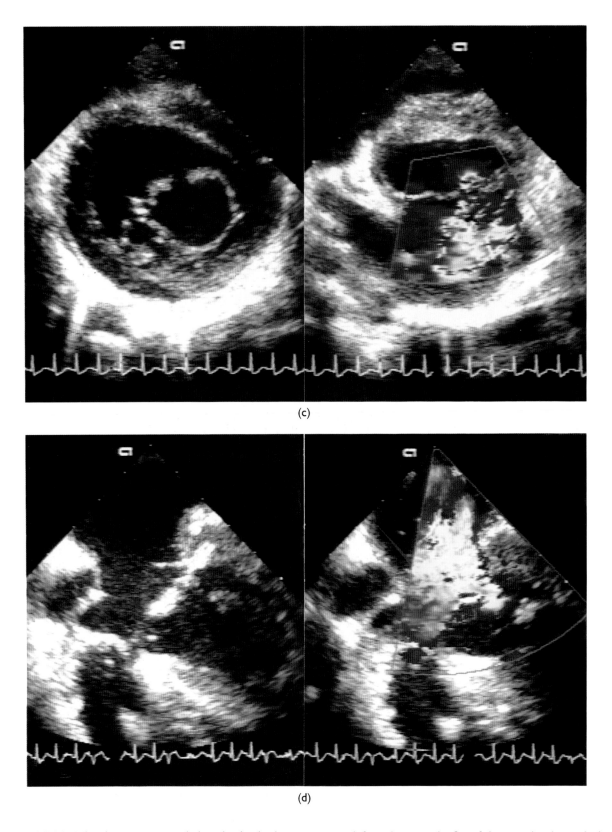

(c)

(d)

Figure 5.14 (c) *The short-axis epicardial study clearly demonstrates a cleft in the aortic leaflet of the mitral valve, which was confirmed by colour flow mapping.* **(d)** *Post-bypass transesophageal study following attempted mitral valve repair (including suture of the cleft and resection of part of the mural leaflet). Imaging showed a persistent mobile structure adjacent to the mural leaflet (thought to be leaflet tissue rather than a suture) and colour flow mapping demonstrated severe residual regurgitation. The patient underwent valve replacement on a second period of cardiopulmonary bypass.*

both ventricular systole and diastole; the peak velocities (about 0.5 m/s) and time velocity integrals of these two phases are approximately equal. In patients with severe mitral regurgitation, there is no forward flow from the pulmonary veins during ventricular systole, or even holosystolic retrograde flow (Fig. 5.15) coinciding with the increased 'v' wave on the left atrial pressure trace (44). These Doppler findings correlate well with angiographic evidence of grade III or grade IV mitral regurgitation, but they are non-specific, since reduced systolic flow is also found in patients with high left atrial pressures from other causes (45) and in patients with atrial fibrillation.

Comparison with surgical inspection

Reconstruction of the mitral valve was performed successfully for many years before intraoperative echocardiography was introduced, and new imaging techniques will never supplant direct visual inspection of the valve. Nonetheless, pre-bypass echocardiographic assessment may be invaluable, because it provides 'physiological' information about anatomy and function in the beating, rather than the cardiopleged, heart. It may also lessen the duration of cardiopulmonary bypass, by reducing the time needed for inspection and surgical planning.

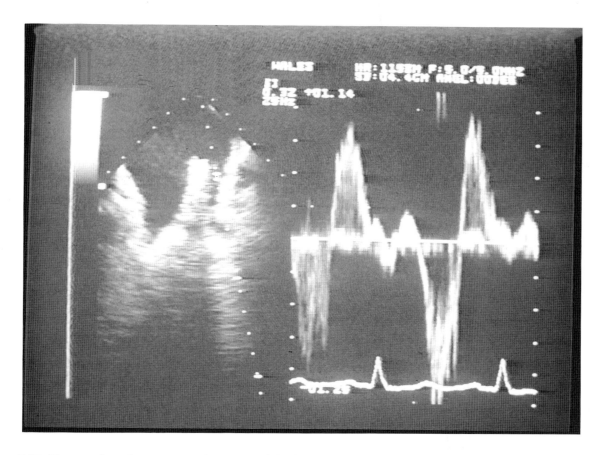

Figure 5.15 *Transesophageal cross-sectional image (on left) demonstrating the positioning of the pulsed Doppler sample volume within the left upper pulmonary vein, about 1 cm from its orifice. In this patient with severe mitral regurgitation, there is systolic retrograde flow into the pulmonary veins.*

After opening the atrium, the surgeon assesses the mobility of the mitral leaflets by inserting nerve hooks under the primary cords, and then applying approximately equal tension to the edges of both leaflets. The reference point is a part of the valve which looks normal. A valve fault is identified when this manoeuvre makes apposition of the edges of the leaflets appear asymmetrical. However, it may be very difficult in a flaccid heart to determine whether there is prolapse of one leaflet or retraction of the opposite one. Another disadvantage of inspection is that it may reveal surgical 'prolapse' (by no means synonymous with echocardiographic prolapse) which is in fact an incidental finding rather than the cause of regurgitation. Not all 'prolapse' needs to be treated.

The assessment of residual regurgitation by filling the ventricle with fluid while the heart is still arrested, or before the left atrium is closed, is frequently inaccurate. Both false positive and false negative findings have been reported (39).

Post-bypass study

After cardiopulmonary bypass, the pattern of closure of the mitral leaflets is reassessed using the same techniques as before surgery. Any prosthetic material such as sutures within the mitral valve or its annulus, or any foreign material at another site where an additional procedure has been performed, may block the transmission of ultrasound. For this reason, epicardial colour flow mapping may not demonstrate flow within the left atrium, and transesophageal echocardiography is the best technique for identifying residual mitral regurgitation (Fig. 5.16). Post-bypass colour flow maps correlate well with the results of follow-up left ventriculography (46). If severe regurgitation is detected, the repair should be revised (see Fig. 5.14(d)). The transesophageal approach is also more useful for aligning pulsed or continuous wave Doppler across the valve, to measure diastolic velocities in patients being treated for mitral stenosis.

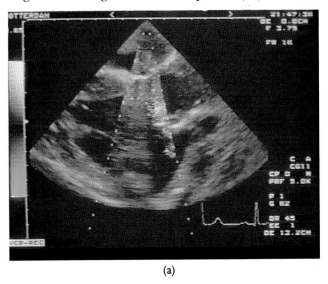

(a)

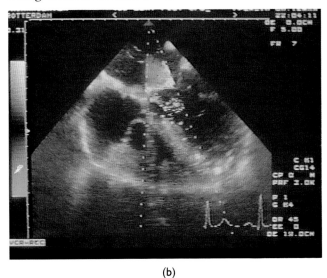

(b)

Figure 5.16 *Comparison of* **(a)** *epicardial long-axis, and* **(b)** *transesophageal four-chamber, colour flow maps following repair of a ventricular septal defect. From the epicardial approach, the prosthetic patch masks all flow within the left atrium. The transesophageal study, however, shows residual eccentric mitral regurgitation directed medially from the orifice of the valve.*

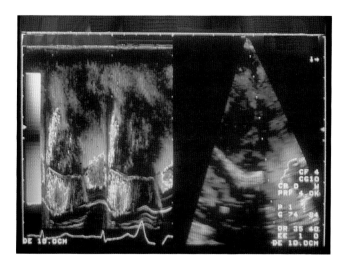

Figure 5.17 *Post-bypass colour flow mapping after a quadrangular resection of the mural leaflet. In diastole (right hand panel) there is asymmetrical acceleration of flow through the orifice. Systolic maps showed some mitral regurgitation extending to the middle of the left atrium, but the colour M-mode recording (left hand panel) documented that this was confined to early systole and therefore 'normal' after mitral reconstructive surgery.*

After a quadrangular resection, the mural leaflet of the mitral valve may appear immobile. Coaptation is achieved by increased excursion of the aortic leaflet, and by the surgical narrowing of the atrioventricular junction. Mild regurgitation is common after surgery, perhaps related to a slower rate of closure of the leaflets due to their comparative immobility. Such 'normal' regurgitation is transient and confined to early systole, as can be demonstrated by using the colour M-mode display (Fig. 5.17). Significant residual regurgitation usually persists throughout systole. After successful surgery, Doppler echocardiography confirms immediate normalisation of the pattern of pulmonary venous flow (47).

Contrast echocardiography can be used as an alternative technique for quantifying residual regurgitation (48). A small volume of echo contrast material, such as a hand-agitated mixture of saline and blood, or a special echocardiographic contrast agent (49), is injected rapidly into the left ventricle (usually by direct ventricular puncture). Assuming that the contrast is distributed uniformly within the left ventricle, and that it is not injected directly through the mitral orifice in diastole, then the extent and density of contrast appearing in the left atrium is directly proportional to the regurgitant volume. In practice, however, all of these factors are difficult to control, and the ventricular puncture may cause arrhythmias which interfere with the interpretation of the test. This is also complicated by the presence of 'spontaneous' microbubbles of air within the left atrium in at least 50% of patients after cardiopulmonary bypass (50,51). Contrast studies with an agitated solution of gelatin have been advocated as a simple, safe and reliable method for assessing mitral or tricuspid regurgitation after bypass (52), but they have been superseded by colour flow mapping. The main indication for contrast echocardiography during surgery for congenital heart disease is probably the exclusion of residual intracardiac shunts (53).

Left ventricular outflow tract obstruction is a rare complication of mitral valve repair, probably caused in part by narrowing of the angle between the plane of the mitral valve and the aorta and in part by the presence after surgery of excess leaflet tissue within a narrowed annulus (54). The problem should be suspected if colour flow mapping shows pronounced turbulence within the outflow tract and imaging shows associated systolic anterior movement of the aortic leaflet of the mitral valve. It can be confirmed by direct manometry or by performing epicardial continuous wave Doppler studies using a pencil probe placed on the ascending aorta. Since the obstruction is exacerbated by underfilling of the ventricle, it is worthwhile waiting for some time after bypass to ensure that left ventricular filling is normal, before electing to revise the repair. Outflow tract obstruction may resolve without specific treatment (55).

It is unwise to base any decision to reoperate on echocardiographic findings alone. Colour flow maps of mitral regurgitation are particularly influenced by haemodynamic factors, and so if possible the post-bypass study should be postponed until these have returned approximately to their pre-bypass levels. If necessary, dobutamine can be infused to ensure that arterial pressures and left ventricular afterload are as near to their normal values as possible. Even when these precautions are followed, however, echocardiographic indicators should be considered in conjunction with the surgeon's impression of the repair, the results of testing the competence of the valve before coming off bypass, and the haemodynamic performance of the heart.

SURGICAL REPAIR OF TRICUSPID REGURGITATION

Isolated tricuspid regurgitation in infancy may be caused by dysplasia of the tricuspid leaflets or by regurgitation associated with hypoxia at birth (56). Tricuspid or right atrioventricular valves regurgitation occurs as part of more complex disease for example in complete atrioventricular septal defect. Regurgitation caused by dilatation of the right atrioventricular junction can be treated relatively simply by annuloplasty, and intraoperative echocardiography can be used to monitor the results if required.

Tricuspid regurgitation is shown equally well on transesophageal and on epicardial echocardiography. Grading systems can be adapted from precordial colour flow mapping techniques, which are an accurate guide to the severity of tricuspid regurgitation assessed by right ventriculography. Mild regurgitation is present when the width of the jet is <50% of the diameter of the right atrium, moderate regurgitation when the width is about 50%, and severe regurgitation when the jet occupies most of the atrium (57). After bypass, epicardial colour flow mapping is a better indicator of late outcome than either the height of the right atrial 'v' wave or the competence of the valve when the right ventricle is filled with fluid (58).

Surgery for Ebstein's anomaly presents a difficult challenge but reconstruction is feasible (59,60). Prebypass epicardial echocardiography readily demonstrates displacement and tethering of the septal leaflet, and enlargement of the anterosuperior leaflet, but important features such as tethering of the anterosuperior leaflet may be missed if the images are not reviewed in detail (61). Associated abnormalities such as atrial septal defect (Fig. 5.18(a)), ventricular septal defect, or an anomalous muscular shelf causing obstruction within the right ventricle (62), can also be shown. Transverse transesophageal imaging is not sufficiently versatile to show the tricuspid leaflets in the detail which the surgeon requires, and which is obvious on inspection, but in future it may be possible to do this by performing transgastric imaging with a multiplane probe (see Fig. 5.5).

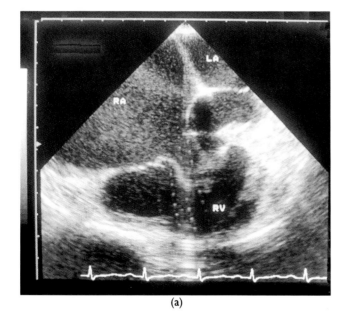

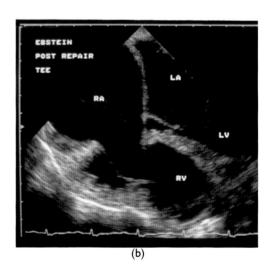

(a) (b)

Figure 5.18 (a) *Transverse transesophageal image obtained before cardiopulmonary bypass, in a patient with Ebstein's anomaly. The right atrium is very enlarged, the septal leaflet of the tricuspid valve is displaced and tethered to the ventricular septum, and there is an additional perimembranous ventricular septal defect.* **(b)** *After bypass, the lateral wall of the right ventricle has been plicated, narrowing the atrioventricular junction. The ventricular septal defect has been closed, and the anterosuperior leaflet of the tricuspid valve has been reattached at the level of the anatomical (and new functional) atrioventricular junction.*

Post-bypass echocardiography has been performed in patients treated by the technique of Carpentier, which entails detaching the anterosuperior and inferior leaflets, then plicating the lateral part of the atrialised portion of the right ventricle, and finally reattaching the leaflets at the level of the true right atrioventricular junction (Fig. 5.18(b)) (61). An immediate improvement in the haemodynamic function of the tricuspid valve was documented in the majority of patients. Residual regurgitation was noted to be at higher velocity than before bypass, owing to improved systolic function of the right ventricle as well as to narrowing of the regurgitant orifice. In one patient, colour flow mapping demonstrated significant residual regurgitation and indicated the need for reoperation (61).

THE VALUE OF INTRAOPERATIVE ECHOCARDIOGRAPHY

Systemic vasodilation is common after cardiopulmonary bypass, and so it is difficult to undertake post-bypass echocardiographic studies under similar loading conditions to those present before bypass. Even when the heart rate and blood pressure are similar, it is likely that stroke volume and cardiac output will be considerably increased. It is not surprising, therefore, that post-bypass epicardial echocardiographic findings do not correlate particularly well with those obtained later in the intensive care unit or before the patient is discharged home. Sreeram et al. found that intraoperative studies correctly identified the vast majority of patients with residual lesions requiring immediate reoperation, but problems such as residual outflow tract obstruction were sometimes missed (63). Persistent regurgitation of the left atrioventricular valve was underestimated in 3 of 11 patients operated for complete atrioventricular septal defect.

The interpretation of intraoperative echocardiographic studies is difficult, particularly in children undergoing complex repairs. During cardiac surgery, time is not available for detailed review and analysis of videotapes. Colour flow maps obtained in neonates or infants with rapid heart rates may be particularly difficult to interpret, and so it is important to use colour M-mode recordings because these enhance both the temporal and the spatial resolution of flow events within the heart. There is a learning curve for performing intraoperative echocardiography, and the cardiac surgeon and the paediatric cardiologist will need to acquire considerable experience together before they will have sufficient confidence to rely on echocardiographic data when deciding whether or not to revise a suboptimal repair.

In spite of these reservations, intraoperative echocardiography is now an established technique during surgery for congenital heart disease. Initial clinical reports (64,65) have been confirmed by large prospective series. In Rotterdam, important or useful new information was found before bypass in 11% of 195 patients (66). Ungerleider et al. found new information in 18% of 328 patients, and additional information helpful for surgical planning in 44% (67). When the post-bypass study showed a significant residual lesion (in 7%), this was a significant predictor of late morbidity and mortality (67).

In the days before intraoperative echocardiography, residual haemodynamic lesions were common after surgery of the atrioventricular valves in children. In some series, a substantial proportion of children required late reoperation (17,68). Now, the diagnosis and surgical plan can be refined by pre-bypass echocardiography. Ungerleider et al. reported that epicardial studies gave additional information in 39% of patients (34), and Roberson et al. found that transesophageal echocardiography was just as accurate (69). After repair, echocardiography is used to review the results and plan a revision if necessary to give an optimal result (34). In one series, post-bypass transesophageal echocardiography altered or refined treatment in 31% of patients with atrioventricular septal defects (69). Similar benefits have been reported from post-bypass echocardiography in adults undergoing mitral valve repair (70,71), with moderate residual regurgitation being a significant predictor of adverse clinical events (70).

REFERENCES

1. STÜMPER OFW, FRASER AG, HO SY, et al. Transoesophageal echocardiographic imaging in the longitudinal axis: a correlative echocardiographic-anatomic study and its clinical implications. *Br Heart J* 1990; **64:** 282–8.

2. FRASER AG, STÜMPER OFW, VAN HERWERDEN LA, HO SY, ANDERSON RH, ROELANDT JRTC. Anatomy of imaging planes used to study the mitral valve: advantages of biplane transesophageal echocardiography. *Circulation* 1990; III-668 (abstract).

3. PENKOSKE PA, NECHES WH, ANDERSON RH, ZUBERBUHLER JR. Further observations on the morphology of atrioventricular septal defects. *J Thor Cardiovasc Surg* 1985; **90:** 611–22.

4. ARISAWA J, MORIMOTO S, IKEZOE J, et al. Cross sectional echocardiographic anatomy of common atrioventricular valve in atrial isomerism. *Br Heart J* 1989; **62:** 291–7.

5. PICCOLI GP, WILKINSON JL, MACARTNEY FJ, GERLIS LM, ANDERSON RH. Morphology and classification of complete atrioventricular defects. *Br Heart J* 1979; **42:** 633–9.

6. ANDERSON RH, ZUBERBUHLER JR, PENKOSKE PA, NECHES WH. Of clefts, commissures, and things. *J Thor Cardiovasc Surg* 1985; **90:** 605–10.

7. SMALL IORN JF, DE LEVAL M, STARK J, et al. Isolated anterior mitral cleft. Two dimensional echocardiographic assessment and differentiation from "clefts" associated with atrioventricular septal defect. *Br Heart J* 1982; **48:** 109–16.

8. DI SEGNI E, BASS JL, LUCAS RV, EINZIG S. Isolated cleft mitral valve: a variety of congenital mitral regurgitation identified by 2-dimensional echocardiography. *Am J Cardiol* 1983; **51:** 927–31.

9. SMALLHORN J, TOMMASINI G, DEANFIELD J, DOUGLAS J, GIBSON D, MACARTNEY F. Congenital mitral stenosis. Anatomical and functional assessment by echocardiography. *Br Heart J* 1981; **45:** 527–34.

10. CARPENTIER A, BRANCHINI B, COUR JC, et al. Congenital malformations of the mitral valve in children. Pathology and surgical treatment. *J Thorac Cardiovasc Surg* 1976; **72:** 854–66.

11. LEVINE RA, HANDSCHUMACHER MD, SANFILIPPO AJ, HAGEGE AA, HARRIGAN P, MARSHALL JE, WEYMAN AE. Three-dimensional echocardiographic reconstruction of the mitral valve, with implications for the diagnosis of mitral valve prolapse. *Circulation* 1989; **80:** 589–98.

12. LEVINE RA, STATHOGIANNIDIS E, NEWELL JB, HARRIGAN P, WEYMAN AE. Reconsideration of echocardiographic standards for mitral valve prolapse: lack of association between leaflet displacement isolated to the apical four chamber view and independent echocardiographic evidence of abnormality. *J Am Coll Cardiol* 1988; **11:** 1010–19.

13. WARTH DC, KING ME, COHEN JM, TESORIERO VL, MARCUS E, WEYMAN AE. Prevalence of mitral valve prolapse in children. *J Am Coll Cardiol* 1985; **5:** 1173–7.

14. ZENKER G, ERBEL R, KRAMER G, et al. Transesophageal two-dimensional echocardiography in young patients with cerebral ischemic events. *Stroke* 1988; **19:** 345–8.

15. STEWART WJ, CURRIE PJ, AGLER DA, COSGROVE DM. Intraoperative epicardial echocardiography: technique, imaging planes, and use in valve repair for mitral regurgitation. *Dynam Cardiovasc Imag* 1987; **3:** 179–86.

16. STÜMPER O, KAULITZ R, SREERAM N, et al. Intraoperative transoesophageal versus epicardial ultrasound in surgery for congenital heart disease. *J Am Soc Echocardiog* 1990; **3:** 392–401.

17. COLES JG, WILLIAMS WG, WATANABE T, et al. Surgical experience with reparative techniques in patients with congenital mitral valvular anomalies. *Circulation* 1987; **76:** III-117–22.

18. COLLINS-NAKAI RL, ROSENTHAL A, CASTANEDA AR, BERNHARD WF, NADAS AS. Congenital mitral stenosis. A review of 20 years' experience. *Circulation* 1977; **56:** 1039–47.

19. CARPENTIER A. Mitral valve reconstruction in children. In: Anderson RH, Macartney FJ, Shinebourne A, Tynan M (eds), *Paediatric cardiology*, vol 5. Edinburgh: Churchill Livingstone, 1983: 361–8.

20. CASALE PM, WHITLOW P, CURRIE PJ, STEWART WJ. Transesophageal echocardiography in percutaneous balloon valvuloplasty for mitral stenosis. *Cleve Clin J Med* 1989; **56:** 597–600.

21. ABASCAL VM, WILKINS GT, O'SHEA JP, et al. Prediction of successful outcome in 130 patients undergoing percutaneous balloon mitral valvotomy. *Circulation* 1990; **82:** 448–56.

22. VAN HERWERDEN LA, FRASER AG, GUSSENHOVEN EJ, ROELANDT JRTC, THE SHK, BOS E. Echocardiographic analysis of regurgitant mitral valves: intraoperative functional anatomy and its relation to valve reconstruction. In: *Epicardial Echocardiography* (MD thesis). Rotterdam: Erasmus University, 1990: 33–52.

23. WILCOX I, FLETCHER PJ, BAILEY BP. Colour Doppler echocardiographic assessment of regurgitant flow in mitral valve prolapse. *Eur Heart J* 1989; **10:** 872–9.

24. SCHLÜTER M, KREMER P, HANRATH P. Transesophageal 2-D echocardiographic feature of flail mitral leaflet due to ruptured chordae tendineae. *Am Heart J* 1984; **108:** 609–10.

25. HASEGAWA I, SAKAMOTO T, HADA Y, et al. Relationship between mitral regurgitation and left ventricular outflow obstruction in hypertrophic cardiomyopathy. *J Am Soc Echocardiogr* 1989; **2:** 177–86.

26. FRASER AG, MCALPINE HM, CHOW L, et al. Abnormal apposition as the cause of mitral regurgitation in patients with intact leaflet coaptation. *Circulation* 1990; III-241 (abstract).

27. NAGATA S, NIMURA Y, SAKAKIBARA H, et al. Mitral valve lesion associated with secundum atrial septal defect. Analysis by real time two dimensional echocardiography. *Br Heart J* 1983; **49:** 51–8.

28. YOSHIDA K, YOSHIKAWA J, YAMAURA Y, et al. Value of acceleration flows and regurgitant jet direction by color Doppler flow mapping in the evaluation of mitral valve prolapse. *Circulation* 1990; **81:** 879–85.

29. MIYATAKE K, YAMAMOTO K, PARK YD, et al. Diagnosis of mitral valve perforation by real-time two-dimensional Doppler flow imaging technique. *J Am Coll Cardiol* 1986; **8:** 1235–9.

30. BANSAL RC, GRAHAM BM, JUTZY KR, SHAKUDO M, SHAH PM. Left ventricular outflow tract to left atrial communication secondary to rupture of mitral-aortic intervalvular fibrosa in infective endocarditis: diagnosis by transesophageal echocardiography and color flow imaging. *J Am Coll Cardiol* 1990; **15:** 499–504.

31. OKITA Y, MIKI S, KUSUHARA K, et al. Early and late results of reconstructive operation for congenital mitral regurgitation in pediatric age group. *J Thorac Cardiovasc Surg* 1988; **96:** 294–8.

32. FRASER AG, VAN HERWERDEN LA, VAN DAELE MERM, SUTHERLAND GR. Is a combination of epicardial and transoesophageal echocardiography the best technique to monitor mitral valve repair? *Eur Heart J* 1989; **10** (abstract suppl): 33.

33. RICE MJ, SEWARD JB, EDWARDS WD, et al. Straddling atrioventricular valve: two-dimensional echocardiographic diagnosis, classification and surgical implications. *Am J Cardiol* 1985; **55:** 505–13.

34. UNGERLEIDER RM, KISSLO JA, GREELEY WJ, VAN TRIGT P, SABISTON DC. Intraoperative prebypass and postbypass epicardial color flow imaging in the repair of atrioventricular septal defects. *J Thorac Cardiovasc Surg* 1989; **98:** 90–100.

35. STEVENSON JG. Two-dimensional color Doppler estimation of the severity of atrioventricular valve regurgitation: important effects of instrument gain setting, pulse repetition frequency, and carrier frequency. *J Am Soc Echo* 1989; **2:** 1–10.

36. WONG M, MATSUMURA M, SUZUKI K, O MOTO R. Technical and biologic sources of variability in the mapping of aortic, mitral and tricuspid color flow jets. *Am J Cardiol* 1987; **60:** 847–51.

37. SHEIKH KH, BENGTSON JR, RANKIN JS, DE BRUIJN N, KISSLO J. Intraoperative transesophageal Doppler color flow imaging used to guide patient selection and operative treatment of ischemic mitral regurgitation. *Circulation* 1991; **84:** 594–604.

38. GRAYBURN PA, PRYOR SL, LEVINE BD, KLEIN MN, TAYLOR AL. Day to day variability of Doppler color flow jets in mitral regurgitation. *J Am Coll Cardiol* 1989; **14:** 936–40.

39. CZER LSC, MAURER G, BOLGER AF, et al. Intraoperative evaluation of mitral regurgitation by Doppler color flow mapping. *Circulation* 1987; **76:** III-108–16.

40. SPAIN MG, SMITH MD, GRAYBURN PA, HARLAMERT EA, DEMARIA AN. Quantitative assessment of mitral regurgitation by Doppler color flow imaging: angiographic and hemodynamic correlations. *J Am Coll Cardiol* 1989; **13:** 585–90.

41. HELMCKE F, NANDA NC, HSIUNG MC, et al. Color Doppler assessment of mitral regurgitation with orthogonal planes. *Circulation* 1987; **75:** 175–83.

42. KLEINMAN JP, CZER LS, DEROBERTIS M, CHAUX A, MAURER G. A quantitative comparison of transesophageal and epicardial color Doppler echocardiography in the intraoperative assessment of mitral regurgitation. *Am J Cardiol* 1989; **64:** 1168–72.

43. CHEN C, THOMAS JD, ANCONINA J, et al. Impact of impinging wall jet on color Doppler quantification of mitral regurgitation. *Circulation* 1991; **84:** 712–20.

44. KLEIN AL, OBARSKI TP, STEWART WJ, et al. Transesophageal Doppler echocardiography of pulmonary venous flow: a new marker of mitral regurgitation severity. *J Am Coll Cardiol* 1991; **18:** 518–26.

45. KUECHERER HF, MUHIUDEEN IA, KUSUMOTO FM, et al. Estimation of mean left atrial pressure from transesophageal pulsed Doppler echocardiography of pulmonary venous flow. *Circulation* 1990; **82:** 1127–39.

46. REICHERT SLA, VISSER CA, MOULIJN AC, et al. Intraoperative transesophageal color-coded Doppler echocardiography for evaluation of residual regurgitation after mitral valve repair. *J Thorac Cardiovasc Surg* 1990; **110:** 756–61.

47. FRASER AG, TUCCILLO B, VAN DER BORDEN S, VAN HERWERDEN LA, SUTHERLAND GR. Pulmonary venous flow in mitral regurgitation and after successful valve reconstruction. *J Am Coll Cardiol* 1990; **15:** 74A (abstract).

48. GOLDMAN ME, MINDICH BP, TEICHHOLZ LE, BURGESS N, STAVILLE K, FUSTER V. Intraoperative contrast echocardiography to evaluate mitral valve operations. *J Am Coll Cardiol* 1984; **4:** 1035–40.

49. FEINSTEIN SB, CHEIRIF J, TEN CATE FJ, et al. Safety and efficacy of a new transpulmonary ultrasound contrast agent: initial multicenter clinical results. *J Am Coll Cardiol* 1990; **17:** 316–24.

50. DUFF HJ, BUDA AJ, KRAMER R, STRAUSS HD, DAVID TE, BERMAN ND. Detection of entrapped intracardiac air with intraoperative echocardiography. *Am J Cardiol* 1980; **46:** 255–60.

51. RODIGAS PC, MEYER FJ, HAASLER GB, DUBROFF JM, SPOTNITZ HM. Intraoperative 2-dimensional echocardiography: ejection of microbubbles from the left ventricle after cardiac surgery. *Am J Cardiol* 1982; **50:** 1130–2.

52. DAHM M, IVERSEN S, SCHMID FX, DREXLER M, ERBEL R, OELERT H. Intraoperative evaluation of reconstruction of the atrioventricular valves by transesophageal echocardiography. *Thorac Cardiovasc Surg* 1987; **35:** 140–2.

53. STÜMPER OFW, FRASER AG, ELZENGA N, et al. Assessment of ventricular septal defect closure by intraoperative epicardial ultrasound. *J Am Coll Cardiol* 1990; **16:** 1672–9.

54. MIHAILEANU S, MARINO JP, CHAUVAUD S, et al. Left ventricular outflow obstruction after mitral valve repair (Carpentier's technique). Proposed mechanisms of disease. *Circulation* 1988; **78:** I-78–I-84.

55. VAN HERWERDEN LA, FRASER AG, BOS E. Left ventricular outflow tract obstruction after mitral valve repair assessed with intraoperative echocardiography: non-interventional treatment. *J Thorac Cardiovasc Surg* 1991; **102:** 461–3.

56. BECKER AE, BECKER MJ, EDWARDS JE. Pathologic spectrum

of dysplasia of the tricuspid valve. *Arch Pathol* 1971; **9:** 167–78.

57. SUZUKI Y, KAMBARA H, KADOTA K, et al. Detection and evaluation of tricuspid regurgitation using a real-time, two-dimensional, color-coded, Doppler flow imaging system: comparison with contrast two-dimensional echocardiography and right ventriculography. *Am J Cardiol* 1986; **57:** 811–15.

58. CZER LSC, MAURER G, BOLGER A, et al. Tricuspid valve repair. Operative and follow-up evaluation by Doppler color flow mapping. *J Thorac Cardiovasc Surg* 1989; **98:** 101–11.

59. DANIELSON GK, FUSTER V. Surgical repair of Ebstein's anomaly. *Ann Surg* 1982; **196:** 499–503.

60. CARPENTIER A, CHAUVAUD S, MACE L, et al. A new reconstructive operation for Ebstein's anomaly of the tricuspid valve. *J Thorac Cardiovasc Surg* 1988; **96:** 92–101.

61. QUAEGEBEUR JM, SREERAM N, FRASER AG, et al. Surgery for Ebstein's anomaly: the clinical and echocardiographic evaluation of a new technique. *J Am Coll Cardiol* 1991; **17:** 722–8.

62. LEUNG MP, BAKER EJ, ANDERSON RH, ZUBERBUHLER JR. Cineangiographic spectrum of Ebstein's malformation: its relevance to clinical presentation and outcome. *J Am Coll Cardiol* 1988; **11:** 154–61.

63. SREERAM N, KAULITZ R, STÜMPER OFW, HESS J, QUAEGEBEUR JM, SUTHERLAND GR. Comparative roles of intraoperative epicardial and early postoperative transthoracic echocardiography in the assessment of surgical repair of congenital heart defects. *J Am Coll Cardiol* 1990; **16:** 913–20.

64. CYRAN SE, KIMBALL TR, MEYER RA, et al. Efficacy of intraoperative transesophageal echocardiography in children with congenital heart disease. *Am J Cardiol* 1989; **63:** 594–8.

65. KYO S, TAKAMOTO S, MATSUMURA M, et al. Immediate and early postoperative evaluation of results of cardiac surgery by transesophageal two-dimensional Doppler echocardiography. *Circulation* 1987; **76** (suppl V): V-113–21.

66. GUSSENHOVEN EJ, VAN HERWERDEN LA, ROELANDT J, LIGTVOET KM, BOS E, WITSENBURG M. Intraoperative two-dimensional echocardiography in congenital heart disease. *J Am Coll Cardiol* 1987; **9:** 565–7.

67. UNGERLEIDER RM, GREELEY WJ, SHEIKH KH, et al. Routine use of intraoperative epicardial echocardiography and Doppler color flow imaging to guide and evaluate repair of congenital heart lesions. A prospective study. *J Thorac Cardiovasc Surg* 1990; **100:** 297–309.

68. LAMBERTI JJ, JENSEN TS, GREHL TM, et al. Late reoperation for systemic atrioventricular valve regurgitation after repair of congenital heart defects. *Ann Thorac Surg* 1989; **47:** 517–22.

69. ROBERSON DA, MUHIUDEEN IA, SILVERMAN NH, TURLEY K, HAAS GS, CAHALAN MK. Intraoperative transesophageal echocardiography of atrioventricular septal defect. *J Am Coll Cardiol* 1991; **18:** 537–45.

70. SHEIKH KH, DE BRUIJN NP, RANKIN JS, et al. The utility of transesophageal echocardiography and Doppler color flow imaging in patients undergoing cardiac surgery. *J Am Coll Cardiol* 1990; **15:** 363–72.

71. STEWART WJ, CURRIE PJ, SALCEDO EE, et al. Intraoperative Doppler color flow mapping for decision-making in valve repair for mitral regurgitation: technique and results in 100 patients. *Circulation* 1990; **81:** 556–66.

Prosthetic valves

A. G. Fraser

INTRODUCTION

The introduction of transesophageal echocardiography was a major advance in the investigation of patients with prosthetic heart valves (1). Although diastolic flow through a prosthetic mitral or tricuspid valve can be assessed very well using precordial Doppler echocardiography from an apical window, regurgitation cannot be demonstrated by this approach since prosthetic valves at these sites mask distant structures and colour flow maps within the atria (2). When cardiac ultrasound is being employed to assess a prosthetic heart valve fully, it is necessary to use at least two opposing echocardiographic approaches. Prosthetic aortic valves can be studied from the apex and the suprasternal notch, but the posterior aspect of prosthetic mitral and tricuspid valves can be interrogated properly by ultrasound only from the esophagus. Even using transesophageal echocardiography, however, it may be difficult or impossible to study prosthetic valves within conduits, because of masking by the material of the conduit.

Not surprisingly, it has been shown that the transesophageal approach is much more sensitive than precordial ones for studying regurgitation of prosthetic valves and for identifying other complications such as infection or thrombosis (1,3). Nonetheless, complete assessment of any prosthetic valve also requires a careful and detailed precordial study, which should be performed before the transesophageal one. This brief account will concentrate on some of those aspects most relevant to children with prosthetic valves.

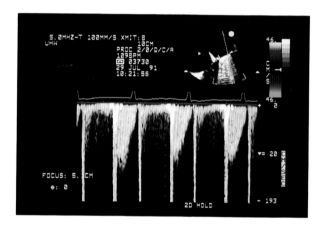

Figure 5.19 *Continuous wave Doppler recording of normal flow across a mitral valve prosthesis, obtained by selecting the plane which allowed optimal alignment, using a biplane transesophageal probe.*

NORMAL PROSTHETIC VALVE FUNCTION

The function of a prosthetic valve should be assessed first by obtaining a good-quality Doppler profile of flow across the valve when it is open.

For mitral and tricuspid prostheses, this is usually achieved using apical pulsed or continuous wave Doppler. If there are no adequate precordial windows, as may happen occasionally in children owing to a congenital abnormality or to deformity of the chest after cardiac surgery, then Doppler traces can be recorded during a transesophageal study if the transducer has facilities for continuous wave Doppler (Fig. 5.19). Alignment to flow through the major orifice of a single-tilting-disc valve (such as the Medtronic Hall or Björk–Shiley prostheses), or through either of the 'lateral' orifices of a bileaflet valve (such as the St Jude or Carbomedics prostheses) is greatly facilitated if a biplane probe is used; often, more exact alignment is possible in a longitudinal plane. Care should be taken, when studying a bileaflet valve, not to interrogate flow through its smaller central orifice. There may be relative stasis of flow between the leaflets of the valve, causing a localised area of reduced pressure and increased local pressure gradients (4). Increased velocities of flow may be recorded, and these may be interpreted erroneously as evidence of prosthetic valvar obstruction.

The Doppler velocities across a prosthetic valve should be measured so that the pressure gradient can be estimated. In general, the peak drop in pressure can be estimated by applying the modified Bernoulli equation (5–7). However, this may be misleading in patients with prosthetic aortic valves and poor left ventricular function (8). The effective orifice area of a prosthetic mitral or tricuspid valve can be calculated by measuring the pressure half-time and applying the Holen–Hatle equation (9–11), but this approach has not been validated for all prostheses. Pressure half-time is influenced by many factors in addition to the size of the valve orifice (12–14). An alternative method of estimating the effective orifice area of a prosthetic valve, which can be applied to both mitral and aortic prostheses, is the use of the continuity equation (13,15). This entails the measurement of velocities and cross-sectional area at an additional site within the heart, so that volumetric flow can be calculated. Assuming that the same flow also crosses the prosthetic valve, means that the area of the valve can be estimated if the peak velocity of flow across it can be recorded. Obviously, this approach cannot be used successfully for a prosthetic aortic or mitral valve if there is an intracardiac shunt at ventricular level. Another disadvantage is that the interobserver variability of echocardiographic measurements of flow at the aortic or mitral valve is considerable (about 10%) (16).

Standard values for Doppler-derived parameters of normally-functioning prosthetic valves have been reviewed (17). If possible, methods should be used which have been validated for the particular model of valve. Surprisingly often, however, the reporting of data is incomplete and in many series only a few patients with small valve sizes are included. All prosthetic valves are obstructive, compared with healthy native valves; 'acceptable' values for normal mitral prostheses are a peak early diastolic gradient of $\leqq$ 10 mmHg and a mean gradient of $\leqq$ 5 mmHg. For a prosthesis in the aortic position, normal values in adults are a peak instantaneous gradient of $\leqq$ 40 mmHg, approximately, and a mean gradient of $\leqq$ 20 mmHg. The peak velocity of flow is influenced by cardiac output, and so studies should be performed in resting patients. In an individual child, it is difficult to rely on published data to be certain whether or not an implanted valve is functioning normally. Instead, the function of every valve should be assessed carefully, soon after it has been implanted, to establish each patient's own baseline or 'control' values. A complicating factor in children is that the estimated gradient across a prosthesis may increase as the child grows older, because cardiac output increases while the dimensions of the prosthesis do not. It may be difficult to distinguish between such 'physiological' obstruction, and pathological complications in the valve. If possible, therefore, methods should be used (such as the continuity equation) which are relatively independent of changes in cardiac output. Occasionally, it may still be necessary to resort to cardiac catheterisation to determine whether or not a prosthetic valve is functionally satisfactorily (18).

All normal prosthetic valves leak (19). Seating of the disc into the prosthetic annulus occurs when there is a retrograde pressure gradient; indeed, without this, the valve would not close. Thus some early systolic regurgitation is invariable, while a prosthetic mitral or tricuspid valve closes. The pattern of regurgitation varies according to the design of the valve; but if a prosthesis is studied in multiple planes, for example using a biplane transesophageal probe, then a regurgitant jet is usually found arising from each orifice of the valve. It may be impossible to demonstrate all of the regurgitant jets from a particular valve, in a single imaging plane. 'Normal' regurgitant jets tend to be short in length, and relatively laminar (Fig. 5.20). Even when jets are relatively long, precise timing of flow, which is best performed using colour M-mode echocardiography, will show that they are very transient (Fig. 5.21). Some valves also leak throughout systole or diastole (depending on the site of insertion, but whenever they are closed), either as an inescapable

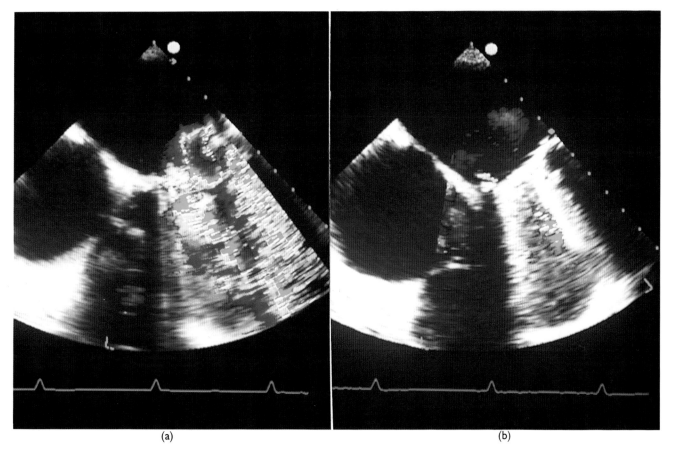

(a)   (b)

Figure 5.20 *Colour flow maps obtained in* **(a)** *diastole and* **(b)** *systole in a patient with a normally functioning single-tilting-disc mitral valve prosthesis. Eccentric flow into the major aperture of the valve is observed in diastole, and in systole a short, laminar, regurgitant jet is observed. This arises from within the annulus of the valve.*

consequence of the design of the valve (such as through the central hole in the disc of a Medtronic Hall valve) or as a planned haemodynamic feature of the valve to allow its surfaces to be 'washed' by the regurgitant blood in order to reduce the risk of thrombosis. In normal prosthetic valves, however, the total volume of such regurgitation is less than 5 millilitres per beat. Prosthetic regurgitation in an individual patient can only be interpreted if the normal pattern for that particular valve is known. For example, patients with a St Jude prosthesis will usually have at least three separate regurgitant jets detectable on colour flow mapping (20).

ATRIOVENTRICULAR VALVE REPLACEMENT

It is not usually necessary to check that a prosthetic valve is functioning satisfactorily, immediately after it has been inserted, and so intraoperative echocardiography is not performed routinely in adults undergoing elective valve replacement. The only indication in such patients would be if the surgeon experiences a problem such as difficulty in weaning

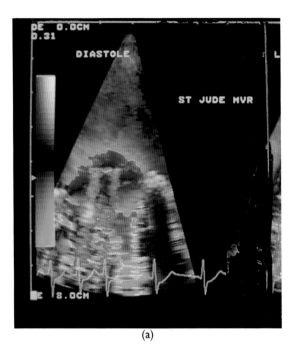

(a)

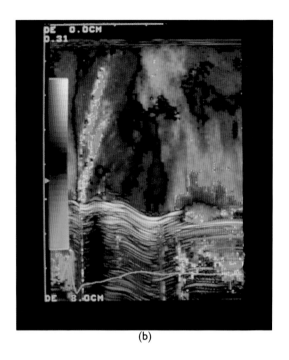

(b)

Figure 5.21 (a) *Colour flow map obtained in a patient with a St Jude mitral valve replacement, showing acceleration of flow (with aliasing) converging into the three orifices of this valve.* **(b)** *A colour M-mode echocardiogram recorded through one of the orifices demonstrates transient early systolic regurgitation. Although this jet reaches almost to the posterior wall of the left atrium, it is 'normal' because it is so transient.*

the patient from cardiopulmonary bypass, and then transesophageal or epicardial echocardiography may be very useful in establishing the diagnosis (such as left ventricular dysfunction, intraoperative infarction, right ventricular failure, obstructed motion of the disc(s) of the valve, or a paraprosthetic leak or partial dehiscence). In children, most mitral valve replacements are performed for atrioventricular septal defect or rheumatic heart disease, and then the surgeon will attempt to reconstruct the valve before resorting to replacement. Thus it is likely that a transesophageal probe will have been used to assess the initial result. This can then be used again to study the prosthetic valve immediately after it has been inserted. The function of the valve can be measured, 'baseline' regurgitant jets can be documented, and the absence of paraprosthetic leaks can be confirmed.

SUSPECTED PROSTHETIC VALVE DYSFUNCTION

Transesophageal echocardiography is invaluable for asssessing patients with suspected dysfunction of a prosthetic valve. As already mentioned, it is the best technique for demonstrating paraprosthetic regurgitation. Biplane studies are preferred, since they are more sensitive and can be used to localise a jet quite precisely (Fig. 5.22). Obstruction of a mitral pros-

thesis is usually suspected on clinical grounds, and then confirmed by precordial Doppler echocardiography, but the transesophageal approach is extremely useful for confirming this diagnosis and demonstrating its mechanism. A large thrombus on the atrial surface of a mitral valve is shown readily. Bioprosthetic valves are now implanted in children only in exceptional circumstances, but when they are, transesophageal echocardiography is again superior to the precordial approach (21). Torn leaflets, or calcification within prosthetic leaflets, may be identified.

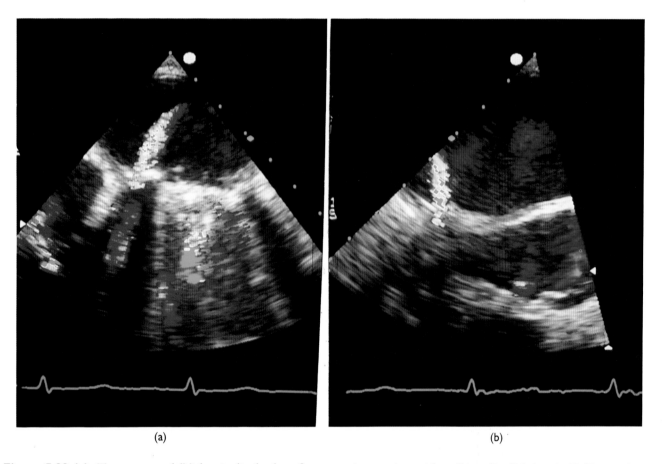

(a)   (b)

Figure 5.22 (a) *Transverse and* **(b)** *longitudinal colour flow maps in a patient with a tilting-disc (Medtronic Hall) mitral valve replacement. Both images were obtained in systole. There is a paraprosthetic leak arising from the middle of the medial border of the prosthesis.*

In patients with prosthetic valves and suspected systemic embolism, transesophageal echocardiography is more sensitive than precordial imaging for detecting a possible intracardiac source. It is the best technique for demonstrating masses within the left atrium (22), and the only reliable non-invasive method for diagnosing thrombus within the left atrial appendage (23). Thrombus may be demonstrated on the atrial surface of a mitral prosthesis even when there is no clinical or Doppler evidence of obstruction of the valve (Fig. 5.23).

In patients with a prosthetic mitral of tricuspid valve, transesophageal echocardiography may also show spontaneous echocardiographic contrast within either atrium (see Fig. 5.23). This phenomenon is observed as a swirling pattern of particulate echoes within any cardiac cavity (often likened to smoke). It is related inversely to velocities of flow

(24) and occurs in conditions of low shear stress (25). Spontaneous echo contrast arises rapidly when flow is slow or stagnating (for example, within the left atrium when the mitral valve is occluded by a balloon), and it may be observed only in a very localised region of a cardiac chamber (such as the left atrial appendage, or next to an to atrial septal aneurysm). It has been suggested that the predominant mechanism giving rise to these appearances is red cell (rather than platelet) aggregation (26), but both processes may be involved. Spontaneous echo contrast is probably not a cause of embolism *per se*, but it is definitely a marker of increased thromboembolic risk (25,27,28). All patients with spontaneous echo contrast in the left atrium, and a prosthetic mitral valve, should certainly be anticoagulated.

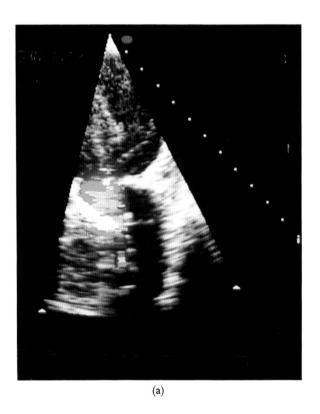

(a)

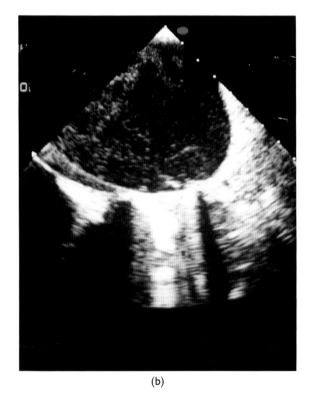

(b)

Figure 5.23 *This patient presented with cerebral embolism following mitral valve replacement.* **(a)** *Colour flow mapping and* **(b)** *Doppler studies showed an unobstructed prosthesis. There was spontaneous echocardiographic contrast within the left atrium, however, and imaging demonstrated small mobile masses (arrow) on the atrial surface of the valve, which were assumed to be thrombi.*

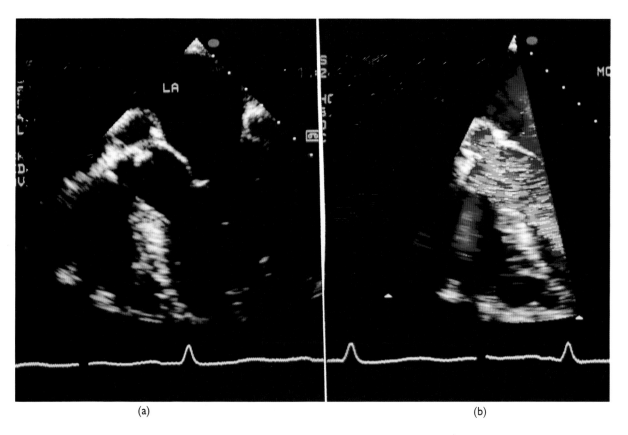

Figure 5.24 (a) *Transesophageal tranverse-axis image and* **(b)** *diastolic colour flow map obtained at the level of the left ventricular outflow tract in a patient with an aortic valve replacement (in fact, a bioprosthesis). There is a mycotic aneurysm of the posterior aortic root, which was the cause of severe paraprosthetic aortic regurgitation.*

The diagnosis of infective endocarditis is made clinically and on the basis of investigations such as positive blood cultures. It cannot be excluded by transesophageal echocardiography, although this approach is more sensitive than precordial echocardiography (29,30). Nonetheless, transesophageal echocardiography is extremely helpful for confirming the diagnosis of infective endocarditis, since it can demonstrate vegetations or other masses of $\geqq$ 1–2 mm in diameter. In patients with a prosthetic valve, it is not possible with certainty to differentiate echocardiographically between infective vegetations and other causes of masses around the valve, such as thrombus or pannus. Sutures may be shown but they can be distinguished easily because of their relative immobility, uniform size, and regularly spaced locations around the sewing ring of a valve. The transesophageal approach is particularly useful for demonstrating or excluding complications associated with infection of a prosthetic valve, such as a paraprosthetic leak (Fig. 5.24), or mycotic abscess or aneurysm.

REFERENCES

1. NANDA NC, COOPER JW, MAHAN EF, FAN P. Echocardiographic assessment of prosthetic values. *Circulation* 1991; **84** (suppl I): I-228–I-239.

2. SPRECHER DL, ADAMICK A, ADAMS D, KISSLO J. *In vitro* color flow and continuous wave Doppler ultrasound masking of flow by prosthetic valves. *J Am Coll Cardiol* 1987; **9:** 1306–10.

3. VAN DEN BRINK R, VISSER CA, BASART DCG, DÜREN DR, DE JONG AP, DUNNING AJ. Comparison of transthoracic and transesophageal color Doppler flow imaging in patients with a mechanical prosthesis in the mitral position. *Am J Cardiol* 1989; **63:** 1471–4.

4. BAUMGARTNER H, KHAN S, DEROBERTIS M, CZER LSC, MAURER G. Discrepancies between Doppler and catheter gradients in aortic prosthetic valves in vitro. A manifestation of localized gradients and pressure recovery. *Circulation* 190; **82:** 1467–75.

5. BURSTOW DJ, NISHIMURA RA, BAILEY KR, et al. Continuous wave Doppler echocardiographic measurement of prosthetic valve gradients. A simultaneous Doppler–catheter correlative study. *Circulation* 1989; **80:** 504–14.

6. WILKINS GT, GILLAM LD, KRITZER GL, LEVINE RA, PALACIOS IF, WEYMAN AE. Validation of continuous wave Doppler echocardiographic measurements of mitral and tricuspid prosthetic valve gradients: a simultaneous Doppler–catheter study. *Circulation* 1986; **74:** 786–95.

7. ENRIQUEZ-SARANO M, ROGER V, VAHANIAN A, VITOUX B, CAZAUX O, ACAR J. Mesure des gradients transvalvulaires par le Doppler. Enregistrements simultanes Doppler-catheterisme chez 78 patients. *Arch Mal Coeur* 1987; **80:** 1593–601.

8. REN JF, CHANDRASEKARAN K, MINTZ GS, ROSS J, PENNOCK RS, FRANKL WS. Effect of depressed left ventricular function on hemodynamics of a normal St Jude Medical prosthesis in the aortic valve position. *Am J Cardiol* 1990; **65:** 1004–9.

9. HATLE L, ANGELSEN B, TROMSDAL A. Non-invasive assessment of atrioventricular pressure half-time by Doppler ultrasound. *Circulation* 1979; **60:** 1096–1104.

10. HATLE L, BRUBAKK A, TROMSDAL A, ANGELSEN B. Noninvasive assessment of pressure drop in mitral stenosis by Doppler ultrasound. *Br Heart J* 1978; **40:** 131.

11. HOLEN J, SIMONSEN S. Determination of pressure gradient in mitral stenosis with Doppler echocardiography. *Br Heart J* 1979; **41:** 529.

12. CHAMBERS J, McLOUGHLIN N, RAPSON A, JACKSON G. Effect of changes in heart rate on pressure half-time in normally functioning mitral valve prostheses. *Br Heart J* 1988; **60:** 502–6.

13. DUMENSIL JG, HONOS GN, LEMIEUX M, BEAUCHEMIN J. Validation and applications of mitral prosthetic valvular areas calculated by Doppler echocardiography. *Am J Cardiol* 1990; **65:** 1443–8.

14. WRANNE B, ASK P, LOYD D. Analysis of different methods of assessing the stenotic mitral valve area with emphasis on the pressure half-time concept. *Am J Cardiol* 1990; **66:** 614–20.

15. CHAFIZADEH ER, ZOGHBI WA. Doppler echocardiographic assessment of the St Jude Medical prosthetic valve in the aortic position using the continuity equation. *Circulation* 1991; **83:** 213–23.

16. ILICETO S, D'AMBROSIO G, AMICO A, et al. Errors in measurements of stroke volume for invasive and echo-Doppler evaluations of valvular regurgitant fractions. Clinical evaluation and computer simulation. *Eur Heart J* 1990; **11:** 355–60.

17. REISNER SA, MELTZER RS. Normal values of prosthetic valve Doppler echocardiographic parameters: a review. *J Am Soc Echo* 1988; **1:** 201–10.

18. SCHOENFELD MH, PALACIOS IF, HUTTER AM, JACOBY SS, BLOCK PC. Underestimation of prosthetic mitral valve areas: role of transseptal catheterization in avoiding unnecessary repeat mitral valve surgery. *J Am Coll Cardiol* 1985; **5:** 1387–92.

19. MOHR-KAHALY S, KUPFERWASSER I, ERBEL R, OELERT G, MEYER J. Regurgitant flow in apparently normal valve prostheses: improved detection and semi-quantitative analysis by transesophageal two-dimensional colour-coded Doppler echocardiography. *J Am Soc Echo* 1990; **3:** 187–95.

20. LANGE HW, OLSON JD, PEDERSEN WR, et al. Transesophageal color Doppler echocardiography of the normal St Jude Medical mitral valve prosthesis. *Am Heart J* 1991; **122:** 489–94.

21. ALAM M, SERWIN JB, POLANCO GA, SUN I, SILVERMAN HA. Transesophageal echocardiographic features of normal and dysfunctioning bioprosthetic valves. *Am Heart J* 1991; **121:** 1149–55.

22. MÜGGE A, DANIEL WG, HAVERICH A, LICHTLEN PR. Diagnosis of noninfective cardiac mass lesions by two-dimensional echocardiography. Comparison of the transthoracic and transesophageal approaches. *Circulation* 1991; **83:** 70–8.

23. ASCHENBERG W, SCHLÜTER M, KREMER P, SCHRÖDER E, SIGLOW V, BLEIFELD W. Transesophageal two-dimensional echocardiography for the detection of left atrial appendage thrombus. *J Am Coll Cardiol* 1986; **7:** 163–6.

24. MACHI J, SIGEL B, BEITLER JC, COELHO JCU, JUSTIN JR. Relation of in vivo blood flow to ultrasound echogenicity. *J Clin Ultrasound* 1983; **11:** 3–10.

25. BEPPU S, NIMURA Y, SAKAKIBARA H, et al. Smoke-like echo in left atrial cavity in mitral valve disease: its features and significance. *J Am Coll Cardiol* 1985; **6:** 744–9.

26. SIGEL B, COELHO JCU, SPIGOS DG, et al. Ultrasonography of blood during stasis and coagulation. *Invest Radiol* 1981; **17:** 71–6.

27. DANIEL WG, NELLESSEN U, SCHRÖDER E, et al. Left atrial spontaneous echo contrast in mitral valve disease: an indicator for an increased thromboembolic risk. *J Am Coll Cardiol* 1988; **11:** 1204–11.

28. BLACK IW, HOPKINS AP, LEE LCL, WALSH WF,

JACOBSON BM. Left atrial spontaneous echo contrast: a clinical and echocardiographic analysis. *J Am Coll Cardiol* 1991; **18:** 398–404.

29. TAAMS MA, GUSSENHOVEN EJ, BOS E, et al. Enhanced morphological diagnosis in infective endocarditis by transoesophageal echocardiography. *Br Heart J* 1990; **63:** 109–13.

30. ERBEL R, ROHMANN S, DREXLER M, et al. Improved diagnostic value of echocardiography in patients with infective endocarditis by transoesophageal approach. A prospective study. *Eur Heart J* 1988; **9:** 45–53.

Evaluation of Mustard and Senning procedures

O. Stümper

INTRODUCTION

Since its introduction in 1964 the Mustard procedure (1) has become the preferred surgical approach for correction of transposition of the great arteries. The operation involves rerouting the systemic venous blood to the left ventricle and the pulmonary venous blood to the right ventricle. In the original Mustard procedure this was achieved by the use of a prosthetic patch. Modifications of this procedure included patch augmentation by additional use of pericardium, or construction of the intra-atrial baffle solely by the use of atrial tissue, i.e. the Senning procedure (2). Although the long-term survival is high after these procedures (3–6), numerous potential late complications make close follow-up of such patients necessary. Well recognised complications include the development of right ventricular dysfunction, tricuspid insufficiency, and arrhythmias. Furthermore, subacute or progressive obstruction of both the systemic venous or pulmonary venous pathways may occur, as well as progressive left ventricular outflow obstruction (3–9).

Assessment of the immediate and long-term results of Mustard and Senning procedures has for long relied on cardiac catheterisation and angiography to demonstrate the functioning of the systemic and pulmonary venous pathways. The introduction of precordial ultrasound imaging and pulsed Doppler interrogation has allowed non-invasive definition of haemodynamic lesions in the follow-up of this patient group (10–12). Nonethe-

less, in clinical practice, transthoracic ultrasound studies are frequently limited. The structures to be evaluated lie in the far field, and the presence of prosthetic patch material produces significant ultrasound masking. In addition, the superior aspects of the atrial chambers are only poorly visualised. These limitations are even more pronounced in the adolescent and adult patient in whom there are generally poor precordial and subcostal ultrasound windows.

Magnetic resonance imaging was proposed by Rees and colleagues for the evaluation of the Mustard procedure (13). However, because of the complex anatomy of the interatrial baffle, such studies are time consuming. Contiguous slices of the oblique baffle are difficult to obtain and thus the definite exclusion of baffle obstruction can rarely be obtained by this technique. Calcific baffle obstructions will generally not be visualised by magnetic resonance imaging. Information on baffle function, such as in the exclusion of baffle obstruction or baffle leakage, can only be obtained by spin-echo techniques, which currently are available in only a few centres. Finally, a significant proportion of these patients have to be excluded from magnetic resonance studies because of the presence of permanent pacemakers. In addition, atrial fibrillation, present in a subset of patients, dramatically reduces the image resolution of this gated technique.

Transesophageal echocardiography, on the other hand, has proved to be a most versatile alternative technique in the follow-up of these patients (14). Because of the proximity of the transducer to the atrial chambers and its excellent visualisation of the postero-superior aspects of the heart, the technique can provide detailed insights into atrial baffle morphology and function. Prior to a look at the transesophageal evaluation of specific abnormalities of the Mustard and Senning circulation, the standard transesophageal transverse imaging sections of a normal atrial baffle will be described in detail.

STANDARD IMAGING PLANES

Transverse axis transesophageal imaging produces unique views of the complex architecture of the interatrial baffle. A detailed understanding of these sections is mandatory for a rapid assessment of atrial baffle morphology and function. Thus, a standard transesophageal examination protocol will be outlined at this point.

The probe is initially advanced to the stomach to obtain a right lateral view of the liver which demonstrates the inferior caval vein and the hepatic veins. With slight counterclockwise rotation, together with gradual withdrawal of the probe, the drainage of the inferior caval vein to the systemic venous atrium is then visualised (Fig. 5.25). The baffle suture line encircles the orifice of the inferior caval vein anteriorly. Posteriorly the baffle is sutured to the wall of the right atrium (Fig. 5.26).

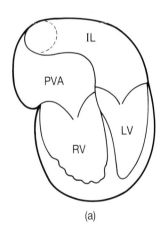

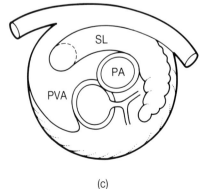

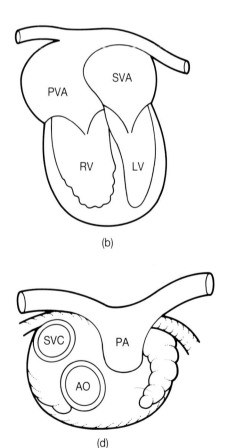

Figure 5.25 *Diagram of standard transverse axis sections obtained in patients with a Mustard circulation.* **(a)** *Low four-chamber cut.* **(b)** *Four-chamber view.* **(c)** *Level of the ventricular outflow tracts.* **(d)** *Arterial valve level. Abbreviations: IL = inferior limb; PVA = pulmonary venous atrium; SL = superior limb; SVA = superior venous atrium.*

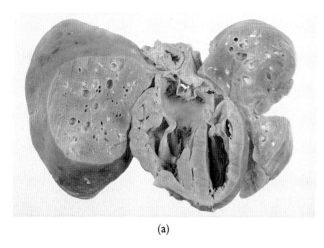

(a)

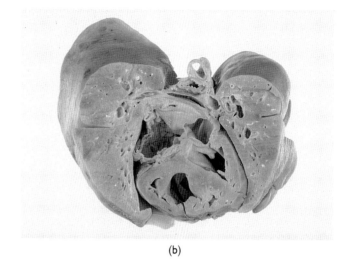

(b)

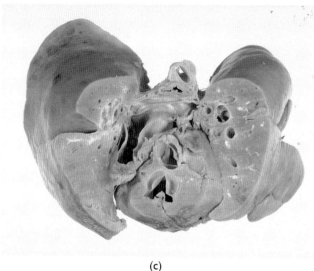

(c)

Figure 5.26 *Anatomic sections demonstrating the most relevant transverse planes in a Mustard heart.* **(a)** *Section simulating a low four-chamber view, which demonstrates the orientation of the inferior limb of the systemic venous atrium and the baffle suture line around the anterior border of the inferior caval vein.* **(b)** *Section demonstrating the midportion of the systemic venous atrium and the distal portion of the pulmonary venous atrium.* **(c)** *Section showing the orientation of the superior limb of the systemic venous atrium, and its relation to the proximal portion of the pulmonary venous atrium, the left sided pulmonary veins and the pulmonary trunk.*

Careful cross-sectional imaging together with colour flow mapping studies should be carried out in this position, as baffle leakage is frequent at this site. Using further counterclockwise rotation of the probe, the entire inferior limb of the systemic venous atrium is readily demonstrated on cross-sectional imaging. Anteriorly the attachment of the baffle to the remnant of the septum primum is seen. The site of drainage of the coronary sinus should be noted in all patients; in the majority it will have been left to drain into the pulmonary venous atrium.

Following a complete assessment of the inferior limb of the systemic venous atrium, the mitral valve morphology and function should be evaluated using a series of transverse axis views. Posterior to the mitral valve the supramitral portion of the systemic venous atrium is visualised. On these views the proximal portion of the pulmonary venous atrium is seen closest to the transducer (i.e. at the top of the screen). Further counterclockwise rotation of the probe then allows inspection of the left lateral portion of the sutureline of the patch. In most cases the left atrial appendage will be found to be incorporated into the systemic venous atrium with the patch sutured to the crest of atrial tissue which separates the left atrial appendage from the left sided pulmonary veins. Both left pulmonary veins are assessed in the standard manner. Clockwise rotation of the probe, at the level of the left atrial appendage, will then allow a complete visualisation of the superior limb of the systemic venous atrium. This is a rather oblique channel which lies immediately posterior to the left ventricular outflow tract and the pulmonary valve (Fig. 5.26(c)). In its midportion the presence of any remnant of the atrial septum should be noted on cross-sectional imaging studies. Further clockwise rotation of the probe with gradual withdrawal will demonstrate the superior caval vein and the suture line of the baffle with this structure. The pulmonary trunk and its bifurcation will be visualised in the same imaging planes.

The pulmonary venous atrium is assessed using a reversed sequence of the above-mentioned imaging planes. The right upper pulmonary vein is visualised in its typical location just posterior to the superior caval vein. Thereafter, using counter-clockwise rotation of the probe the superior aspect of the posterior pulmonary venous atrium is assessed and both left sided pulmonary veins are again demonstrated. Rotation of the probe, so as to scan the right lateral aspects of the atrial chambers, will then visualise the connection between the posterior and the anterior portion of the pulmonary venous atrium. Finally, the right lower pulmonary vein is best visualised just posterior to the site where the inferior limb of the systemic venous atrium is demonstrated. The tricuspid valve morphology and function is assessed thereafter using standard views.

Detailed colour flow mapping and pulsed wave Doppler studies should complement the initial imaging study. Colour flow mapping should particularly be used for the rapid identification of baffle leakage, and the detection of obstructed intra-atrial flow patterns. In our experience, turbulent flow patterns within the baffle limbs are a common finding when assessing atrial baffle function. The use of high pulse repetition frequencies during colour flow mapping studies are preferred, so as to decrease the sensitivity of the technique in the demonstration of even minor degrees of turbulent flow. Pulsed wave Doppler studies should also represent a routine integral part of the complete evaluation of atrial baffle function. Sampling sites should include individual pulmonary veins, the superior limb and inferior limb of the systemic venous atrium, the communication between the proximal and the distal pulmonary venous atrium and the tricuspid valve.

When compared with single-plane transesophageal imaging, the recent advent of biplane transesophageal imaging has added relatively little to the evaluation of the Mustard or Senning procedure. However, a couple of benefits, which make the technique a useful adjunct, are noteworthy. When there is obstruction of the systemic venous atrium, collateral channels, such as the azygos and hemiazygos system, will be found dilated. Adequate visualisation and Doppler evaluation of these vessels is largely facilitated by longitudinal axis imaging. With respect to the assessment of atrial baffle morphology, the longitudinal imaging plane frequently allows a better appreciation of the internal dimensions of obstructed limbs of the systemic venous atrium, since these are visualised in cross-section. The height of the mid portion of the pulmonary venous atrium can be ascertained only on longitudinal imaging planes. Finally, in some cases with baffle leakage, the leak is better demonstrated on longitudinal planes than on standard transverse axis planes.

Baffle leakage

Residual interatrial shunting is a frequent finding following either the Mustard or Senning procedure. In several studies the incidence of such lesions has been reported to vary between 25 and 90% (4,5). The majority of these baffle leaks are clinically inapparent. However, a number of patients will suffer from marked desaturation in particular during exercise.

Definition of the size, number and location of these defects is essential for the planning of any subsequent surgical correction. Preoperative evaluation is still most commonly performed by cardiac catheterisation and angiocardiography. However, this technique meets with various limitations and difficulties. Firstly, oximetry is too crude a method to detect small interatrial shunts and to determine their precise site. In addition, oximetric studies performed under heavy sedation or general anaesthesia (when oxygen consumption is low) frequently fail to detect any shunting despite marked desaturation during exercise. Secondly, a multitude of contrast injections and projections frequently have to be used during angiographic studies to delineate the exact site of the communication(s). Moreover, a full appreciation of the complex baffle anatomy is difficult on angiographic films. Precordial ultrasound techniques are limited by the poor penetration of the Doppler beam, and thus only rarely provide sufficient colour flow mapping information to unequivocally demonstrate or exclude these lesions.

Transesophageal ultrasound studies have several definite advantages (14). The proximity of the ultrasound transducer to the atrial baffle allows high-quality colour flow mapping information to be obtained. The entire baffle suture line can be scanned, thus allowing the rapid identification of even multiple and small defects (Fig. 5.27). In addition, the complex baffle architecture is readily appreciated, and it is possible to define the site(s) of baffle leakage relative to the adjacent structures, thus providing invaluable information to the surgeon and for detailed planning of subsequent transcatheter defect occlusion.

Of 37 patients entered into a prospective study of the comparative value of these three diagnostic

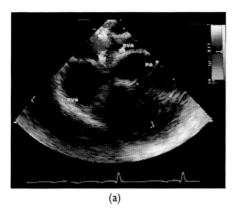 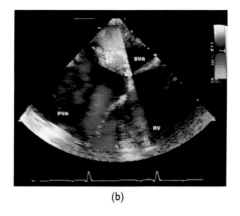

(a) (b)

Figure 5.27 *Transoephageal definition of multiple sites of baffle leakage following the Mustard procedure. Both leaks were missed during prior precordial ultrasound studies.* **(a)** *Small baffle leak at the mid portion of the antero-superior sutureline of the baffle.* **(b)** *Wide patch dehiscence in the area of the left lateral sutureline of the patch towards the left sided pulmonary veins.*

modalities in the evaluation of the Mustard circulation, 19 were documented by transesophageal ultrasound studies to have baffle leakage. In 11 of these 19 patients multiple leaks were identified and their locations determined accurately. In contrast, only 5 of these 19 patients (26%) were identified by precordial ultrasound techniques, and only 15 (79%) were identified during angiographic studies using up to five contrast injections. Multiple leaks were not identified by precordial ultrasound in any patient, and in only one by angiography. On the basis of these results we have altered our diagnostic approach to patients in whom baffle leakage is clinically suspected. Exercise testing under saturation monitoring reveals the clinical significance of any right-to-left shunting resulting from baffle leakage. The subsequent transesophageal study is then used to document the precise number and location of the defects. On the basis of this information patients are selected for either surgical or transcatheter closure.

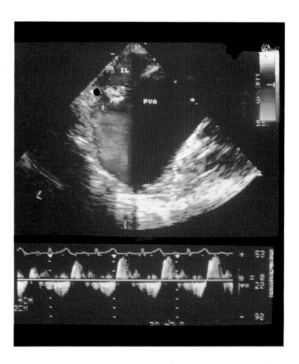

Figure 5.28 *Colour flow mapping study of a small baffle leak at the sutureline of the baffle anterior to the inferior caval vein. Pulsed wave Doppler sampling at the site of communication reveals characteristic early diastolic left-to-right shunting.*

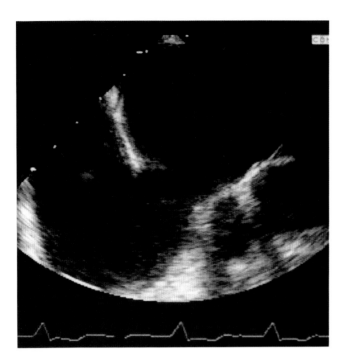

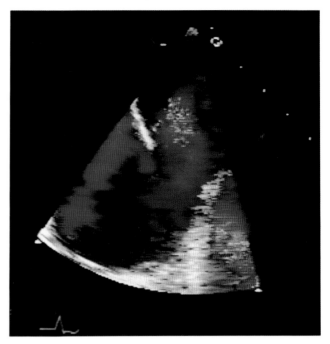

Figure 5.29 *Wide dehiscence of the baffle sutureline along the anterior attachment to the septum primum.*

Frequent sites of baffle leakage include, firstly, the anterior aspect of the baffle suture line with the inferior caval vein (Fig. 5.28), secondly the area where the baffle is sutured to the crux of the heart (Fig. 5.29), thirdly the left lateral aspect of the suture line, that is near the left sided pulmonary veins, and, lastly, the right lateral suture line at the junction with the superior caval vein (Fig. 5.30). In addition, in patients with severe obstruction of either limb of the systemic venous atrium, a small baffle leakage at the site of obstruction can be noted in the majority of patients.

Although transesophageal echocardiography would appear to be the diagnostic technique of choice in the assessment of baffle leakage, there are certain limitations and potential pitfalls which have to be borne in mind. Frequently the prosthetic patch used for the construction of a Mustard baffle is heavily calcified. This may lead to echo dropouts on cross-sectional imaging, which may be mistaken for a discontinuity of the baffle suture line. Thus, colour flow mapping studies, with clear-cut evidence of shunt flow, are required for a definitive diagnosis. Secondly, the finding of turbulent flow patterns on either side of the patch should not be interpreted as a proof of baffle leakage. It is a rather frequent finding and may be caused by knots of the suture material. Depending on the flow map and settings used during the study, these turbulent flow areas may then appear to communicate with one another. In cases where ambiguity persists even following adequate changes of the settings of the ultrasound machine and slight alterations in transducer position, peripheral contrast injections may provide the definitive diagnosis.

Pulsed wave Doppler evaluation of the transbaffle shunt flows is extremely rewarding. In patients with completely unobstructed systemic and pulmonary venous pathways normally there will be a bidirectional shunt. However, in face of elevated right ventricular end diastolic pressures and subsequent elevation of mean pulmonary venous atrial pressures a functional left-to-right shunt will be encountered. Thus flow is predominantly directed towards the systemic venous atrium. In a subset of patients with baffle obstruction, relative location of the leak to the obstruction appears to be the only determinant for the direction of shunt flow. Leaks proximal to an obstruction result in almost continuous shunt flow towards the unobstructed pathway. In the presence of such findings, subsequent evaluation of the severity of baffle obstruction should be largely guided by an assessment of the minimal internal dimensions of the obstructed pathway. In particular, it is noteworthy that in the presence of a more proximal baffle leak, pulsed wave Doppler interrogation across the obstruction may fail to demonstrate continuous turbulent flow patterns, a sign which is otherwise diagnostic of severe obstruction (see below). The calculation of pressure gradients from the pulsed wave Doppler waveforms obtained across baffle leaks should be interpreted with caution, because of the inherent limitations of the Bernoulli equation when used to evaluate venous and turbulent flow patterns.

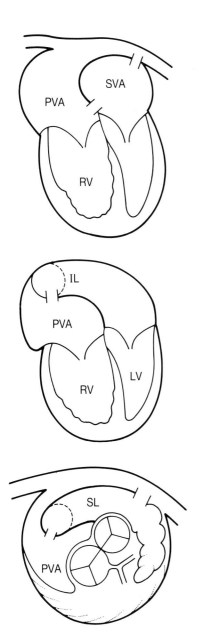

Figure 5.30 *Diagram of frequent sites of baffle leaks following the Mustard procedure. Abbreviations as in Fig. 5.25.*

OBSTRUCTIONS OF THE PULMONARY VENOUS PATHWAYS

Obstructions of the pulmonary venous pathways are a relatively uncommon finding following the Mustard procedure. However, their incidence in large series of patients has been reported to be as high as 5–7% (6,7,15). The majority of these obstructions develop in the late follow-up period, and are confined to the communication between the proximal and the distal chamber of the pulmonary venous atrium. Other rarer sites of obstruction include the stenosis of an individual pulmonary vein (most often the left sided ones). These latter lesions appear to be related to suboptimal placement of the baffle suture line relative to the pulmonary venous orifices.

Precordial ultrasound techniques previously have been shown to be highly sensitive in the detection of obstructions of the mid portion of the pulmonary venous atrium (16,17). Our own experience using the precordial approach to assess these lesions would confirm these reports. However, there are several aspects of this range of lesions which are better evaluated by transesophageal echocardiography. Whereas precordial imaging most often fails to adequately demonstrate the posterior portion of the pulmonary venous atrium (near the pulmonary venous drainage), this routinely can be achieved by transesophageal imaging. This in turn allows a more detailed documentation of atrial baffle morphology and thus allows a better definition of any potential obstruction. The insights provided by the technique revealed that there appear to be two types of mid pulmonary venous atrium obstruction. The most common type is a discrete narrowing of the communication between the posterior and anterior portion of the pulmonary venous atrium. This type of lesion is readily identified by the demonstration of a shelf-like ridge on cross-sectional imaging (Fig. 5.31). In such lesions the right lateral and posterior wall of the narrowing is related to the crest of the atrial septum which the surgeon cannot excise completely. The second type of obstruction is a rather tubular narrowing produced by approximation of both the inferior and superior limbs of the systemic venous atrium, together with a small posterior portion of the pulmonary venous atrium (Fig. 5.32). The clinical significance of the differentiation between these two types of obstructions is that the first one is potentially amenable to balloon dilatation, whereas the second type of obstruction is better approached by surgical patch enlargement of the pulmonary venous atrium.

Transesophageal pulsed Doppler evaluation of the function of the pulmonary venous atrium can be performed with a better angle of incidence than that commonly obtained during a precordial ultrasound study (see Fig. 5.31). This in turn allows a better estimation of any intra-baffle gradient. In a series of patients studied with these lesions at our institutions, there was very good correlation between the transesophageal and the catheter-derived gradient. Although the peak velocities of flow between the proximal and distal chambers of the pulmonary venous atrium may frequently exceed 1.5 m/s, this does not represent obstruction. The major criterion for obstruction should rather be the finding of continuous high-velocity flow patterns, that do not reach baseline throughout the cardiac cycle (Fig. 5.32). Considering the progressive nature of these lesions, it may be justified to refer such patients for early balloon dilatation in cases where the transesophageal study has documented a favourable anatomy for such a procedure.

Obstructions of individual pulmonary veins are a rare finding in the late postoperative period. Such lesions are almost impossible to exclude by precordial ultrasound techniques, since the presence of the large prosthetic patch will almost always preclude both adequate visualisation and Doppler interrogation of the individual pulmonary veins from the precordium. In contrast, this can be performed routinely by the transesophageal ultrasound approach (18). Again, the finding of continuous turbulent flow patterns which do not reach baseline during the cardiac cycle are conclusive in the diagnosis of pulmonary vein obstruction. Cross-sectional imaging can then be used to delineate the cause of the obstruction, which in turn should be helpful in selecting the appropriate therapeutic procedure.

OBSTRUCTION OF THE SYSTEMIC VENOUS PATHWAYS

Obstructions within the systemic venous atrium are a relatively common finding following the Mustard procedure in particular. Previous reports have stated the incidence to vary between 3 and 17%. Obstructive lesions within the superior limb of the systemic venous atrium are much more frequently encountered than those within the inferior limb. They may be subacute, occurring in the immediate postopera-

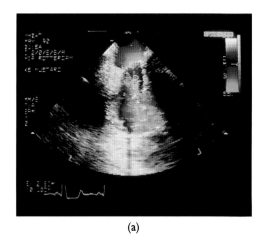
(a)

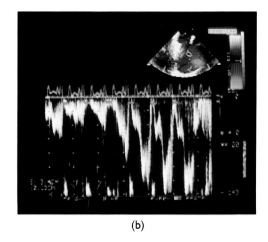
(b)

Figure 5.31 (a) *Mild obstruction of the mid portion of the pulmonary venous atrium, which is produced by a shelf-like ridge of the remnant of the posterior portion of the atrial septum.* **(b)** *The corresponding pulsed wave Doppler study, by shifting the sampling volume, allows the operator to document precisely the level of obstruction. The persistence of phasic flow patterns that reach baseline during the cardiac cycle excludes significant obstruction despite increased maximal flow velocities.*

tive period, or, more commonly, may be chronic and progressive lesions (19,20). In a recent series of patients reported by Turley and associates (21), 25% of the patients suffered from obstruction of the superior limb of the systemic venous atrium, and 40% of these patients required reoperation.

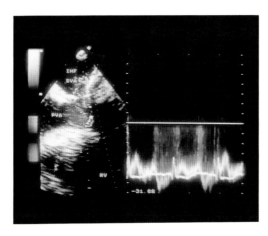

Figure 5.32 *Tunnel-like obstruction of the pulmonary venous atrium, which is produced by approximation of both the superior and inferior limbs of the systemic venous atrium. The pulsed wave Doppler study reveals continuous turbulent high-velocity flow patterns, indicating significant obstruction.*

Precordial ultrasound techniques have been used extensively in the exclusion and in the assessment of this spectrum of lesions. In particular pulsed wave Doppler studies, using both the precordial and the suprasternal approaches, have been reported to be a sensitive technique in the detection of superior limb obstruction (22). In addition, contrast echocardiographic studies have been used in the diagnosis of superior baffle limb obstruction (23). The diagnosis was made when contrast material was detected first appearing within the inferior baffle limb (via the azygos system) following injection into a peripheral arm vein. Although these techniques have proved valuable in daily clinical practice, there are major inherent limitations and drawbacks to be considered. In particular, the exact site and the morphology of superior limb obstructions can hardly ever be documented in detail by precordial studies beyond infancy. This is related to the poor demonstration of this region of the heart by precordial

ultrasound techniques. This is further aggravated by difficulties imposed by both the presence of fibrous tissue adhesions following sternotomy and the presence of prosthetic patch material in the area of interest. Cardiac catheterisation and angiography are still considered to be the definitive diagnostic technique. Angiography can provide adequate visualisation of both the dimensions, albeit not the morphology, of the stenotic segment and the magnitude of the collateral circulation. The value of catheter-derived pressure gradients between the different levels of the systemic venous atrium in the presence of adequate collateral circulation is, however, questionable. Finally, catheter balloon angioplasty, which can be performed during the same procedure, offers a therapeutic approach to these lesions (24).

Transesophageal ultrasound offers several advantages in excluding or diagnosing this range of lesions. By using the examination technique outlined above, the transesophageal approach can provide a complete evaluation of the morphology of the entire systemic venous pathways. In adolescent and adult patients the technique can be used as a routine outpatient screening technique, whereas clinical evidence of baffle dysfunction should guide in the indication for study in children. Transesophageal imaging, in our experience, is the best technique to document the mechanism and the precise morphology of systemic pathway obstruction. This is particularly true for obstructions within the superior limb of the systemic venous atrium. In a high proportion of such patients the obstruction will be visualised to be at the site of the atrial septum. The surgeon frequently cannot fully resect the superior portion of the atrial septum because of its proximity to the sinus node artery. A remnant of this structure consequently is often visualised near the junction of the superior limb and the supramitral portion of the systemic venous atrium (Fig. 5.33). It appears that progressive pathway obstruction is most frequently encountered at this site. Such lesions are initially discrete shelf-like ridges which are associated with phasic but turbulent flow patterns. Higher degrees of obstruction are defined by increasing narrowing of this area as defined on cross-sectional imaging. Flow patterns as assessed by pulsed wave Doppler interrogation may become continuous. However, in the presence of a sufficient collateral circulation or in the presence of a more proximal baffle leak, flow patterns may remain phasic. Complete occlusion of the pathway is readily identified on combined cross-sectional imaging and colour flow mapping studies. This will be caused in the majority of cases by a tunnel-shaped lesion of varying extent (Fig. 5.34). A further type of obstruction is the presence of either discrete or widespread calcification within the systemic venous pathways (Fig. 5.35). Finally, we encountered two patients in our series who suffered from dynamic obstruction of the superior limb of the systemic venous atrium, which was caused by a moderate to severe tricuspid regurgitation jet which partially compressed the superior limb during ventricular systole.

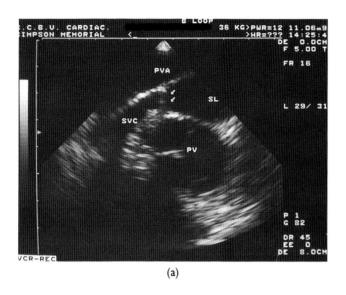

(a)

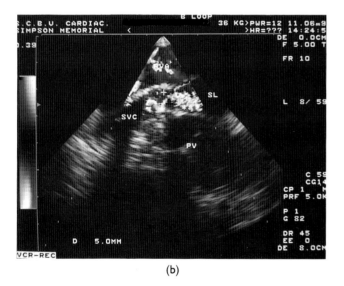

(b)

Figure 5.33 (a) *Discrete obstruction within the superior limb of the systemic venous atrium, caused by the remaining superior portion of the atrial septum (arrows).* **(b)** *The corresponding colour flow mapping study confirms the level of obstruction. The maximal diameter of the communication measures 5 mm. Pulsed wave Doppler studies demonstrated continuous turbulent flow.*

The alignment of the transesophageal pulsed wave Doppler beam to the direction of flow within the systemic venous atrium is generally poor, and no attempts to predict the resulting pressure gradient between the various levels should be undertaken. This, in our opinion, is of little importance since, in the presence of a venous collateral circulation, the meaning of actual pressure gradients remains questionable. Given clinical symptoms of obstruction, it is rather the underlying morphology of the lesion which should determine the indication and the selection (angioplasty or surgery) of subsequent therapeutic steps. In view of the progressive nature of these lesions a more aggressive approach may be justified.

LEFT VENTRICULAR OUTFLOW OBSTRUCTION

Left ventricular outflow obstruction is a frequent finding in complete transposition. Its incidence has been reported to be some 20% for cases with an intact ventricular septum and some 30% in those with a ventricular septal defect (25,26). Thus, in the long-term follow-up of the Mustard or Senning patient this spectrum of lesions is often encountered. Precordial ultrasound techniques, in our experience, are often inadequate in defining the exact nature and the precise morphology of these lesions following either the Mustard or Senning procedure. This is related in particular to the shape and the orientation of the left ventricle and its outflow tract in such hearts. In contrast, the transesophageal approach provides unique views of this area of the heart (see Chapter 3.6). In patients with an intact ventricular septum the obstruction is most often produced by bulging of either the membranous or muscular ventricular septum, resulting in a dynamic obstruction (Fig. 5.36). These lesions may develop in the long-term follow-up period only, and are probably related to the longstanding systemic pressure of the right ventricle. In cases with severe obstruction and impingement of the septum against the anterior leaflet of the mitral valve the secondary formation of a fibromuscular ridge or membrane may be encountered. The precise underlying anatomy of this range of complex lesions is generally readily documented on transverse axis imaging studies; however in selected cases the addition of longitudinal plane amaging is most valuable.

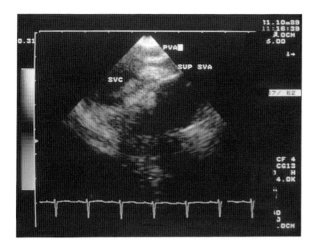

Figure 5.34 *Long-standing tunnel-shaped obstruction at the same site as in Fig. 5.33, leaving only a pinhole communication.*

In those patients with a ventricular septal defect, the obstruction may be produced by either localised or tunnel-shaped fibromuscular lesions, by a deviation of the outlet septum or by an abnormal subvalvar apparatus of the mitral valve (27). The latter range of lesions is frequently produced by implantation of chordae of the anterior leaflet of the mitral valve to the septal surface of the left ventricle (Fig. 5.37). The range of information to be gained by the technique would suggest that transesophageal imaging should be the tool of first choice in planning the therapeutic approach.

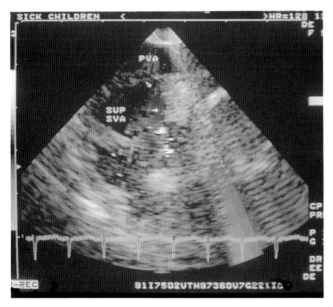

Figure 5.35 *Widespread calcific obstructive lesion (arrows) of the superior limb of the systemic venous atrium, which led to marked enlargement of the superior caval vein and the proximal portion of the superior limb. No antegrade flow could be recorded across this lesion.*

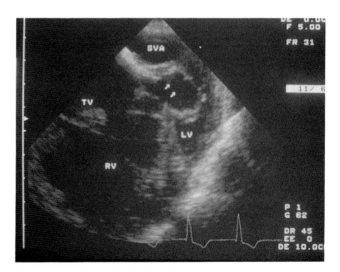

Figure 5.36 *Dynamic obstruction of the left ventricular outflow tract in an adult patient following the Mustard procedure. The obstruction is produced by an aneurysm of the perimembranous and muscular ventricular septum. Any involvement of the mitral valve apparatus in this lesion could be excluded during real-time imaging.*

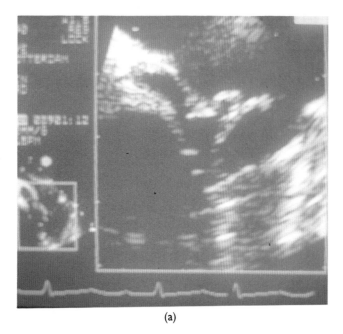

(a)

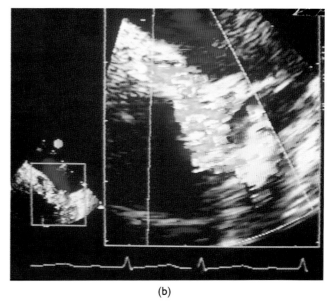

(b)

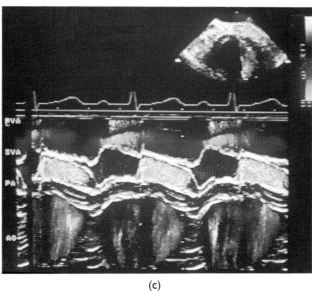

(c)

Figure 5.37 *Transesophageal study in a patient with left ventricular outflow obstruction following the Mustard procedure.* **(a)** *Cross-sectional imaging demonstrates additional chordal attachments of the anterior leaflet of the mitral valve to the interventricular septum.* **(b)** *Colour flow mapping rapidly identifies the level of obstruction.* **(c)** *Corresponding colour M-mode study at the level of the arterial valves.*

RIGHT VENTRICULAR DYSFUNCTION

Variable degrees of right ventricular dysfunction are a common finding following atrial correction procedures for transposition of the great arteries. The morphologically right ventricle in transposition does not appear to be capable of performing at a similar level as the left ventricle in the systemic circulation. Progressive right ventricular dysfunction appears to be the major cause of reduced exercise performance in the late postoperative period.

Transthoracic ultrasound techniques are limited in the assessment of systolic right ventricular function because of the lack of a suitable algorithm to calculate right ventricular volume and work indices. Not surprisingly, the same holds true for transesophageal ultrasound studies. In contrast, magnetic resonance imaging has been reported to be a most valuable and accurate technique in the non-invasive quantitative assessment of systolic right ventricular function in these patients (13).

However, with the growing insights into cardiac function, there is now an increased interest in the assessment of diastolic events. In fact, deterioration of diastolic function may precede systolic dysfunction, and thus the early detection of such changes may be of more than only prognostic value. By offering the possibility of acquisition of high-quality pulsed wave Doppler recordings of both pulmonary venous and tricuspid valve flow patterns, transesophageal Doppler ultrasound studies potentially offer a new and somewhat unique approach in the evaluation of diastolic right ventricular function (18). Although our current experience is still limited it appears that such a technique may become an early and sensitive indicator for reduced right ventricular function. When combined with either pharmacologic stress testing, or esophageal pacing, the technique could be used to determine changes in ventricular function during various degrees of exercise. Such studies are currently under way. Initial results suggest that this approach can clearly differentiate true right ventricular dysfunction from exacerbation of subclinical haemodynamic lesions (e.g. relative baffle obstructions) as the cause for poor late postoperative exercise performance.

REFERENCES

1. MUSTARD WT, KEITH JD, TRUSLER GA, FOWLER R, KIDD L. The surgical management of transposition of the great vessels. *J Thorac Cardiovasc Surg* 1964; **48:** 953–8.
2. SENNING A. Surgical correction of transposition of the great arteries. *Surgery* 1959; **45:** 966–70.
3. WARNES C, SOMERVILLE J. Transposition of the great arteries: late results in adolescents and adults after the Mustard procedure. *Br Heart J* 1987; **58:** 148–55.
4. DARVELL FJ, ROSSI IR, ROSSI ML, et al. Intermediate to late term results of Mustard's procedure for complete transposition of the great arteries with an intact ventricular septum. *Br Heart J* 1988; **59:** 468–73.
5. WILLIAMS WG, TRUSLER GA, KIRKLIN JW, BLACKSTONE RM. Early and late results of a protocol for simple transposition leading to an atrial switch (Mustard) repair. *J Thorac Cardiovasc Surg* 1988; **95:** 717–26.
6. PARK SC, NECHES WH, MATHEWS RA, et al. Hemodynamic function after the Mustard operation for transposition of the great arteries. *Am J Cardiol* 1983; **51:** 1514–19.
7. MARX GR, HOUGEN TJ, NORWOOD WI, FYLER DC, CASTANEDA AR, NADAS AS. Transposition of the great arteries with intact ventricular septum: results of Mustard and Senning operations in 123 consecutive patients. *JACC* 1983; **1**(2): 476–83.
8. RUBAY JE, DE HALLEUX C, JAUMIN P, et al. Long-term follow-up of the Senning operation for transposition of the great arteries in children under 3 months of age. *J Thorac Cardiovasc Surg* 1987; **94:** 75–81.
9. EGLOFF CP, FREED MD, DICK M, NORWOOD WI, CASTANEDA AR. Early and late results with the Mustard operation in infancy. *Ann Thorac Surg* 1978; **26:** 474–84.
10. AZIZ KU, PAUL MH, BHARARTI S, et al. Two dimensional echocardiographic evaluation of Mustard operation for d-transposition of the great arteries. *Am J Cardiol* 1981; **47:** 654–64.
11. CHIN AJ, SANDERS SP, WILLIAMS RG, LANG P, NORWOOD WI, CASTANEDA AR. Two-dimensional echocardiographic assessment of caval and pulmonary venous pathway after the Senning operation. *Am J Cardiol* 1983; **53:** 118–26.
12. VICK GW, MURPHY DJ, LUDOMIRSKY A, et al. Pulmonary venous and systemic ventricular inflow obstruction in patients with congenital heart disease: detection by combined two-dimensional and Doppler echocardiography. *J Am Coll Cardiol* 1987; **9:** 580–7.
13. REES S, SOMERVILLE J, WARNES C, et al. Comparison of magnetic resonance imaging with echocardiography and radionuclide angiography in assessing cardiac function and anatomy following Mustard's operation for transposition of the great arteries. *Am J Cardiol* 1988; **61:** 1316–22.
14. KAULITZ R, STÜMPER O, GEUSKENS R, et al. The comparative values of the precordial and transesophageal approaches in the ultrasound evaluation of atrial baffle function following an atrial correction procedure. *J Am Coll Cardiol* 1990; **16:** 686–94.
15. DRISCOLL DJ, NIHILL MR, VARGO TA, MULLINS CHE, MCN AMARA DG. Late development of pulmonary venous obstruction following Mustard's operation using a Dacron baffle. *Circulation* 1977; **55:** 484–8.
16. SMALLHORN JF, GOW R, FREEDOM RM, et al. Pulsed Doppler echocardiographic assessment of the pulmonary venous pathway after the Mustard or Senning procedure for transposition of great arteries. *Circulation* 1986; **73:** 765–74.
17. VICK GW, MURPHY DJ, LUDOMIRSKY A, et al. Pulmonary venous and systemic ventricular inflow obstruction in patients with congenital heart disease: detection by combined two-dimensional and Doppler echocardiography. *J Am Coll Cardiol* 1987; **9:** 580–7.
18. KAULITZ R, STÜMPER O, FRASER AG, KREIS A, TUCILLO B, SUTHERLAND GR. The potential value of transoesophageal evaluation of individual pulmonary vein flow after an atrial baffle procedure. *Int J Cardiol* 1990; **28:** 299–308.
19. STARK J, SILOVE ED, TAYLOR JFN, GRAHAM GR. Obstruction to systemic venous return following the Mustard's operation for transposition of the great arteries. *J Thorac Cardiovasc Surg* 1974; **68:** 742–9.
20. WYSE RKH, HAWORTH SG, TAYLOR JFN, MACARTNEY FJ. Obstruction of superior vena caval pathway after Mustard's repair. *Br Heart J* 1979; **42:** 162–7.
21. TURLEY K, HANLEY FL, VERRIER ED, MERRICK SH, EBERT PA. The Mustard procedure in infants less than 100 days of age. *J Thorac Cardiovasc Surg* 1988; **96:** 849–853.
22. STEVENSON JG, KAWABORI J, GUNTHEROTH WG, DOOLEY TK, DILLARD D. Pulsed Doppler echocardiographic detection of obstruction of systemic

venous return after repair of transposition of the great arteries. *Circulation* 1979; **60:** 1091–5.

23. SILVERMAN NH, SNIDER AR, COLO J, EBERT PA, TURLEY K. Superior vena caval obstruction after Mustard's operation: detection by two-dimensional contrast echocardiography. *Circulation* 1981; **64:** 392–6.

24. LOCK JE, BASS JL, CASTANEDA-ZUNIGA W, FUHRMAN BP, RASHKIND WJ, LUCAS RV. Dilation angioplasty of congenital or operative narrowings of venous channels. *Circulation* 1984; **70:** 457–64.

25. SANSA M, TONKIN IL, BARGERON LM, ELLIOT LP. Left ventricular outflow tract obstruction in transposition of the great arteries: an angiographic study of 74 patients. *Am J Cardiol* 1979; **44:** 88–95.

26. VANGILS FA, MOULAERT AJ, OPPENHEIMER-DEKKER A, WENINK CG. Transposition of the great arteries with ventricular septal defect and pulmonary stenosis. *Br Heart J* 1978; **40:** 494–501.

27. AMMIRATI A, ARTEGA M, GARCIA-PELAEZ I, et al. Congenital mitral valve anomalies in transposition of the great arteries. *Jpn Heart J* 1989; **30:** 187–95.

Evaluation of Fontan-type procedures

O. Stümper and J. Hess

INTRODUCTION

In 1971 Fontan and Baudet described the first case of surgical correction of tricuspid atresia (1). The right ventricle was bypassed by a communication between the right atrium and the pulmonary artery; a principle which since then has become known as the Fontan procedure. Today various modifications of the original procedure are applied to treat a wide spectrum of complex cyanotic congenital heart disease (2–5). Although the type of surgical repair must be tailored to suit the individual patient, it is appropriate at this point to describe the most commonly used modifications of the Fontan procedure (Fig. 5.38).

Atriopulmonary connections are currently the most widely used type of procedure for patients with tricuspid atresia. These can be established by either direct anastomosis or by insertion of a conduit between the systemic venous atrium (right atrium) and the pulmonary artery system. Direct anastomoses can be constructed either anterior (using the right atrial appendage) or posterior to the aorta (Fig. 5.38(d)). In selected cases the native pulmonary valve can be incorporated into an anterior connection, the so-called Kreutzer procedure (6) (Fig. 5.38(e)). In older patients, a homograft or a bioprosthetic valve may have been incorporated within either a direct or a conduit connection, independent of its location (7,8). The use of such valves has now largely been abandoned. Following atriopulmonary connections the systemic venous blood enters the pulmonary artery system directly from the atria without a pumping chamber.

The second group of procedures to be considered are those in which a communication between the right atrial chamber and the (rudimentary) right ventricle is established (Fig. 5.38(f). Such procedures are only applicable in patients with tricuspid atresia and normally related great vessels in whom the right ventricular outflow tract and the pulmonary valve are non-stenotic. The communication is established either by a direct anastomosis of the right atrial appendage to the subpulmonary outlet chamber, or by insertion of a valved or non-valved conduit (9). Although the incorporation of a ventricular chamber may be beneficial to drive pulmonary blood flow, in clinical experience there has been little evidence that these procedures are advantageous over atriopulmonary connections.

Recently these two principal groups of procedures have been extended by a further approach which is termed 'total cavopulmonary connection' (10). A prosthetic patch is sutured into the right atrial cavity so as to produce an intracardiac channel which directs inferior caval venous blood to the pulmonary artery. The superior caval vein is anastomosed to the right pulmonary artery in an end-to-side fashion (Fig. 5.38(c)). Since its introduction in 1988, this procedure has been shown to be applicable to a range of patients with complex congenital heart disease other than tricuspid atresia. In addition, further modifications have been developed. The most important one includes fenestration of the prosthetic patch, which allows for controlled right-to-left shunting in patients with borderline pulmonary vascular resistance (11). This

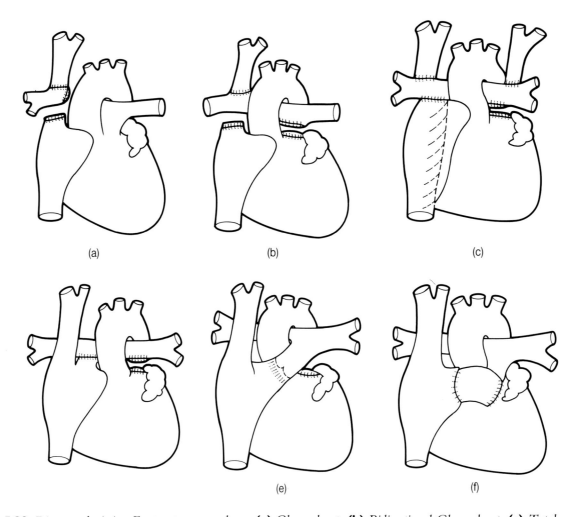

Figure 5.38 *Diagram depicting Fontan-type procedures.* **(a)** *Glenn shunt.* **(b)** *Bidirectional Glenn shunt.* **(c)** *Total cavopulmonary connection.* **(d)** *Direct atriopulmonary connection.* **(e)** *Kreutzer procedure.* **(f)** *Atrioventricular connection.*

procedure is often referred to as a 'fenestrated Fontan'. The baffle fenestration is subsequently closed by transcatheter device placement once the patient is completely stabilised.

Before the introduction of the Fontan concept in the repair of tricuspid atresia, a superior vena cava to pulmonary artery end-to-end anastomosis was designed by Glenn (12) for palliation of a range of cyanotic congenital cardiac defects, including the univentricular heart (Fig. 5.38(a)). These shunts provided adequate palliation in a large number of

patients. However, the reported frequent development of arteriovenous fistulae (13) has resulted in a dramatic decrease in the use of this approach. With the introduction of the bidirectional cavopulmonary shunt (14), which is an end-to-side anastomosis between the superior caval vein and the right pulmonary artery (Fig. 5.38(b)), there is now a renewed interest in this technique (15). This latter shunt constitutes an integral part in the creation of a total cavopulmonary connection.

Although the early and late results of Fontan-type procedures have improved considerably over the past decade (16), a large proportion of these patients will have residual or acquired haemodynamic lesions (17–19). Whereas some of these lesions are residua from a suboptimal surgical repair, others may develop during the late follow-up and may lead to either acute or progressive clinical deterioration. Therefore close follow-up of all patients who underwent a Fontan-type procedure is required.

Transthoracic imaging and Doppler ultrasound studies are widely used to assess the functional results of these patients (20,21). However, in particular in the adolescent and adult patient population such studies are limited by a multitude of factors. Firstly, in the presence of considerable liver enlargement, the subcostal ultrasound window is no longer accessible. Secondly, the posterior and superior aspects of the heart, and thus the site of the majority of Fontan connections, is only poorly visualised by parasternal imaging. Thus, in patients in whom Fontan dysfunction is clinically suspected, cardiac catheterisation will often be resorted to in order to obtain more diagnostic information. Magnetic resonance imaging has been proposed by several investigators to be an alternative to transthoracic ultrasound evaluation. However, to the best of our knowledge no detailed study so far has been reported on the value of this technique. In fact, several

considerations may suggest that magnetic resonance imaging encounters severe limitations in the assessment of the Fontan circulation. The major one is that calcific obstructions are not adequately visualised, thus precluding identification of one of the major causes of late obstruction to pulmonary blood flow in patients with conduit connections. In addition, haemodynamic data derived from spin echo techniques is currently available in only a few centres.

The potential value of transesophageal echocardiography in the follow-up of patients who have undergone a Fontan-type procedure lies in the enhanced evaluation of cardiac structures closest to the esophagus when compared with the transthoracic approach. This in most cases permits improved visualisation of the various types of Fontan connections and identification or exclusion of the majority of residual or acquired haemodynamic lesions (22).

RESIDUAL ATRIAL SHUNTING

Persistent arterial desaturation following a Fontan-type procedure is a frequent finding (17). In the majority of cases this will be caused by a residual communication between the atrial chambers at the site of the former atrial septal defect, or by multiple leaks at the suture line of the patch used to create a total cavopulmonary connection. Following all Fontan-type procedures the systemic venous pressures are invariably elevated. Usually there is a mean gradient of about 5–8 mmHg between the right and the left atrium even in the absence of obstruction to pulmonary blood flow. Thus, in cases with residual atrial communications there will be a continuous right-to-left shunt. Such shunts increase in magnitude during exercise.

Precordial imaging and colour flow mapping studies are frequently less than optimal techniques for use in the definition of residual atrial shunting. In particular it remains the exception to demonstrate the number, size and exact location of the defects by this technique. The addition of contrast echocardiographic studies, in our experience, most often adds only little new information. In the presence of marked enlargement of the liver, the contrast effect achieved in the right atrium following injection into a leg vein is frequently inadequate to allow an accurate diagnosis. In the presence of a Glenn shunt, systemic venous blood of the upper body half preferentially enters the pulmonary artery system di-

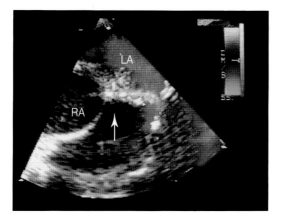

Figure 5.39 *Residual defect at the sutureline of the patch with the atrial septum (arrow) in a child with total cavopulmonary connection. Multiple defects are excluded by scanning the entire sutureline in a series of transesophageal views.*

rectly, and thus cannot produce an adequate contrast effect within the right atrial chamber.

In comparison, transesophageal imaging studies allow complete visualisation of the entire atrial septum or, in patients with a total cavopulmonary connection, of the entire sutureline of the interatrial patch. Thus, either gross patch dehiscence or large residual defects are easily recognisable on cross-sectional imaging. However, the majority of defects will be caused by rather small communications, which are not easily recognisable by cross-sectional imaging alone. Such smaller defects are rapidly identified on transesophageal colour flow mapping studies (Fig. 5.39). Multiple defects, their size and

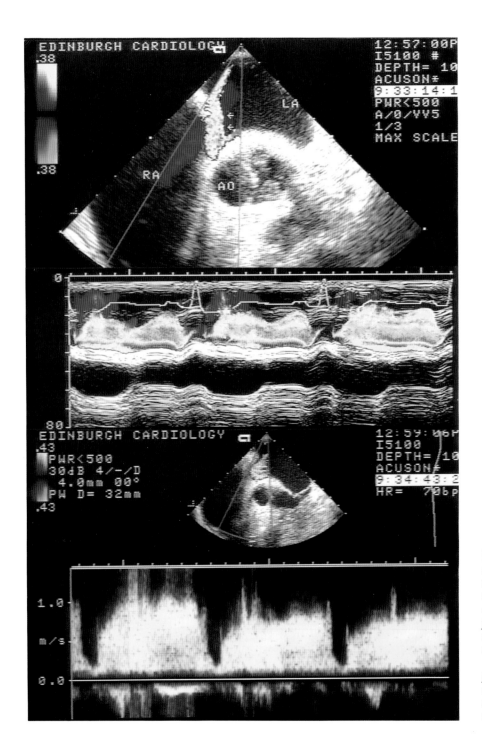

Figure 5.40 *Residual atrial septal defect in an adult patient who was noted to suffer from persistent arterial desaturation following an atriopulmonary connection with ASD patch closure for tricuspid atresia. The defect is localised in the antero-superior portion of the atrial septum. The colour M-mode study and the pulsed wave Doppler trace document continuous turbulent right-to-left shunting, which ceases only following right atrial relaxation.*

their exact locations can all be identified, thus providing invaluable information for the accurate planning of subsequent treatment. The suitability for transcatheter device closure of individual defects can be readily assessed on combined cross-sectional imaging and colour flow mapping studies, and this therapeutic approach may become the technique of first choice (Fig. 5.40).

The range of information which may be obtained by transesophageal ultrasound studies in the assessment of these lesions is likely to alter the diagnostic and therapeutic approach. The clinical significance of residual atrial shunting is best assessed during exercise testing in combination with pulse oximetry for quantification of the degree of arterial desaturation. Transesophageal ultrasound studies should then be carried out to define the precise location of residual shunting. This allows better planning of the optimal therapeutic approach. Device closure of residual defects appears to be feasible in the vast majority of patients who have a dilated right atrial chamber. In patients with a total cavopulmonary connection, and in particular in children, surgical closure may be the preferred technique, because of the potential risk of baffle obstruction. However, excellent results in this latter patient group have been reported previously (11).

THROMBOTIC LESIONS

Prior reports based on transthoracic ultrasound imaging have suggested that excessive right atrial thrombus formation is a rare finding in the late postoperative follow-up period following a Fontan procedure (23). In the majority of cases thrombus formation was associated with a recent history of atrial fibrillation, obstruction to pulmonary blood flow or both. Frequently it is not possible to decide which the initial lesion had been. The exclusion of thrombotic lesions on transthoracic ultrasound imaging is hampered by a generally poor image quality; in our experience only massive thrombi are detected. Similar limitations would appear to apply for the detection of thrombi by angiography. Magnetic resonance imaging has the potential to detect intra-atrial thrombus formation at an early stage using spin echo sequences. Differentiation from slow moving blood can be achieved by using cine sequences (24). However, current limitations in terms of availability preclude magnetic resonance imaging being considered a first line investigational technique.

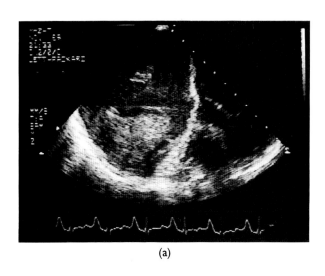

(a)

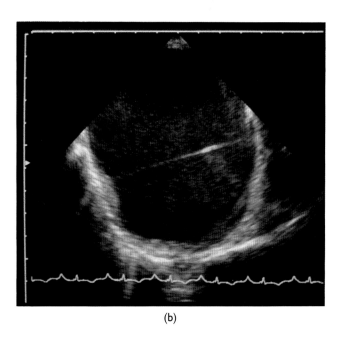

(b)

Figure 5.41 (a) *Massive right atrial thrombus detected by transesophageal imaging. The prior precordial study remained ambiguous about the presence of atrial thrombi. The majority of thrombi are found in an anterior compartment of the right atrial chamber, in particular when there is a prominent Eustachian valve.* **(b)** *Repeat transesophageal study in the same patient after thrombolytic therapy demonstrating complete resolution of the thrombus. Note persistence of spontaneous echocardiographic contrast within the entire right atrial cavity.*

Transesophageal cross-sectional imaging is a highly sensitive technique for the detection of atrial thrombus formation following Fontan-type procedures (Fig. 5.41). By scanning the entire right atrial cavity in a series of short axis cuts, even small thrombi are readily identified. Such thrombi can be either free floating, entirely attached to the right atrial wall (mural thrombus), or attached by only a fine stalk. Using transesophageal cross-sectional imaging studies in a series of Fontan patients, the incidence of thrombus formation was found to be much higher than that previously reported (22). This should lead to reconsideration of the need for routine anticoagulation of Fontan patients. In general, slow flow within the atrial chamber is suspected to be the precursor of thrombus formation. Slow flow or eventually stasis within the atrial chambers is aggravated by the loss of sinus rhythm, which in turn is likely to promote thrombus formation. However, thrombi may be encountered also in patients in sinus rhythm, or in those with total cavopulmonary connections, in whom there should be sufficient laminar flow within the reduced 'atrial' chamber (Fig. 5.42). Thus, there would appear to be further factors contributing to an increased potential for thrombus formation following a Fontan-type procedure. It has been suggested that one of these factors may be changes in the activity and concentration of various coagulation factors (25).

The appearance of a spontaneous contrast echo effect within the atrial chambers has been most commonly described in particular in patients with either severe mitral valve stenosis or with severe left ventricular myopathies (26). This phenomenon is much more often recognised since the introduction of high-resolution transesophageal imaging. Although the exact aetiology is not yet fully explained (microaggregation of blood cells?), it appears that the finding is indicative of an increased thromboembolic risk. Following all the modifications of the Fontan procedure, spontaneous contrast appearance within the right atrial cavity is a frequent finding (Fig. 5.41 (G)). This may be related to a combination of factors discussed above. Further detailed studies are required to elucidate the clinical significance of this finding, and whether antiplatelet therapy may benefit the long-term prognosis.

Patients with massive thrombus formation within the right atrium and those with thrombus embolisation into the pulmonary artery system may present acutely in the late follow-up period. Our current diagnostic approach to patients in whom such lesions are suspected is to perform a detailed transesophageal study. Thrombi within the right atrium are readily identified on cross-sectional imaging. Embolisation into the pulmonary artery system may sometimes be visualised directly by scanning the branch pulmonary arteries. In other cases detailed Doppler studies of both the flow patterns within the branch pulmonary arteries and the corresponding pulmonary veins will allow the identification of this life-threatening complication (22). Thrombolytic treatment with right atrial infusion of streptokinase should be considered in such cases (22,27). Following a completed course of streptokinase repeat transesophageal studies can be used effectively to document the results both on thrombus morphology and pulmonary blood flow.

OBSTRUCTION TO PULMONARY BLOOD FLOW

Obstruction to pulmonary blood flow may either occur in the immediate postoperative period or may present as a slowly progressive lesion in the late follow-up (18,28,29), which ultimately requires reoperation. In particular, both long-standing Dacron conduits and prosthetic valves incorporated in atriopulmonary connections are at high risk of becoming obstructed in the long-term. Progressive calcification and pronounced neointimal thickening are among the underlying pathophysiologic factors.

Precordial ultrasound techniques often fail to

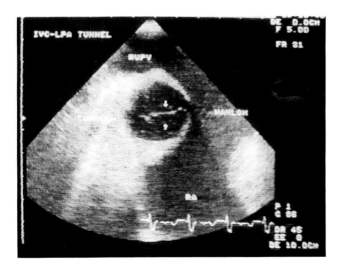

Figure 5.42 *Discrete thrombus formation (arrows) in a patient following total cavopulmonary connection.*

Table 5.1 *Comparison between transthoracic (PE) and transesophageal (TEE) ultrasound studies in the evaluation of Fontan and Glenn connections*

Connection	PE		TEE	
Anterior connections	73%		60%	
Atriopulmonary		7/9		6/9
Atrioventricular		4/6		3/6
Posterior connections	33%		96%	
Direct atriopulmonary		2/7		7/7
Valved atriopulmonary		0/3		2/3
Total cavopulmonary connection		6/14		14/14
Glenn shunts	18%		88%	
Right sided		3/13		12/13
Left sided		0/4		3/4
Total (n = 56)	39%		84%	

identify obstruction within the various types of Fontan connections. Posterior connections, such as in atriopulmonary connections, are especially difficult to visualise using the transthoracic approach. Thus, cardiac catheterisation is often performed to effect the diagnosis or definite exclusion of obstruction. Compared with transthoracic ultrasound, transesophageal studies provide a more detailed insight into both the morphology and function of the various types of Fontan connections. In a prospective study only 39% of Fontan and Glenn connections could be evaluated by transthoracic ultrasound studies whereas transverse axis transesophageal studies allowed a detailed assessment in 84% of these. Major advantages for transesophageal studies were found in the evaluation of posterior connections – 96% of all posterior connections could be evaluated by transesophageal studies as opposed to only 33% by transthoracic studies. Both techniques were comparable in the assessment of anterior Fontan connections (Table 5.1). The advantage of transesophageal studies is even more pronounced in the adolescent and adult population, where it is rarely possible to obtain adequate precordial imaging and Doppler information. Finally, with the introduction of biplane transesophageal imaging the assessment of anterior Fontan connections has now been improved, although some limitations persist because of the large distances between the oesophagus and these retrosternal connections.

In most cases direct atriopulmonary connections can be assessed adequately by transesophageal cross-sectional imaging, when scanning high esophageal views of the right aspect of the heart (Fig. 5.43).

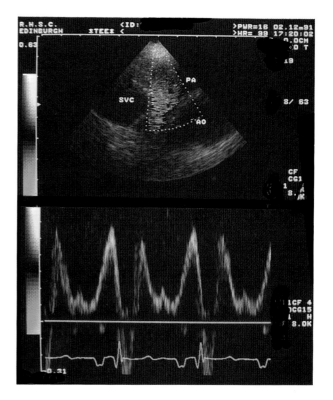

Figure 5.43 *Transesophageal demonstration of a direct posterior atriopulmonary anastomosis in a patient with tricuspid atresia. The communication is located interposed between the superior caval vein and the proximal ascending aorta. The internal dimensions of the anastomosis can be assessed on cross-sectional imaging. Slight probe rotation allows for the demonstration of the adjacent segments of the pulmonary artery. The colour flow mapping and pulsed wave Doppler study (sampling at the site of connection) reveal unobstructed flow patterns.*

Even in younger children the size of the anastomosis and the size of the adjacent pulmonary arteries can be evaluated in more detail than by precordial ultrasound techniques (30). Distortion of one of the pulmonary arteries at the site of the anastomosis is also readily identified. By scanning the course of the right and the left pulmonary arteries, more peripheral stenoses of the pulmonary arteries, such as occur after previous systemic – pulmonary shunts, can sometimes be visualised. However, because of the interposition of the bronchial tree between the esophagus and the pulmonary arteries, there are obvious limitations to the technique. Clearly angiography will remain the diagnostic technique of choice in the assessment of these peripheral pulmonary artery lesions.

In cases where a prosthetic conduit has been inserted, transesophageal imaging provides the internal dimensions of the conduit largely irrespective of conduit calcification (Fig. 5.44). This should prove to be a definitive advantage over magnetic resonance imaging. In addition, the presence of dissected neointima flaps as the underlying cause of the obstruction (31) should be readily identified by this technique. In those patients who have had a bioprosthetic or a homograft valve inserted, the transesophageal imaging study frequently reveals that the valve leaflets stay partially open throughout the cardiac cycle, and thus do not prevent retrograde flow during atrial relaxation. Finally, thrombotic or endocarditic lesions on the valve leaflets are likely to be excluded best by transesophageal imaging.

Although transesophageal cross-sectional imaging on its own already provides a spectrum of information on the integrity of the various types of Fontan connections, it is only its combination with both colour flow mapping and pulsed wave Doppler studies that allows the diagnosis or definitive exclusion of obstruction to pulmonary blood flow. Colour flow mapping studies will demon-

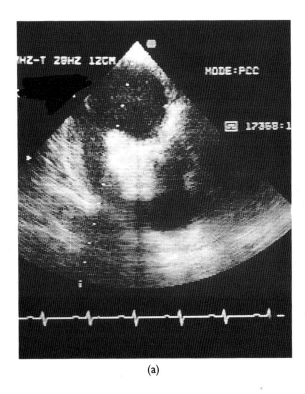

(a)

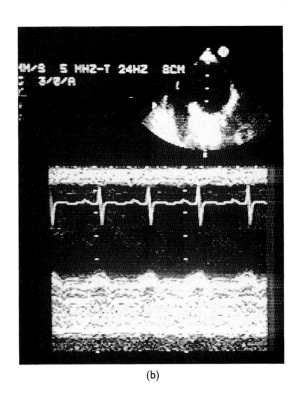

(b)

Figure 5.44 (a) *Transverse axis cross-sectional imaging in a patient with a conduit connection from the right atrium to the right ventricle. Both the atrial and the ventricular anastomosis are well visualised, as is the lumen of the conduit.* **(b)** *Assessment of right atrial function in the same patient by means of an M-mode recording reveals good atrial contraction without a significant fractional shortening.*

strate continuous turbulent flow patterns at the site of obstruction (Fig. 5.45(a)). The precise nature of the flow abnormality should then be confirmed by pulsed wave Doppler sampling. Where obstruction is present these tracings will reveal continuous turbulent flow whose velocity never reaches zero during the cardiac or respiratory cycle (Fig. 5.45(b)). Because of limited applicability of the Bernoulli equation to venous flow patterns and a generally poor alignment to the flow, it is, however, not possible to determine accurately the resulting pressure gradient by this technique. This is best obtained by cardiac catheterisation.

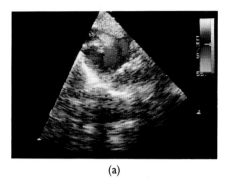

(a)

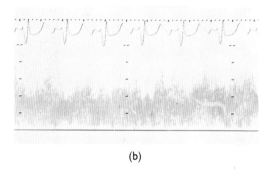

(b)

Figure 5.45 (a) *High transesophageal transverse axis view in a patient following a total cavopulmonary connection. The right superior caval vein (encoded in blue) was left to drain into the right atrium. On colour flow mapping there is continuous turbulent flow towards the right pulmonary artery, suggesting obstruction.* **(b)** *The subsequent pulsed wave Doppler study with sampling in the area of maximal turbulence reveals continuous turbulent flow patterns that do not reach baseline through the cardiac or respiratory cycle, and thus confirm obstruction.*

When evaluating cavopulmonary shunts, transesophageal transverse axis imaging allows the demonstration of the site of shunt anastomosis and a segment of the distal pulmonary artery in the vast majority of cases. This is irrespective of whether the shunt was created on the right or the left side of the patient. A right sided shunt is visualised by the same technique used in the assessment of the right superior caval vein. A left sided shunt between a left persistent superior caval vein and the left pulmonary artery, in our experience, is best documented after visualisation of the left pulmonary artery anterior to the descending aorta. Counter-clockwise rotation of the probe together with slight withdrawal will then identify the site of connection. Additional longitudinal axis imaging may be helpful for this step of the investigation, but current experience is limited.

MISCELLANEOUS HAEMODYNAMIC LESIONS

Although obstruction to pulmonary blood flow and atrial thrombus formation are among the most serious immediate or long-term haemodynamic sequelae following Fontan-type procedures, a range of other haemodynamic lesions may be encountered which impair functional capacity and may require either early or late reoperation.

Atrioventricular valve incompetence is frequently found following Fontan procedures. In particular, in patients who were operated at an older age, the longstanding left ventricular volume overload may result in valve annulus dilatation with resultant atrioventricular valve regurgitation. In those

Fontan patients with complex underlying cardiac lesions (e.g. common atrioventricular valves or double-inlet ventricles) atrioventricular valve regurgitation is frequently present preoperatively. As with transesophageal ultrasound evaluation of acquired atrioventricular valve disease, use of the technique in the Fontan situation to determine the mechanism and the severity of valvar regurgitation is extremely rewarding, and is much more sensitive than transthoracic ultrasound techniques (22,30). In those desperate cases with moderate to severe postoperative valvar regurgitation, transesophageal ultrasound studies should be considered the optimal diagnostic technique for an evaluation of valve morphology and should enhance both the selection of patients and the detailed planning of reconstructive surgical procedures. Valve replacement in the Fontan situation must be avoided at all costs, since it inevitably increases left atrial pressures and therefore the afterload of the pulmonary circulation. Consequently this is followed by a further rise in right atrial pressures and a likely decrease in cardiac output.

Obstruction to the systemic circulation is a further complication, which is more likely to be encountered in the immediate postoperative period. It is especially in patients with discordant ventriculo-arterial connections, with the aorta arising from a rudimentary outlet chamber, that the ventricular septal defect may become restrictive. In children with good precordial ultrasound windows, transthoracic ultrasound studies are clearly superior to transverse axis transesophageal studies in the exclusion of these lesions, since relatively poor visualisation of the subaortic chamber is obtained from within the esophagus. In addition, transesophageal Doppler investigations are generally limited because of a poor angle of incidence. Our initial experience with longitudinal plane imaging in these lesions has been promising but is limited.

Regurgitation of the aortic valve is a rare finding in this group of patients. However this may be encountered following a Damus–Kaye–Stansel operation (end-to-side anastomosis between the pulmonary artery and the ascending aorta). Transverse axis imaging is most often inadequate in the evaluation of these procedures, and detailed studies can only be performed using biplane equipment.

Coronary artery fistulae are a further rare finding following a Fontan procedure. However, following total cavopulmonary connection we encountered three patients with small fistulae between the right coronary artery and the pulmonary venous atrium (Fig. 5.46). These had not been present preoperatively and thus presumably were related to the surgical procedure, i.e. the technique of atriotomy for placement of the atrial baffle. In all cases these fistulae did not have any haemodynamic significance, but follow-up of such lesions appears to be indicated.

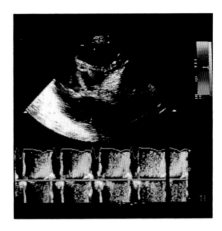

Figure 5.46 *Transesophageal detection of a small fistulous communication between a branch of the right coronary artery and the new left atrium in a patient following total cavopulmonary connection. Flow occurs mainly during diastole. In addition there is a tiny residual atrial shunt at the lateral sutureline of the patch (asterisk) and extensive pericardial effusion (PE).*

Pericardial effusions are a frequent problem in the early postoperative period, but these may also develop during the late follow-up period. The majority of anterior or apical effusions will be readily identified during transthoracic ultrasound studies. Localised or organised effusions located in particular in the posterior aspects of the pericardial cradle are often better identified by transesophageal studies.

Echocardiographic evaluation of ventricular function in the Fontan circulation remains a problem area. Transthoracic ultrasound studies are frequently hampered by poor image quality and thus are limited. The major limitation for transesophageal studies in the evaluation of ventricular function in Fontan patients lies in the marked degree of hepatomegaly, which is almost always present. This precludes the acquisition of high-quality transgastric short axis images of the ventricular chambers. Moreover, in patients with complex intracardiac anatomy, such as double-inlet ventricles, the question remains whether the established standard methods used in the assessment of ventricular function may be applicable. Thus, assessment of systolic ventricular function is currently limited at its best to the exclusion of regional wall motion abnormalities. However, with a better understanding of diastolic ventricular function in the normal heart, it is likely that there will also be a major advance in the evaluation of diastolic ventricular function of Fontan patients. Undoubtedly, diastolic ventricular function would appear to be the more relevant aspect of ventricular function in the presence of a predominant passive pulmonary circulation which occurs in the Fontan circulation. Recently, Penny and associates (31) have reported a striking degree of incoordinate ventricular relaxation immediately after the Fontan operation. In addition, they reported a marked difference in ventricular filling patterns in a subset of their patients. These initial findings would support the idea that routine evaluation of both pulmonary venous and atrioventricular valve inflow patterns, which allows the assessment of diastolic function (32–34), may be rewarding in the early detection of ventricular dysfunction. Clearly transesophageal echocardiography would be a powerful tool for such studies.

PULSED WAVE DOPPLER EVALUATION

Transthoracic pulsed wave Doppler evaluation of patients with Fontan-type procedures is most often limited because of the increased cardiac dimensions and the posterior location of the areas of interest. Hepatomegaly, which is almost always present in these patients, precludes the acquisition of high-quality signals from the subcostal window. Transesophageal ultrasound studies, on the other hand, allow detailed visualisation and high-quality interrogation of both pulmonary artery and pulmonary venous flow patterns, and thus potentially provide a more detailed insight into the underlying haemodynamic characteristics of the different modifications of the Fontan procedure.

At our institutions, routine sampling sites for pulsed wave Doppler interrogation in patients with

Fontan procedures include, firstly, the distal segments of the branch pulmonary arteries, secondly, the corresponding pulmonary veins (ultimately all four), and, thirdly, the systemic atrioventricular valve inflow patterns. With the increasing availability of biplane imaging technology, flow patterns within both the inferior and superior caval veins should also be assessed. In theory such a technique should allow a complete Doppler evaluation of the Fontan circulation. However, several limitations have to be borne in mind. Firstly, if studies are performed with the patient lying in a lateral position, inevitably there is preferential blood flow to the contralateral lung. Naturally, the same holds true for Doppler evaluation of pulmonary blood flow by precordial ultrasound techniques. Secondly, in children studies will be performed most often under general anaesthesia and using positive pressure ventilation, which inevitably leads to a significant change in the patterns of pulmonary perfusion. Thus, spontaneous breathing should be maintained during all such studies. Nonetheless, with the aid of transesophageal pulsed wave Doppler interrogation it is possible to define clearly pulmonary flow patterns distal to any coexisting collateral circulation or distal to established Glenn shunts, and away from the right atrial chamber. In addition, the unique possibility of assessing the flow patterns in all four of the pulmonary veins greatly improves the identification of regional differences of pulmonary blood flow, as may be present following pulmonary thromboembolism.

When assessing pulmonary venous flow patterns following each of the different modifications of the Fontan circulation, it is striking that these are almost uniform. In patients with sinus rhythm there is commonly some degree of reversed flow following left atrial contraction. This retrograde flow is not transmitted backwards to the pulmonary artery. Forward flow occurs with a biphasic flow pattern; the larger peak most often occurring during ventricular systole. In patients with atrial fibrillation, pulmonary venous flow patterns are highly variable and reflect the incoordinate interaction between the left atrial and ventricular chamber.

Frequently the upper pulmonary venous flow patterns demonstrate higher flow velocities, suggesting a higher amount of total blood flow. In patients with low cardiac output the diastolic flow integral normally exceeds the systolic flow integral. However, this finding appears to be unsuitable for quantification. The documentation of only to-and-fro flow within a pulmonary vein (Fig. 5.47) in our experience, is highly suggestive of largely diminished or absent blood flow within the corresponding pulmonary artery, such as occurs with pulmonary thromboembolism or severe pulmonary artery obstruction. Such a finding should then lead to a more detailed exclusion of the range of the potential underlying lesions.

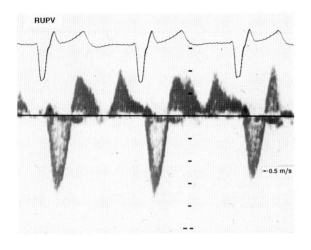

Figure 5.47 *Pulsed wave Doppler sampling within the right upper pulmonary vein in a patient with complete occlusion of the right pulmonary artery. There is only to and fro flow within the corresponding pulmonary vein. The flow integrals for forward and retrograde flow approximate to zero.*

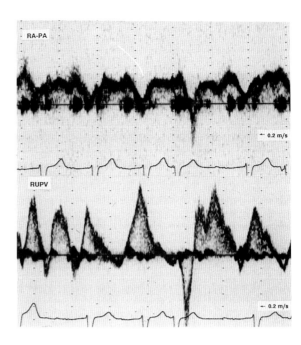

Figure 5.48 *Matched pulsed wave Doppler recordings of pulmonary artery (at the site of the anastomosis) and pulmonary venous flow patterns in a patient with atrial fibrillation. Both flow patterns are largely independent from one another and only major pressure rises within the left atrium are transmitted backwards to the pulmonary artery (arrows).*

Correlation of the pulmonary artery and pulmonary venous flow patterns potentially allows a better understanding of the driving forces of the Fontan circulation (22). It has long been discussed to what extent the systemic ventricular function contributes to pulmonary blood flow. This discussion culminated in the postulation of a 'suction effect' of the left ventricle to drive the Fontan circulation. A predominant contribution of the right atrial pumping function represented the opposing concept (35,36). Against a major contribution of the left ventricle is the fact that pulmonary artery flow patterns are relatively independent from the corresponding pulmonary venous flow patterns. Only major pressure differences within the left atrium are transmitted retrogradely to the pulmonary artery bed and hence the right atrium (Fig. 5.48). In patients with a total cavopulmonary connection, where there is no right atrial chamber, the pulmonary artery flow patterns should more closely resemble pulmonary venous flow patterns if the concept of a suctioning ventricle should hold true.

However, in such patients pulmonary artery flow patterns change only little during the cardiac cycle. Major variations are found only with respiration. Forward flow decreases with expiration and peaks during inspiration, i.e. with the maximum in negative intrathoracic pressure (Fig. 5.49). Similar observations are made in patients with Glenn shunts when the pulsed Doppler sampling volume is placed within the pulmonary arteries distal to the shunt (Fig. 5.50). These findings have recently been confirmed by Penny and associates (37). In addition, they reported the effect of various manoeuvres on pulmonary blood flow. During a Mueller manoeuvre (inspiration against the closed glottis) pulmonary blood flow was found to be largely increased, whereas with a Valsalva manoeuvre pulmonary blood flow approximated zero and eventually reversed.

These observations in patients with total cavopulmonary connection suggest that the right atrial pumping function is not essential to drive the Fontan circulation. However, in patients with atriopulmonary connections, and especially those with a hypertrophied right atrium, pulmonary artery flow patterns most often demonstrate a biphasic flow pattern (see Fig. 5.43). The marked forward flow that occurs following atrial contraction was for long interpreted to document the importance of right atrial activity. Nonetheless, retrograde flow almost always occurs with atrial relaxation. It is noteworthy that this flow component is pronounced in patients with high pulmonary arterial pressures (Fig. 5.51). In addition, it can be found in the majority of patients with valved atriopulmonary connections, suggesting that such valves do not function in the low-pressure venous circulation. The second component of forward flow is most likely passive flow, and again varies largely with respiration. These observations suggest that right atrial activity modulates pulmonary artery flow patterns. In patients with atrioventricular types of Fontan connections, the right ventricle serves merely as a conduit during ventricular systole. During ventricular diastole it represents a poorly compliant chamber which is filled by both passive antegrade flow from the right atrium and retrograde flow from the pulmonary artery (Fig. 5.52).

Thus, pulmonary artery flow in the Fontan circulation is a predominantly passive process. Variations in pulmonary artery flow patterns occur with the effects of respiration, the contraction and the relaxation of any chamber incorporated into the circulation.

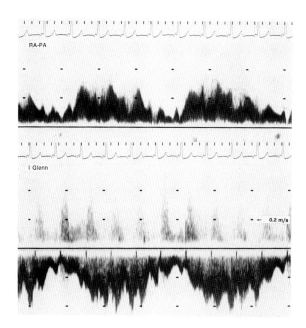

Figure 5.50 *Pulsed wave Doppler recordings in the proximal left pulmonary artery and distally to a left Glenn shunt in a patient after total cavopulmonary connection. In the distal pulmonary arteries antegrade flow is away from the transducer.*

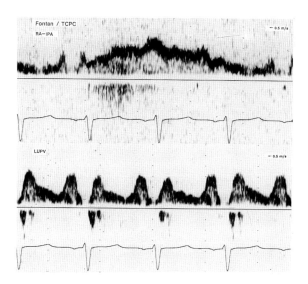

Figure 5.49 *Matched Doppler recordings within the proximal left pulmonary artery and the left upper pulmonary vein in a patient after total cavopulmonary connection.*

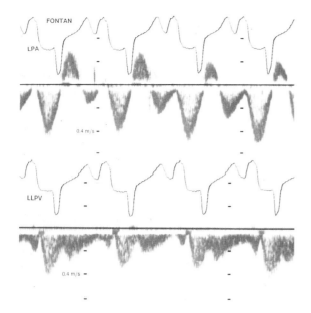

Figure 5.51 *Pulmonary artery and pulmonary venous flow patterns in a patient with atriopulmonary connection and raised pulmonary resistance. Sampling in the distal left pulmonary artery reveals prominent retrograde flow following atrial relaxation. The second peak of forward flow (away from the transducer) is largely dependent on respiration (arrow). Pulmonary venous return peaks during diastole, indicative of low cardiac output. Because of cardiac malrotation antegrade pulmonary venous flow is away from the transducer.*

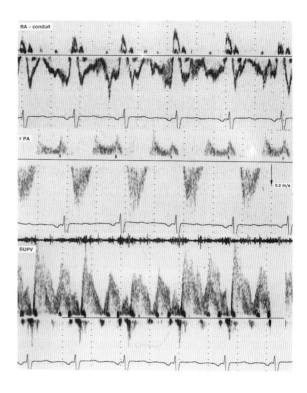

Figure 5.52 *Pulsed wave Doppler evaluation in a patient following a valved atrioventricular connection. Sampling sites include the anastomosis between the right atrium and the conduit, the distal right pulmonary artery, and the right upper pulmonary vein.*

REFERENCES

1. FONTAN F, BAUDET E. Surgical repair of tricuspid atresia. *Thorax* 1971; **26:** 240–8.
2. ANNECHINO FP, BRUNELLI F, BORHI A, ABBRUZZESE P, MERLO M, PARENZAN L. Fontan repair for tricuspid atresia – experience with 50 consecutive patients. *Ann Thorac Surg* 1988; **45:** 430–6.
3. DELEON SY, ILBAWI MN, IDRISS FS, et al. Fontan type operation for complex lesions – Surgical considerations to improve survival. *J Thorac Cardiovasc Surg* 1986; **92:** 1029–37.
4. STELLIN G, MAZZUCCO A, BORTOLOTTI U, et al. Tricuspid atresia versus other complex lesions. *J Thorac Cardiovasc Surg* 1988; **96:** 204–11.
5. MAYER JE, HELGASON H, JONAS RA, et al. Extending the limits for modified Fontan procedures. *J Thorac Cardiovasc Surg* 1986; **92:** 1021–8.
6. KREUTZER GO, VARGAS FJ, SCHLICHTER AJ, et al. Atriopulmonary anastomosis. *J Thorac Cardiovasc Surg* 1982; **83:** 427–36.
7. EIJGELAAR A, HESS J, HARDJOWIJNO R, KARLICZEK GF, RATING W, HOMAN VD HEIDE JN. Experience with the Fontan operation. *Thorac Cardiovasc Surg* 1982; **30:** 63–8.
8. PRENGER KB, HESS J, CROMME-DIJKHUIS AH, EIJGELAAR A. Porcine-valved dacron conduits in Fontan procedures. *Ann Thorac Surg* 1988; **46:** 526–30.
9. COLES JG, LEUNG M, KIELMANOWICZ P, et al. Repair of tricuspid atresia: utility of right ventricular incorporation. *Ann Thorac Surg* 1988; **45:** 384–9.
10. DELEVAL MR, KILNER P, GEWILLIG M, BULL C. Total cavopulmonary connection: a logical alternative to atriopulmonary connection for complex Fontan operations. Experimental studies and early clinical experience. *J Thorac Cardiovasc Surg* 1988; **96:** 682–95.
11. BRIDGES ND, LOCK JE, CASTANEDA AR. Baffle fenestration with subsequent transcatheter closure.

Modification of the Fontan operation for patients at increased risk. *Circulation* 1990; **82:** 1681–9.

12. GLENN WWL. Circulatory bypass of the right side of the heart: IV: Shunt between superior vena cava and distal right pulmonary artery – report of clinical application. *New Engl J Med* 1958; **259:** 117–20.

13. BARGERON LM, KARP RB, BARCIA A, KIRKLIN JW, HUNT D, DEVERALL PB. Late deterioration of patients after superior vena cava to right pulmonary artery anastomosis. *Am J Cardiol* 1972; **30:** 211–16.

14. HOPKINS RA, ARMSTRONG BE, SERWER GA, PETERSON RJ, NEWLAND OLDHAM H. Physiological rationale for a bidirectional cavopulmonary shunt. *J Thorac Cardiovasc Surg* 1985; **90:** 391–8.

15. BAFFA JM, RYCHIK J, GULLQUIST SD, et al. Outcome following bidirectional cavo-pulmonary anastomosis prior to modified Fontan procedure. *J Am Coll Cardiol* 1991; **17:** 33A (abstract).

16. FONTAN F, KIRKLIN JW, FERNANDEZ G, et al. Outcome after a 'perfect' Fontan operation. *Circulation* 1990; **81:** 1520–36.

17. LEUNG MP, BENSON LN, SMALLHORN JF, WILLIAMS WG, TRUSLER GA, FREEDOM RM. Abnormal cardiac signs after Fontan type of operation: indicators of residua and sequelae. *Br Heart J* 1989; **61:** 52–8.

18. FERNANDEZ G, COSTA F, FONTAN F, NAFTEL DC, BLACKSTONE EH, KIRKLIN JW. Prevalence of reoperation for pathway obstruction after the Fontan operation. *Ann Thorac Surg* 1989; **48:** 654–9.

19. GEWILLIG MH, LUNDSTRÖM UR, BULL C, WYSE RKH, DEANFIELD JE. Exercise response in patients with congenital heart disease after Fontan repair: Patterns and determinants of performance. *J Am Coll Cardiol* 1990; **15:** 1424–32.

20. HAGLER DJ, SEWARD JB, TAJIK AJ, RITTER DG. Functional assessment of the Fontan operation: combined M-mode, two-dimensional and Doppler echocardiographic studies. *J Am Coll Cardiol* 1984; **4:** 756–64.

21. DISESSA TG, CHILD JS, PERLOFF JK, et al. Systemic venous and pulmonary arterial flow patterns after Fontan's procedure for tricuspid atresia or single ventricle. *Circulation* 1984; **70:** 898–902.

22. STÜMPER O, SUTHERLAND GR, GEUSKENS R, ROELANDT JRTC, BOS E, HESS J. Transesophageal echocardiography in the evaluation and management of the Fontan circulation. *J Am Coll Cardiol* 1991; **17:** 1152–60.

23. DOBELL ARC, TRUSLER GA, SMALLHORN JF, WILLIAMS WG. Atrial thrombi formation after the Fontan operation. *Ann Thorac Surg* 1986; **42:** 664–7.

24. DINSMORE RE, WEDEEN V, ROSEN B, WISMER GL, MILLER SW, BRANDY TJ. Phase-offset technique to distinguish slow blood flow and thrombus on MR images. *Am J Roentgenol* 1987; **148:** 634–6.

25. CROMMER-DIJKHUIS AH, HENKENS CMA, BIJLEVELD CMA, HILLIGE HL, BOM VJJ, VD MEER J. Coagulation factor abnormalities as possible riskfactor after Fontan operations. *Lancet* 1990; **336:** 1687–90.

26. DANIEL WG, NELLESSEN U, SCHRÖDER E, et al. Left atrial spontaneous echo contrast in mitral valve disease: an indicator for an increased thromboembolic risk. *J Am Coll Cardiol* 1988; **11:** 1204–11.

27. MAHONY L, NIKAIDOH H, FIXLER DE. Thrombolytic treatment with streptokinase for late intraatrial thrombosis after modified Fontan procedure. *Am J Cardiol* 1988; **62:** 343–4.

28. GIROD DA, FONTAN F, DEVILLE C, OTTENKAMP J, CHOUSSAT A. Long-term results after the Fontan operation for tricuspid atresia. *Circulation* 1987; **75:** 605–10.

29. DEVIVIE R, RUPPRATH G. Long-term results after Fontan procedure and its modifications. *J Thorac Cardiovasc Surg* 1986; **91:** 690–7.

30. WONG P, DYCK JD, SMALLHORN JF, MUSEWE NN, BARKER GA, WILLIAMS WG. Transesophageal echocardiography in the pediatric patient following Fontan surgery. *Circulation* 1991; **82**(suppl II): 439 (abstract).

31. PENNY DJ, LINCOLN C, H XIAO, RIGBY ML, REDINGTON AN. The acute effects of transition to the Fontan circulation on systemic ventricular function. *Eur Heart J* 1991; **12** (abstract): 373.

32. KEREN G, SHEREZ J, MEGIDISH R, LEVITT B, LANIADO ?. Pulmonary venous flow patterns – its relationship to cardiac dynamics: A pulsed Doppler echocardiographic study. *Circulation* 1985; **71:** 1105–12.

33. APPLETON CP, HATLE LK, POPP RL. Relation of transmitral flow velocity patterns to left ventricular diastolic function: new insights from a combined hemodynamic and Doppler echocardiographic study. *J Am Coll Cardiol* 1988; **12:** 426–40.

34. NISHIMURA RA, ABEL MD, HATLE LK, TAJIK AJ. Relation of pulmonary vein to mitral flow velocities by transesophageal doppler echocardiography. *Circulation* 1990; **81:** 1488–97.

35. MATSUDA H, KAWASHIMA Y, TAKANO H, MIYAMOTO K, MORI T. Experimental evaluation of atrial function in right atrium-pulmonary artery conduit operations for tricuspid atresia. *J Thorac Cardiovasc Surg* 1981; **81:** 762–7.

36. NAKAZAWA M, NAKANISHI T, OKUDA H, et al. Dynamics of right heart flow patterns in patients after Fontan procedure. *Circulation* 1984; **69:** 306–12.

37. PENNY DJ, HAYEK Z, SHINEBOURNE EA, REDINGTON AN. The effects of intrathoracic pressure on pulmonary blood flow after right heart bypass. *Eur Heart J* 1991; **12**(suppl): 373 (abstract).

CHAPTER 6

Summary

O. Stümper and G. R. Sutherland

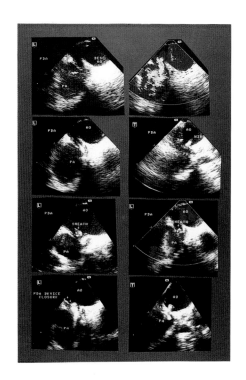

Transesophageal echocardiography has become an established investigative technique in the adult patient with acquired heart disease. However, until recently its role in patients with congenital heart disease has remained limited. It was only with the introduction of dedicated paediatric transesophageal probes that safe studies could be performed in large series of infants and children. This has led to a more detailed understanding of the anatomy and function of congenital heart disease as assessed by transesophageal ultrasound studies. In addition, the advantages and limitations of the technique in the assessment of specific lesions, when compared with other established imaging techniques, have become apparent. Thus, transesophageal echocardiography over the past years has become a valuable additional diagnostic and monitoring technique in the evaluation of congenital heart disease both in the paediatric and adult patient population. Current indications for transesophageal ultrasound studies are listed in Table 6.1.

The major advantage of the transesophageal ultrasound approach lies in the provision of superior quality images of the posterior cardiac structures when compared with transthoracic ultrasound studies. Therefore its diagnostic impact is most apparent in the older patient with poor precordial ultrasound windows or in post-surgical patients whose precordial imaging is poor as a result of a midline sternotomy. The major disadvantages of the technique include, firstly, its semi-invasive character (in particular in children), secondly, the need for heavy sedation or general anaesthesia in the younger patient population, and thirdly, the limited number of imaging planes and the limited amount of haemodynamic information that can be derived from such studies. With the introduction of biplane transesophageal ultrasound probes and the incorporation of continuous wave Doppler facilities there has been a marked improvement in the range of information to be obtained by such studies, but some limitations persist.

In this book the current technology and techniques of both single and biplane transesophageal echocardiography have been outlined in detail. The assessment of unoperated congenital cardiac lesions is discussed following a sequential chamber approach. The terminology used to describe complex congenital cardiac lesions is summarised in each chapter so as to provide a rapid reference for the adult cardiologist who is not entirely familiar with the range of lesions that may be encountered. Thereafter the transesophageal appearances of specific lesions are discussed in detail together with guidelines for probe manipulation to obtain a rapid diagnosis. Later chapters discuss use of the technique in monitoring of the perioperative period and during interventional cardiac catheterisation, and in evaluation of the patient following surgical correction of congenital cardiac defects. Undoubtedly these latter two clinical settings will become the standard settings for transesophageal ultrasound studies in patients in the paediatric age group with congenital heart disease. In the adolescent and adult age group, the technique will have its major role as a diagnostic technique used in the outpatient clinic.

What are the future prospects for transesophageal imaging in congenital heart disease? Two important technological developments are required to further establish its role in cardiac imaging. Better paediatric probes are required which provide high-resolution imaging across the whole paediatric age range. Such probes should provide biplane imaging. This development would hasten the acceptance of the technique.

For the study of older children and adults, a multiplane approach would seem to be of value. At the time of writing, multiplane technology is not commercially available but is soon to appear on the market. Although an experienced operator can, using the steering mechanisms appropriately, produce the equivalent of multiplane images using a biplane probe, it is likely that these would be more easily and rapidly obtained using a multiplane probe. In addition, the multiplane approach would more readily give the operator the ability to follow structures within the heart more easily. This would be an added advantage in the study of complex three dimensional abnormalities of cardiac morphology. It is currently unlikely that miniaturised paediatric multiplane probes will be widely available in the next year or two because of the size constraints induced by the steering mechanism which is located in the transducer tip.

With the introduction of the above developments, the place of transesophageal echocardiography in the study of congenital heart disease will be further secured. Its appropriate diagnostic role in terms of other cardiac imaging techniques such as ultra-fast CT and MRI remains to be established.

Table 6.1 *Current indications for transesophageal ultrasound studies in patients with congenital heart disease*

Primary diagnosis	Anomalous systemic venous connections
	Anomalous pulmonary venous connections
	Atrial arrangement, atrial isomerism
	Juxtaposition of the atrial appendages
	Atrial septal defects
	Atrioventricular junction abnormalities
	Atrioventricular valve abnormalities
	Left ventricular outflow tract obstruction
Monitoring	
(a) Perioperative	Surgical repair at venous level
	Surgical repair at atrial level
	Atrioventricular valve repair/replacement
	Mustard/Senning procedure
	Fontan-type procedures
	Continuous monitoring during early postoperative period
	Diagnosis and management of early postoperative complications
(b) Interventional catheterisation	Continuous real-time monitoring of cardiac morphology and function
	Guidance of guidewire and balloon catheter position
	Exclusion of immediate complications
	Assessment of immediate morphologic changes
	Assessment of immediate haemodynamic results/changes
	Dilatations of venous pathway obstructions
	Device closure of atrial septal defects
Follow-up	Suspected residual or acquired atrial lesions
	Repair of anomalous venous connections
	Mustard/Senning procedures
	Fontan-type procedures
	Atrioventricular valve repair/replacement

Index